17.95

SHOCK THERAPY

SHOCK THERAPY

A History of Electroconvulsive Treatment in Mental Illness

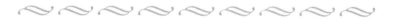

EDWARD SHORTER
DAVID HEALY

Rutgers University Press
NEW BRUNSWICK, NEW JERSEY, AND LONDON

Library of Congress Cataloging-in-Publication Data

Shorter, Edward.
Shock therapy : a history of electroconvulsive treatment in mental illness / Edward
Shorter, David Healy.
p. ; cm.
Includes bibliographical references and index.
ISBN 978-0-8135-4169-3 (hardcover : alk. paper)
1. Electroconvulsive therapy—History. I. Healy, David, MRC Psych. II. Title.
[DNLM: 1. Electroconvulsive Therapy—history. 2. History, 20th Century. 3. Mental
Disorders—therapy. WM 11.1 S559s 2007]
RC485.S56 2007
616.89′122—dc22

                                                                    2006039516

A British Cataloging-in-Publication record for this book is available from the British
Library.

Visit our Web site: http://rutgerspress.rutgers.edu

Manufactured in the United States of America

It was a small band of European émigrés—Italians, Germans and Austrians, and Jews for the most part—who saw the merits in electroconvulsive therapy and sustained its use despite professional antipathy and ostracism, and public and governmental attacks. They are unacknowledged heroes in the twentieth-century history of psychiatry. This book is in their memory.

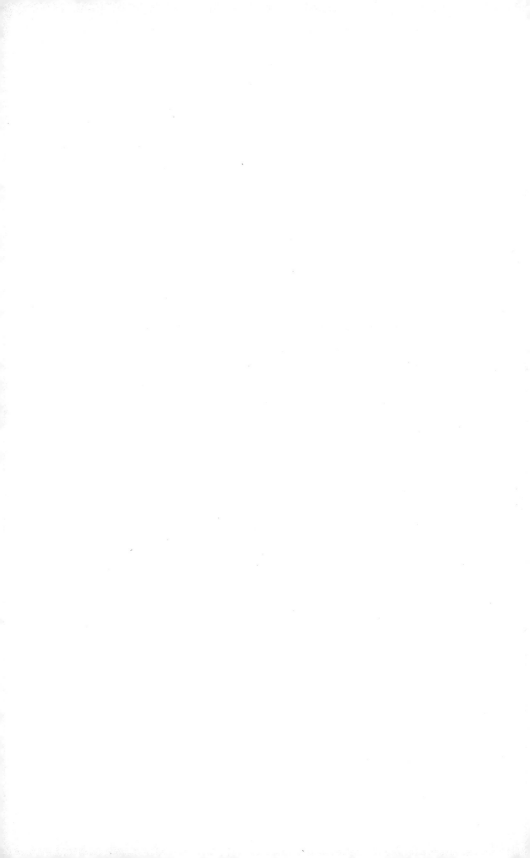

Contents

Illustrations

Acknowledgments

This book owes a special debt to Max Fink. It was Max who encouraged us to tackle the subject, which we initially conceived as a history of electroconvulsive therapy alone. As it became apparent that telling the ECT story properly meant drawing a larger tableau of all the shock treatments, we decided to include the history of insulin coma and Metrazol convulsion as well. But at every step Max helped us by drawing from the depths of his own enormous experience and wisdom. He opened a number of doors for interviews with other pioneers of the field, and, finally, he gave the manuscript a critical reading. This is in no sense Max's book, because we have told the story from our own point of view. But if Max had not said that one of the great untold stories of medical history was out there, just begging to be written, we probably would have glanced elsewhere. We are also grateful to Tom Ban and Gerald Grob for comments on an earlier draft.

A number of people gave generously of their time in interviews. We particularly would like to thank Richard Abrams, Linda Andre, Tom Bolwig, Peter Breggin, Robert Cohen, George Curtis, Herbert Fox, Leonard Roy Frank, Fred Frankel, Alfred Freedman, Mark George, Alexander Glassman, William Karliner, Robert Levine, Louis Linn, Sarah Lisanby, Bruno Magliocco, Sidney Malitz, Helen Mayberg, Jan-Otto Ottosson, John Pippard, Matthew Rudorfer, Harold Sackeim, Thomas Schlaepfer, Conrad Swartz, Michael Alan Taylor, Richard Weiner, and Arthur Zitrin.

This research was supported in part by a grant from the Scion Natural Science Association and by the Canadian Institutes of Health Research. Susan Bélanger helped with the library work and transcribing of interviews, as did Heather Dichter and Ellen Tulchinsky. And Andrea Clark, administrator of the history of medicine program at the University of Toronto, cleared the brush from the authors' path. For all of this assistance we are most thankful.

It has been exhilarating to work with an editor as intellectually engaged and inquiring as Doreen Valentine at Rutgers University Press. To the meticulous copyediting of Beth Gianfagna the authors also owe a good deal.

Edward Shorter
David Healy

SHOCK THERAPY

CHAPTER ONE

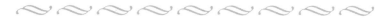

The Penicillin of Psychiatry?

t is 1947. X, a thirty-eight-year-old New York physician and veteran of World War II, has just dropped out of training in internal medicine. He has been diagnosed with lung tuberculosis and has become depressed. He develops feelings of guilt, particularly about his income tax, "complaining that he did not file properly after he sold his house."[1] He confesses to his wife that he has had extramarital affairs "and that he has committed so many crimes that he will never be able to do penance for it." He is fearful of starting up practice on his own, that patients will never come, and is "convinced that he is incompetent and that he does not have any chances of getting out of the mess in which he finds himself."

In the second week of May, X attempts suicide, swallowing a handful of the barbiturate drug, sodium seconal. Taken to Queen's County General Hospital in New York, he awakens twenty-four hours later, deeply depressed and yet bewildered that he could have attempted to end his life. He is transferred to Hillside Hospital, a private psychiatric facility at the eastern end of Queens, where his attendants describe his state as "gloomy, his whole attitude expresses deep despair, his voice [is] soft, his posture . . . stooped, his movements . . . slow, his eyes . . . [look] down at the floor as if he [is] one of the most terrible criminals not being able to carry his burden." He is also concerned about his physical body: his bowel movements, overall weakness, "his inability to move his legs and arms, and . . . pain in his back and in his heart." The staff cannot get him to stay in bed as he keeps "jumping up to go to the mirror and look at his face in order to find the confirmation that he [is] deadly ill." Most alarmingly, he threatens another attempt at suicide, stating that "it would be better to send [me] away immediately since [I am] unable to go on living."

His doctors at Hillside do not send him away. Rather, on the second day of his hospitalization, they start him on electroconvulsive therapy, or ECT. Patient X has eleven separate treatments, and during their course, eight grand mal seizures are induced. Although seizures are considered a hallmark of epilepsy or brain illness, seizures in ECT are beneficial. As early as his second treatment, X begins to brighten. By the end of the series "his depression has cleared up entirely and patient is busy making plans for his future," as his hospital chart notes. He is transferred to one of Hillside's cottages, where he remains for another month, making plans "to go to a mountain resort for the first two months after leaving the hospital, to reopen later his private practice in Washington, D.C." As he is discharged, he looks forward to the future, optimistically planning to "take his car, his wife, and his boy and start out on a trip. He [is] sure that they would all enjoy themselves." The prognosis for X is favorable; ECT seems to have cured his debilitating depressive illness and given him back his life.

Electroconvulsive therapy has been used for nearly seventy years to treat mental illness, and yet its story as a powerful and beneficial medical tool is relatively unknown. As ECT pioneer Max Fink puts it: "except for penicillin for neurosyphilis and niacin for pellagra," ECT for severe mental illness "is the most effective treatment . . . developed in this [the twentieth] century."[2] Since it was first originated in the 1930s, untold numbers of severely depressed, suicidal, or psychotic patients have received ECT and other "shock" therapies, with significant amelioration of their symptoms. Its effectiveness in treating these patients would suggest it as a frontline therapy, but instead it has been employed as a method of last resort. Despite its use as a safe and effective treatment in psychiatry, ECT has been much maligned, and for a period of time spanning the 1960s through the 1980s, it was virtually absent from the list of protocols used to treat mental illness. For many, ECT and its kin somatic therapies, insulin coma and Metrazol convulsion therapy, conjure up images of spasms, fits, shock, coma, and shame. Critics claim ECT produces significant and severe memory loss and brain damage, yet in fact such side effects are either completely unfounded or are short-lived and less profound than stated.

So how can it be that a safe and effective medical procedure should garner such vitriolic negative criticism? Proven and reliable medical treatments typically continue to be practiced until they are replaced by more efficacious ones, new products of research and clinical trials, or better technologies. ECT has produced relief from acute symptoms and saved lives, but its image as a psychiatric tool is stereotyped as dangerous and inhumane. Its recent resurgence in leading psychiatric facilities is striking: What factors have contributed to this renewed acceptance of somatic therapies in contemporary psychiatry? Indeed, new tools and protocols, such as transcranial magnetic stimulation (TMS), vagus nerve stimulation (VNS), and deep brain stimulation (DBS) owe their swift acceptance by clinicians and patients alike to the trajectory of ECT's use in psychiatric medicine. And yet not one of these approaches is convincingly better or safer than ECT at treating profound mental illness.

In order to answer these questions, a careful look at the history of ECT is required—something that has not been undertaken before by either historians or psychiatrists. As writers, we come from both disciplines and can present a fair and comprehensive investigation of ECT and other shock therapies from their development in the 1930s to their use today. Our research convinces us that ECT is an important, responsible, and reliable therapy that deserves to be more widely used. Indeed, so clear are the benefits of ECT for patients who might otherwise commit suicide, or languish for years in the blackness of depression, that there should be little controversy over whether it is safe or effective. Somatic therapies like ECT easily trump anything in the psychopharmaceutical medicine chest as the most effective treatment for such severe illnesses as melancholic depression, catatonia, or manic excitement; it also has a place in the treatment of schizophrenia. We will show that the charge of brain damage from ECT is an urban myth, one first put forth by the developer of a rival therapy, Vienna's Manfred Sakel, who tried hard to subvert his competition. We take seriously the assertion that ECT is associated with memory loss, but in the vast majority of patients, memory is restored within weeks after the last treatment, suggesting that no long-term damage to the brain's memory capacities is sustained.

Why today, seventy years after its discovery, is ECT highly stigmatized, both among patients and many physicians? ECT is, in a sense, the penicillin of psychiatry. We would be baffled if the benefits of penicillin were not widely touted in the patients' world, lauded by the press, and accepted as a matter of fact by medical doctors. Why has this not happened with ECT? The question is especially important because there are a great many people with depression who do not respond to antidepressant drugs. According to a RAND Corporation study in cooperation with the University of California, Los Angeles–Neuropsychiatric Institute, even after several courses of treatment with pharmaceuticals, about half of all patients with depression remain depressed. The population of "nonresponders" is thus very large, and prominent among them are patients with suicidal ideation.[3] So it is an urgent public health matter to find therapies that will quickly show results in these patients, rescuing them from the brink. ECT is highly effective in suicidal ideation and works quickly to yield therapeutic results. A single stimulus or two is all that is typically required to dispel a patient's fixation on committing suicide, and it is clear that ECT should be tried earlier in the treatment program rather than later. Later could be too late.

Unbridled psychiatric illness has a fury that makes it among the most terrible of all diseases. Losing your faculties in the prime of life, immobilizing despair that leaves you wishing for death, delusional thoughts that see the world as alien and threatening—few illnesses are as life-crushing as these. For centuries humankind had been as helpless against them as against the ravages of bacterial infection or heart failure: if nature did not grant a spontaneous recovery, the joy of that person's life was snuffed out. These realities once made the discipline of psychiatry a prospectless enterprise; warehousing the mentally ill was seen as the only solution to safeguarding against harm to themselves or others.

In the decades before patient X was born, the treatment of mental illness represented a vast wasteland of hopelessness. Psychotherapeutic techniques for the minor psychiatric illnesses, called psychoneuroses, had been bounding ahead, particularly with the launching of Freud's psychoanalysis after 1900. Yet for the major psychiatric disorders such as endogenous depression, manic-depressive (bipolar) illness, and schizophrenia, doctors had little to offer. A working definition of schizophrenia crystallized around 1910, and if a patient received a diagnosis of schizophrenia, such as dementia praecox or hebephrenia, physicians simply shook their heads, for there was nothing they could do. "True schizophrenia" was seen as a death sentence, for the patient would be consigned to a life either cloistered at home, there to be locked in a bedroom and harangued by a distraught parent, or placed in an institution the joylessness of which it is difficult today to even imagine.

The therapeutics of psychiatry before the late nineteenth century were limited to sedation. Medicine has always been able to sedate agitated people with alkaloids of plants such as henbane or cannabis. After 1870, the resources of the German organic chemical industry started to make synthetic sedatives such as paraldehyde available. Asylum life was characterized by the stench of that compound, the patients' breath reeking of it. After 1900, considerable progress was achieved in psychopharmacology with the launch of the barbiturates, drugs that provided the respite of sleep to the troubled. Yet for the deep sadness of melancholia, the delusions of psychotic depression, the unceasing restlessness of mania, or the hallucinations of schizophrenia there was no relief. Either patients recovered spontaneously, typically after about eight months of torment, or they remained in a state marked by symptoms of varying degree. Schizophrenic illness is characterized by natural ebbs and flows, although the basic disease does not go away. For the schizophrenic and the melancholic whom the tide was sweeping out to sea, medicine offered no rescue.

Thus, frustration pervaded mainstream psychiatry before the 1930s. Physicians were helpless, families despairing, and the patients themselves subjected to such misery that suicide is a constant theme in patients' records—the psychiatric "charts" that are the main source for historians of mental illness. Older psychiatrists had long made their peace with helplessness. They sought to preserve their patients from self-harm while awaiting a spontaneous recovery and otherwise managed their asylums much as a gamekeeper manages an estate.

In the years after World War I, a younger generation of psychiatrists chafed at their therapeutic impotence and attempted to innovate. Many were inspired by the success of Vienna psychiatrist Julius Wagner von Jauregg who, in 1917, treated neurosyphilis—an illness whose early symptoms were primarily psychiatric in nature—with malarial fever, a highly physical therapy. (Wagner-Jauregg, as his name is often abbreviated, discovered that the spirochete that causes syphilis, including its neuropsychiatric symptoms, is heat-sensitive, and malarial fever arrests its proliferation.) Psychiatrists experimented with new drugs that might offer relief, and some success was achieved among derivatives of the antihistamine family. A series of compounds, most notably the antipsychotic drug chlorpromazine and other members of the phenothiazine class, ushered in a revolution in psychopharmacology by the early 1950s.

At the same time as these early stirrings in psychopharmacology, other psychiatrists tested "physical" therapies, procedures that would act on the brain as the organ of illness in mental disease. The idea behind the physical or somatic therapies was to shock the brain—and the mind—to adjust itself out of an illness state using a physical stimulus. Symptoms of disease were somehow relieved, though contemporaries were very aware that the underlying disease was not actually cured. Today, we think of somatic therapies as rewiring neural circuits in the service of remediating psychiatric symptoms, though the mechanism of their effect is not fully known.

How does one shock the brain? There are various forms of shock therapy, from insulin shock—or insulin coma—to convulsive shock therapy induced by chemical agents or by electricity. Austrian physician Manfred Sakel in 1933 coined the term "shock" therapy in the context of "hypoglycemic [low blood sugar] shock," borrowing from medical and surgical concepts of shock. But the term *shock* is largely a misnomer. Medically speaking, shock occurs when venous blood pressure plummets. ECT and other shock therapies do not cause patients to go into a state of shock. Rather, they experience unconsciousness from a dose of electric current or a chemical stimulus and then undergo a therapeutic convulsion of about a minute's duration, regaining consciousness shortly thereafter. As veteran New York ECT specialist William Karliner, a refugee from Hitler's Europe, commented in 1951: "The term 'shock' is misleading and intimidating. Its meaning is different from that used in surgery and internal medicine. Its use in psychiatry stems from its introduction in insulin coma therapy. It definitely is a misnomer."[4]

Yet shock therapy it is. The term is embedded too deeply in the patients' world and the public perception to change, even in the title of this book. As Richard Abrams, author of a leading ECT textbook, said in an interview in 2004, ECT does not get renamed "brief stimulus therapy" or whatever term might be more exact because "there are some things that will never change! No matter what you tell a patient, if you say I'm going to give you ECT, once you explain it the patient will always say, 'oh, shock therapy.' That will never change. Doesn't matter what you call it. Electrostimulatory, electrocerebral stimulation—the patient always then says 'oh, you mean shock therapy.'"[5]

Most of this book is about the form of shock therapy that causes convulsions—ECT. Why convulsive therapy, giving patients epileptic-like seizures, should be restorative in psychiatric illness remains a mystery even today. "By what path does a stimulus given to the soma reach the domain of the psyche and rehabilitate it to follow patterns that we call normal or quasi normal?" asked psychiatrist Hirsch L. Gordon in 1948. "Why should the lights of consciousness have to be extinguished before one can be relieved of anxiety and false ideas? Must one step on the very threshold of death before his shackles of seclusion and apathy may be cracked so as to save him from his own self imprisonment?"[6] For years, ignorance of the mechanism of ECT was flung in the faces of the ECT specialists, particularly by the psychoanalysts, who believed that they alone understood the mechanisms of the mind. They claimed that any treatment unable to get at the "root causes" could not be contemplated on the grounds that it was empirical. Although we now know a great deal about the relationship of the brain to behavior, we are still largely ignorant of the reasons for success and failure of any psychiatric treatment. Many psychiatric drugs are thought to work by modulating the production of neuronal receptors for specific endogenous brain chemicals. For example, imipramine, an antidepressant launched in the United States in 1959 as Tofranil, is thought to act on the metabolism of the neurotransmitter norepinephrine. ECT, on the other hand, may affect many neurochemical systems at once, especially the endocrine hormones regulated by the hypothalamus and pituitary gland. Importantly, ECT produces a therapeutic effect more quickly than the psychiatric drugs. Also, many more patients respond to it. The difference can be a matter of life and death.

As scientists offer explanations for how various treatments alleviate symptoms of mental illness, the fact remains that these are speculations. We still know neither what causes mental illness nor how to cure it. But denying patients the benefits of an effective therapy on the grounds that it is theoretically poorly understood would be unethical. This theoretical puzzlement has contributed to the stigma that continues to envelop electroconvulsive therapy. So deeply has it been stigmatized that some readers will peruse these pages with astonishment. Shock therapy! We thought that barbarous treatment long out of style! It is as though we had considered a rehabilitation of the ducking stool in the treatment of hyperactivity. The basic reality to grasp here, one thoroughly apparent to psychiatrists of past generations and to a cadre of psychiatrists working today at some of the world's top mental health research hospitals, is that ECT really does work in illnesses where drugs fail. A treatment of last resort may again be a therapy of first choice, particularly for the nonresponder group of psychiatric patients.

As these lines are written, ECT is undergoing a comeback, soaring in popularity within psychiatry and benefiting from well-informed medical journalism that portrays the procedure objectively and not as a series of Hollywood horror images. It is important to understand the history of this valuable treatment, once reviled and disdained and now in the process of rediscovery, because it can make a difference in people's lives. The history of ECT offers us much to consider as psychiatric medicine evolves in the twenty-first century.

CHAPTER TWO

"Some Experiments on the Biological Influencing of the Course of Schizophrenia"

The whole idea of a "convulsive" therapy is dissonant to many doctors and patients. By training, physicians are resistant to the notion that convulsions can be curative and their induction desirable, because they typically associate fits with brain illness or damage. Deliberately causing a patient to have an epileptic seizure, many doctors feel, means opening Pandora's box. Patients, too, instinctively shun the notion that fits can be therapeutic and imagine themselves unconscious and convulsing on a laboratory table as they have seen in films such as *One Flew over the Cuckoo's Nest*. But this image is a misconception. Convulsive therapy is not the same as induced epilepsy. Epilepsy is a neurological condition and considered a disease. Therapeutic convulsions induced by electricity, by contrast, do not harm the brain and can save lives.

Shock Therapy Enters Psychiatry

In medicine, the term *shock* implies hypothermia (low body temperature) and hypotension (low blood pressure). It can occur during exposure to harsh weather conditions, particularly when the body is both wet and cold, or surgically as a result of blood loss. Anaphylactic shock, caused by a sudden discharge of histamine, happens in an allergic reaction to a bee sting. So shock has long been a familiar medical concept.

In 1926, the Parisian psychiatrist Constance Pascal introduced the word *shock* to psychiatry.[1] As a young medical graduate of Romanian origin, she had been in 1908 the first female psychiatrist in France to join the elite Parisian asylum psychiatrists. Nearly twenty years later at the age of forty-nine and in charge of the departmental asylum in Châlons-sur-Marne, she made an important innovation. In her 1926 book on "shock treatment," she deplored the previous therapeutic nihilism of psychiatry: "To have to look on helplessly at the fatal advance of psychosis, to indifferently note demented immobility and the transition to chronicity, is just to endorse fate; accepting the predisposition to delusions and the fatal destiny of constitution also means renouncing the practical applications of the biological sciences that have modified the study of general pathology."[2]

Pascal argued that mental illness originated from "mental anaphylactic reactions." To combat it, one needed to shock the brain and the autonomic nervous system back into equilibrium. This shock should be "capable of preventing, of suspending or of curing these mental anaphylactic manifestions."[3] She argued that the body might be shocked by the injection of various substances such as colloidal gold, milk, or vaccines, or by the kind of fever therapy that Julius Wagner-Jauregg had just introduced in Vienna against neurosyphilis. In French psychiatry in the 1920s, a good deal of research was devoted to such stratagems, although it was Pascal who provided this overarching theoretical rationale. Today, she is virtually unknown, and after World War II her enthusiasm for these peculiar injections was seen as horrific. Though Pascal brought the concept of "shock" to psychiatry, she did not mean it in the sense of convulsions, which she was at pains to avoid with her various therapies.

After decades of providing stagnant custodialism in isolated asylums, the psychiatry of the 1920s tumbled with innovative new somatic or physical therapies. Injecting various substances to modify the action of the autonomic nervous system; to raise or lower vascular tone or body temperature; or even, in a throwback to a thousand years of humoral medicine, to stimulate the action of the bowels was common practice. In some asylums, infected teeth were rooted out on the grounds that they might cause "autointoxication," a kind of systemic poisoning that might involve the brain itself. There was a vogue for colectomy, removing part of the large bowel on the grounds that toxins leaking from the gut might instigate madness. Deep-sleep therapies, using barbiturates to make patients stuporous for weeks on end, gained wide currency.[4]

In those days insulin was often mentioned in the medical press. It was discovered in 1922 at the University of Toronto as the chemical governing the uptake of sugar from the bloodstream and employed, of course, in the treatment of diabetes. But it was soon used to treat nondiabetic illness as well. In psychiatric clinics it was mainly given to undernourished patients to encourage appetite.[5] Under the direction of Wagner-Jauregg, in 1926 Edith Klemperer at the University of Vienna psychiatry clinic gave insulin to a number of patients with delirium tremens, a term used to describe the psychosis and shakes of withdrawal from alcohol.[6] (Later, in her American exile, Klemperer pioneered hypnotherapy.)

At the University of Budapest psychiatry clinic somatotherapies for schizophrenia had been under way since World War I. In 1927, Dezsö Miskolczy in Professor Karl Schaffer's clinic experimented with giving large doses of insulin, and in 1928, Julius Schuster (who had earlier published results on inducing anaphylactic shock) proposed treating psychosis with shock and insulin together.[7] By the late 1920s various researchers came across the idea of deliberately putting psychiatric patients into hypoglycemic insulin comas. Swiss psychiatrist Hans Steck, at the mental hospital in Lausanne-Céry, began in 1929 the "hypoglycemic" treatment of psychosis, though he was careful to avoid producing overly deep comas and convulsions. Steck published, however, in obscure Swiss and French medical journals, and his work was not widely known.[8] In 1931 and 1932 in Basel, John Staehelin and his colleagues carried out insulin metabolism experiments on their schizophrenic patients, noting behavioral changes in the fasting patients who received insulin. Staehelin never published his findings.[9]

Manfred Sakel and Insulin Coma Therapy

In 1934, a man of forty-six was admitted to the university psychiatric clinic in Vienna with symptoms of paranoia. From the city's affluent class, he had recently demonstrated unusual behavior, becoming pathologically miserly and remaining in bed until noon in a darkened room in order to spare himself the cost of lunch. He quarreled with his relatives, who, he believed, wanted to poison him, and subsequently broke off contact with them completely. He held the Austrian National Bank and the federal chancellor responsible for money he had lost in a recent deflation and carried his written complaints personally—to save the cost of postage—to the Finance Ministry and the chancellor's residence. "In the last few days the patient has been very agitated. He says people are constantly trying to provoke him. Somebody visited him who laughed when the patient said they are shooting artillery shells

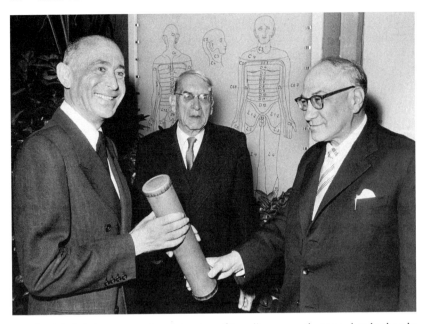

Manfred Sakel (1900–1957), originator of insulin coma therapy, beginning in 1930. Sakel, on left, is accepting an award at a 1957 symposium honoring his discovery, from Hans Hoff, head of the Vienna neuropsychiatric clinic; in the center is former Vienna psychiatry professor Otto Poetzl, with whom Sakel did his early work. ICT was the first of the shock therapies. AP/Wide World Photos.

at him. He believes he was recently hypnotized in a coffee house."[10] On the ward he was terribly fearful about his being a Jew, though he believed everyone else considered him to be a National Socialist. He felt he had to prove that he was not a Nazi. He sought protective custody from the police, thinking everybody wanted to kill him. Also, he claimed to hear his father crying (although his father lived many miles away in Silesia).

Manfred Sakel was the attending psychiatrist, and he and his colleagues at the clinic diagnosed the patient with schizophrenia. On the day following his admission, Sakel injected the patient with 45 units of insulin. Nothing happened. That evening the patient was still paranoid and hallucinotic, and refused his dinner, claiming it was poisoned. The next morning he was given three injections of 40 units of insulin each. He became calmer. At noon he was given an injection of 50 units and went into hypoglycemic shock. Insulin causes the liver and muscles to remove circulating glucose from the blood, which means denying it as well to the brain. In the absence of glucose the brain goes into a coma or stupor, which is called "insulin shock." When this patient awakened spontaneously from the coma, he was rational and apologized for all the trouble that he had caused. But then his condition worsened again. Over the next several days he continued to receive insulin injections.

"On the sixth day of the treatment the patient experiences a strong hypoglycemic reaction with somnolence and the onset of a coma, also with a huge outpouring of sweat." (This is why Sakel referred to such comas as "wet shock.")[11] The patient was calmer after this. The insulin injections continued. "In the third week of the treatment, with no warning signs, the patient experiences a major attack of epilepsy one and a half hours after an injection of 50 units of insulin, displaying tonic-clonic convulsions [muscles flexing and extending] and biting his tongue. . . . He foams at the mouth." Sakel let the fit continue for a while before terminating it with an injection of glucose (trade name, Osmon). After the seizure, the patient had complete amnesia for the preceding events, and his memory loss lasted an hour and a half. But as it returned, including recall of the beginning of the convulsion, he had complete insight into the pathological nature of his previous behavior. In the following days, small insulin injections continued, and in the fourth week of his admission the patient was judged to be normal, showing insight into the nature of his illness, and was released from the clinic able to resume work. Sakel titled the report of this patient's experience "The Treatment of Schizophrenia with Insulin as Well as with Hypoglycemic Shock," acknowledging that he was administering a shock therapy that often led to epileptic-like convulsions.

What was it that Sakel actually discovered, shock therapy or convulsive therapy? Later in life he tried to have it both ways, so as to eclipse his rivals. He claimed that when he started out, he envisioned convulsions as the workhorse of his treatment but that subsequently he came to realize that convulsions were damaging and praised the element of insulin coma. From his clinical notes on this first patient, it is clear that Sakel was not trying to induce a seizure, for the patient's sudden convulsion took him and his assistants off guard. That the patient bit his tongue indicates they had no time to insert a mouth block, and thus failed to anticipate the convulsive effect.

With insulin hypoglycemia, Sakel introduced the first of the major physical therapies of the 1930s—Metrazol and electric convulsive therapy being the other two. One obituarist honored him for "inaugurating the period of active somatic treatment of the many psychiatric patients from whom the chronic population of our mental hospitals is recruited."[12] Unlike Steck in Switzerland, who also pioneered the insulin treatment of psychosis, Sakel believed that he was treating the psychosis itself, rather than just symptoms of it. He aggressively pushed the patients into long series of deep comas, something Steck was loath to do. Many of his patients had convulsions in the course of their insulin comas, and perhaps it was those convulsions that were the therapeutic element in the "Sakel treatment."[13] The whole subject remains quite obscure today. Yet Sakel's insulin coma ushers in a period of active treatment of patients with major psychiatric illnesses, and it is this concept—that one can actually do something for people with schizophrenia, melancholia, and manic-depressive illness—that turns a page in the history of psychiatry.

Manfred Sakel was born Menachem Sokol in 1900 in the small town of Nadverna, Galicia, a province of the Austro-Hungarian Empire. He stemmed from an "old-established rabbinical family that claimed Maimonides . . . as an ancestor," according to an obituary in the *New York Times* (Maimonides was a twelfth-century Jewish philosopher). The "Polish Jews" of Sakel's day were subject to vicious anti-Semitism, and at an early age Sakel acquired a stance of haughty arrogance that accompanied him through life, alienating almost everyone with whom he came in contact.[14] He graduated in medicine from the University of Vienna in 1925, served briefly as a staff physician at an unnamed hospital there, and then in 1927, landed a position as junior staff doctor at Kurt Mendel's exclusive private nervous clinic in the Berlin suburb of Lichterfelde. It had been known as "Dr. Goldstein's Sanatorium" and specialized in the treatment of addictive disorders as well as major psychiatric illnesses (although to reassure prospective clients, it stipulated "no insanity"). Sakel, with his typical tendency to exaggerate his achievements, later referred to himself as the chief physician of the sanatorium, but he was not.

At Lichterfelde, Sakel claimed to develop a complicated theoretical rationale for insulin coma therapy and to have carried out animal research before undertaking his first human experiments. There is no evidence that any of this occurred, and indeed his later versions are at odds with his earlier stories.[15] Heinz Lehmann, later a distinguished psychopharmacologist in Montreal, knew Sakel in 1927, when he was a medical student in Berlin. According to Lehmann: "[Sakel] got his idea when he was treating heroin addicts with insulin in Berlin to help them over their withdrawal symptoms. I don't remember what his rationale was but it calmed them down. Once one of his addicts who was also schizophrenic slipped into a hypoglycemia coma. Sakel was scared but brought him out of the coma quickly with an injection of glucose. To his amazement, the patient showed a considerable improvement of his schizophrenic symptoms."[16] Sakel later told William Karliner (a fellow Viennese who was Sakel's second cousin) that this 1927 patient in Berlin had experienced a very slight convulsion. Sakel had given him insulin for sedation, but the patient felt much better afterward. Based on this experience with the drug addict who was also schizophrenic, Sakel decided to treat schizophrenics simply because he felt they were otherwise hopeless.[17]

The story goes that Sakel realized he was onto something quite promising and wanted to undertake systematic clinical trials, persuading Karl Bonhoeffer, the head of the department of psychiatry at Berlin University, to let him carry them out in the Charité Hospital, the major teaching hospital of Berlin. Bonhoeffer's colleagues revolted at the suggestion, and, for the moment, Sakel's work was stalled.[18] By 1930, however, Sakel published an article in the *Berlin Medical Weekly,* "A New Treatment for Morphine Addiction," that described giving patients insulin. Nothing was said about an insulin coma. Indeed, he said he simultaneously administered grape sugar "because I fear hypoglycemic shock."[19] Three years later, in 1933, Sakel published in a distinguished German psychiatry journal a more extensive piece on his new treatment for morphine addiction. He admitted that some of his patients experienced hypoglycemic "shocks," but he said nothing about inducing them deliberately or about their possible therapeutic value.[20]

In May 1933, Sakel returned to Vienna, apparently as a result of persecution after the Nazi seizure of power. Hans Hoff, a clinician at the psychiatric clinic at the time, recalled Sakel's first insulin case in Vienna. "Professor Wagner-Jauregg had a young lady patient who was suffering from schizophrenia as a result of an unhappy love-affair." Wagner-Jauregg promised the parents that, given treatment with bromides and barbiturates, she would soon be well again. But in fact, after a year in the private clinic where she had been admitted, she was worse. Hoff continued:

The mother told me that she planned to commit suicide together with her daughter. I went to Sakel, who had already tried insulin treatments successfully . . . in some restless schizophrenic patients. He suggested making an attempt with the use of a full insulin shock treatment, in the case of this unhappy girl. Not knowing what the results would be we started the treatment in a private institution. . . . To our surprise, after the second shock the girl seemed very coherent and started to speak with her mother, a thing which she had refused to do during her last six months' stay. However, she had another relapse after a few days, but a few more shocks led to a complete recovery which she has maintained to this day [1958].

Sakel and Hoff then treated a second patient successfully and thereupon went to Otto Poetzl, director of the University of Vienna psychiatric clinic, and informed him of their results. Poetzl offered Sakel all the facilities of the clinic for his work. Beginning in October 1933, under Poetzl's supervision and in collaboration with Karl Dussik and Christine Palisa, Sakel went on to develop his treatment method.[21]

The English neuropsychiatrist Eliot Slater was in Vienna in 1934 and saw Sakel at work. At first, Slater was inclined to be scornful, but he said later: "I am sorry to record the fact that I regarded this pioneer effort, in due time to be the thin end of a wedge which broke a way through an impassable barrier, as so much absurdity. I thought to myself, the Viennese have done it once, with the senseless but successful malarial treatment of GPI [general paralysis of the insane (neurosyphilis)] and they think they can pull off just such another wild shot."[22]

They did indeed pull it off. But was this the beginning of convulsive therapy? Sakel later claimed that it was, on the basis of a lecture on his new treatment he had given to the Vienna Medical Society on November 3, 1933. His talk was summarized in a one-paragraph description in the medical press, which stated that Sakel had thus far treated four cases of psychosis, previously resistant to all therapies, with "deep hypoglycemic shock, even involving coma and epileptic seizures. . . . The results achieved to the present justify the hope that a new direction has been taken in the treatment of schizophrenia and other states of agitation."[23] Julius Wagner-Jauregg, by then a retired professor of psychiatry in Vienna, apparently stormed out of the lecture hall upon hearing these words.[24] After Sakel had finished, a beaming Otto Poetzl stood up and said how encouraged he was by the new therapy: "The nature of the treatment consists of a very deep hypoglycemic shock with epileptic seizures."[25] According to Poetzl in 1933, Sakel's procedure *was* a convulsive therapy.

That Sakel was interested in therapeutic seizures from the start is confirmed by another young foreign visitor to the Vienna psychiatric clinic. In 1934–35, Joseph Wortis, a researcher in the psychiatry department of Bellevue Hospital in New York, visited Sakel and brought insulin therapy with him back to Bellevue. Much later Wortis said to an interested observer that, on the subject of priorities in insulin therapy, there was no doubt that Sakel was trying to induce seizures much before Ladislaus Meduna (the developer of Metrazol therapy, which we discuss later in this chapter) did so: "Meduna visited Sakel's setting in that period. . . . There is no doubt that Sakel later abandoned the induction of seizures, when Meduna developed his treatment, so that Sakel cannot claim priority for convulsive treatment. On the other hand, it was ungracious of Meduna, to say the least, never to acknowledge that Sakel did indeed try for a while to induce seizures for therapeutic benefit."[26]

Sakel himself, as we have said, tried to have it both ways. In 1950, he told the Paris World Psychiatry Congress that he had initially conceived his procedure as a convulsive therapy but then realized that convulsions were damaging to the brain, making the illness worse, and that the procedure was in fact a coma therapy. (Coma and seizures are both forms of "shock." Seizures often occur in comas, but not invariably.) "My official proposal to employ such dramatic shocks with convulsions as a therapy was [in 1933] immediately widely and sensationally publicized in the daily press at home and abroad. My preference for the convulsion, at the time of the lecture, apparently encouraged von Meduna to proceed in his laudable attempt to simplify the shock treatment by confining it to and singling out the convulsion alone for therapeutic use in schizophrenia."[27] On the basis of this supposed switch in his theoretical position, Sakel was able to argue that Meduna had stolen from him the idea of convulsive therapy, but that Meduna's convulsive therapy was harmful. This particular piece of legerdemain took place before Meduna's astonished eyes. (On the podium afterward, Meduna demonstratively refused to shake hands with Sakel.)

Still later, as Sakel realized that electroconvulsive therapy was the wave of the future and insulin coma therapy was being widely abandoned, he had yet another version that would let him claim paternity of the somatic treatments. In 1955, he told the participants at a clinical symposium on insulin at Hillside Hospital, which by this time had moved to the borough of Queens, New York, that "the therapeutic high points of the treatment, contradictory as they may appear, were introduced by me in my first lecture, as coma-hibernation or convulsion. I employed the unspecific name of shock to embrace these two diametrically opposed clinical pictures which the same treatment produced."

He told his colleagues that he disliked the terms "convulsive treatment" and "coma treatment," mere variants on the same principle of shock: "I still think that insulin shock treatment or Sakel treatment is the best name because we do not yet know the mechanics of the treatment."[28]

In the months after the November 1933 lecture, Sakel continued to perfect his technique while earning a living as co-chief physician at the Parksanatorium in the Vienna suburb of Hütteldorf-Hacking.[29] Patients began arriving from far and wide, and when an Australian psychiatrist visited Sakel at his "private sanatorium" in Vienna in 1937, Sakel had seventeen individuals there under insulin treatment.[30] Sakel became world-famous on the basis of a more extensive description of his cure that he published in the *Vienna Medical Weekly* in a thirteen-part series beginning in November 1934.[31] His 1935 book *A New Treatment for Schizophrenia* was basically a reprint of those articles.[32] He made little use of statistics in his initial publications. A controlled trial would have been out of the question, as nobody was doing them in those days. Yet once Sakel hitched himself to the more systematic Karl Theodor Dussik, their joint publications began to deliver some solid numbers. Of the first fifty-eight patients with schizophrenia of recent onset treated in the university psychiatric clinic, 86 percent had remissions that could be described either as full, good, or fit for work; of the forty-six chronic schizophrenic patients, nearly half showed remissions.[33] These were impressive results—indeed, too impressive—for other clinics were unable to confirm them. As such, the whole procedure would be cast in a shadow without strong evidence to support it.

In his papers and lectures, Sakel laid out a method so precisely that the treatment could not help but be named after him. The ideal insulin treatment would have four stages: phase 1 was a complicated series of insulin injections, with exact spacing; phase 2 was the actual shock, that had to be carefully monitored; phase 3 involved suspending the injections to let the patient rest; phase 4 was moderate insulin injections to bring the patient to the verge of shock.[34] These patients were actually brought to the brink of death, which is the next step beyond hypoglycemic coma. "The procedure is complicated, difficult and dangerous," said Joseph Wortis. Indeed, during Wortis's two-month stay in Vienna he witnessed one death and eighteen successful discharges out of twenty-five patients. "The justification for the losses," Wortis reasoned, "has been the remarkable results in the remaining cases of an otherwise almost hopeless disease."[35]

Sakel insisted that the insulin treatment should be performed

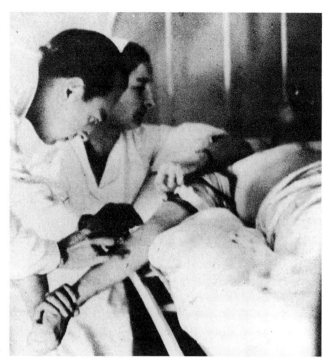

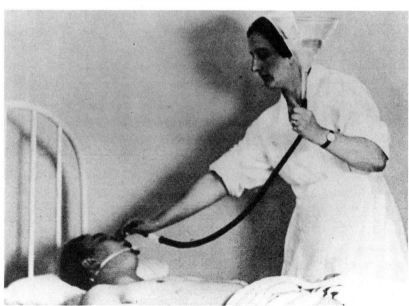

(Top) Injection of glucose to end insulin coma in the Rome university psychiatric clinic, 1937. (Above) Interrupting insulin coma with glucose in a nasogastric tube, Rome university psychiatric clinic, 1937. *Sapere*, no. 72 (December 31, 1937).

exactly as he laid it out, in all of its stages and dosages. Was this science or grandiosity? Researcher Deborah Doroshow sees all the punctilio as an exercise in "branding": "He consistently insisted upon a rigid protocol for its administration. . . . He dogmatically stressed certain key terms, categories, and tests, firmly establishing what would be known as the 'Sakel method' of administering ICT [insulin coma therapy]. . . . He could dismiss disappointing clinical results by arguing that the investigator in question had not properly adhered to the method."[36]

Meanwhile, Sakel's own behavior became increasingly obsessional and grandiose. Max Müller, a prominent early advocate of the insulin treatment on staff at Münsingen mental hospital in Berne, visited Sakel in Vienna in 1934 and remembered his "paranoid insinuations about the wickedness of a world that would not recognize his accomplishments."[37] On another occasion Sakel expressed concern to Joseph Wortis that dark international forces were conspiring to deny him the Nobel Prize—and to give it instead to Meduna—because Sakel was Jewish: "What is happening is a systematic infernal anti-Semitic campaign, supported by moneyed sources from abroad, dedicated to averting the danger that a Jew might ultimately win the Prize. The general European situation has sobered me up a bit. But the quieter I comport myself, the more openly the others proceed and choose the racially pure Meduna as the most suitable opponent."[38] (Sakel apparently did not know that Meduna himself was Jewish.) There is evidence that Sakel suffered from manic-depressive illness based on at least one clearly documented episode of serious depression.[39] His public displays of grandiosity were frequent, such as what occurred on stage at the Paris World Psychiatry Congress in 1950 when he accused Meduna of stealing his ideas. His paranoia might thus make sense in the context of a serious psychiatric illness.

Sakel did, however, have some rational reasons to be apprehensive. He was, after all, a Jew living in Austria during Hitler's rise to power. The Vienna psychiatric establishment had, by and large, turned its back on him, and Julius Wagner-Jauregg—known to be anti-Semitic—found Sakel utterly distasteful. Fearful of Wagner-Jauregg, Karl Theodor Dussik, a junior psychiatrist responsible for editing a favorable lecture on insulin by the new professor, Poetzl, "toned down" the overall optimism for the drug.[40] Aubrey Lewis, a professor of psychiatry at the Maudsley Hospital in London, said after a visit to Vienna in 1937: "It appears . . . that some of the early publicity which Sakel managed to obtain for himself caused a great deal of resentment among the more responsible people in Vienna, who felt that Sakel, and Poetzl's clinic incidentally, were almost starting a 'racket.'"[41] Sakel was the object of a particularly nasty attack by Josef Berze, the recently retired director of the Viennese provincial mental hospital Am Steinhof, in the *Vienna Medical Weekly* of December 2, 1933: Berze criticized the insulin treatment as useless—its supposed effects solely the product of suggestion— and dangerous to boot. Interestingly, Berze, a Catholic who after 1938 consulted for the Nazi Eugenics Tribunal of Vienna, misspelled Sakel's name throughout the article as "Sackel."[42]

Through the haze of unpleasantness that surrounds Sakel's personality, it is impossible not to recognize his historic importance as the originator of an effective active treatment in psychiatry.[43] As English psychiatrist Isabel Wilson commented after her careful inspection of Sakel's methods in 1936: "One of the most striking effects of the whole therapy is the occurrence of lucidity. This does not by any means always occur, but when it does, it is very remarkable." Swiss psychiatrist Max Müller told Wilson: "Very interesting is the attitude of the patients themselves to these events—they describe spontaneously that they felt better in hypoglycaemia; that their thoughts ordered themselves; that they suddenly had quite other relationships to their environment."[44] For all the virtues of the antipsychotic drugs that came along in the 1950s, few patients felt that clarity and lucidity were their main psychological benefits.

There was indeed something special about the insulin therapy. It meant that for the many languishing in the back wards of mental hospitals, there was now hope. And it offered encouragement to the discipline of psychiatry as well, previously a custodial specialty intended to keep society safe from the patients and the patients from hurting one another. With insulin therapy, psychiatry became a discipline actually able to make the patients better. As émigré psychiatrist Lothar Kalinowsky, German-born, Italian-trained, and by the beginning of World War II safely arrived at the New York State Psychiatric Institute, later said: "We can state today that whatever ways psychiatric therapy may take in the future it was the insulin treatment that made psychiatrists therapeutic-minded."[45]

Ladislaus Meduna and Induced Seizures: Metrazol Therapy

Sakel's claims aside, convulsive therapy really begins with a young neuropathologist in Budapest who made a chance observation under the

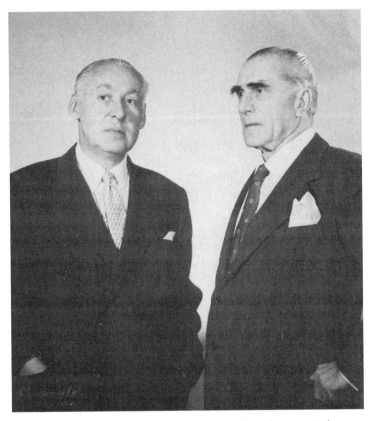

Ladislaus Meduna (1896–1964), originator of convulsive therapy, Budapest, 1935, who, with Ugo Cerletti (1877–1963), introduced electroconvulsive therapy at the Rome university psychiatric clinic in 1938. Meduna used pharmacological agents to initiate the seizures. *Convulsive Therapy* 1, no. 2 (1985): 120. Courtesy of Max Fink.

microscope. His work was entirely unrelated to Sakel's, and it is doubtful that he even knew about Sakel before the publication of Sakel's 1934 article, by which time Meduna was well launched onto his own path. The story demonstrates that convulsive therapy was not just "empirical," something that works without one knowing why, but had a rigorously scientific justification.[46]

László Meduna was born in Budapest in 1896 into a middle-class milieu.[47] He styled himself as Ladislaus von Meduna outside of Hungary and, he said, used the noble predicate "von" only to deceive the anti-Semitic German medical editors of the 1930s into believing that he was not Jewish. He was by all accounts an affable and easygoing man, and quite unpretentious—in polar contrast to the posturing Sakel. Descended from a family of Sephardic Jews, his grandfather had owned a meatpacking plant, but Meduna himself had been educated for eight years in a Catholic boarding school. On graduating from high school in 1914, he went directly into medical school. The war then intervened, and he served in an artillery unit, returning after the end of hostilities to school and graduating with a medical degree in 1921. The following year he entered the Interacademic Institute for Brain Research in Budapest, directed by Karl Schaffer, a neuropathologist and neurologist.

"Karl Schaffer was a psychiatrist sui generis," Meduna later said. Schaffer had started out as a neuroanatomist, drifted toward neuropathology, and then—like Theodor Meynert in Vienna and many other neuropathologists in those days when pathological anatomy was the basis of knowledge about mental disease—ended up in psychiatry. Schaffer had firm ideas about schizophrenia: believing it an endogenous, or inborn, psychosis, he thought it was fixed in the patient's germ plasm and would remain with the patient for the rest of his or her days. "Since [Schaffer] considered schizophrenia to be an endogenous hereditary disease, he held that it could not be cured," said Meduna later. "As the ectoderm [one of the primary germ layers from which other organs, including the central nervous system, are developed] of the embryo was already sick and as the disease was transferred by the chromosomes, any idea that this disease could be cured was to him nonsensical."[48]

Research in histopathology meant learning the techniques for slicing thin sections of nervous tissue with a microtome, then preserving and staining them so they could be examined under the microscope. "In one room of the Brain Research Institute all four walls were covered with shelves heavy-laden with jars containing brains."[49] Meduna latched onto the pineal gland (which produces melatonin in the brain), worked up the techniques for investigating it under the "mike," and was soon promoted to assistant professor. In the years from 1923 to 1930, he slowly began to develop an interest in central-nervous pathology as well as anatomy. In 1927, Karl Schaffer took the post of professor of psychiatry in the faculty of medicine and moved the Interacademic Institute to the department of psychiatry. Yet Schaffer's students did not know any psychiatry: they were pathologists.

Meduna and his colleagues went with Schaffer to the department of psychiatry, in a "small hospital of 240 beds. . . . We met the crew of the former Professor of psychiatry. They were a strange lot to our eyes and no doubt so were we to them. We did not recognize a schizophrenic patient at that time when we saw one; on the other hand, they knew as little about the brain as we knew about schizophrenia. All in all, we, the neuro-anatomists and brain research men, had a friendly and tender pity for those psychiatrists who did not know anything about the brain, while the psychiatrists looked at us with ironical derision whenever we blundered in diagnosis."[50]

In the late 1920s, Meduna became head of the outpatient department and saw many epileptic patients. Sometimes at autopsy "there were tremendous changes in the brain . . . just the opposite of those found in schizophrenia." Meduna had always been fascinated by "the beautiful slides which we could make of epileptic brains . . . and I accepted Schaffer's explanations of the great abundance of glia hyperplasia [excessive growth of a kind of support cell in the brain called glia cells]." What struck Meduna, however, was the contrast between the excessive growth of glia cells in epilepsy and "the apparent torpor of the glia system in the schizophrenic brains. . . . Thus, fairly early, I developed an idea of some sort of antagonism between the behavior of the glia system in epilepsy and the behavior of this system in schizophrenia."[51] (The finding of glia disappearance in schizophrenia came in 1931 from Béla Hechst, Meduna's colleague at the university psychiatric clinic in Budapest.[52] It is likely these findings were discussed among colleagues long before publication.)

In his previous research, Meduna sketched out the notion of there being two kinds of changes in microglia cells depending on the disease. In 1927, he studied alterations in glia in rabbit brains and wrote: "In terms of the morphological changes in the microglia there are two groups that diverge sharply from each other, of which degenerative atrophy represents mainly the intrinsic illness of the microglia, while the changes associated with swelling represent the disruption of the normal relationship between the microglia and the ganglion cells."[53] So he had clearly in mind the opposing of the two illness types, as studied through the glia, established through laboratory research at the animal level.

By 1930, Meduna's thinking veered so wildly from the ideas of his superior, Karl Schaffer, that he began doing his research in secret. To obtain human tissue, he persuaded a surgeon to do brain biopsies of patients with focal (that is, localized to a particular spot) epilepsy. The area of the brain causing the symptoms was surgically removed, and Meduna examined the tissue microscopically. He also looked at brain tissue samples from schizophrenics. "I could not help but notice at that time the contrast in the behavior of those elements of the nervous system in schizophrenia and in epilepsy: almost complete abolition of the function of the glia cells in schizophrenia and an increased proliferation in epilepsy. . . . I published this work in 1932 without knowing at that time that this would become the origin of the shock treatment."[54]

At this point Meduna began to pursue epidemiological data to nail down his case that epilepsy and schizophrenia antagonized each other. That epilepsy was uncommon in populations of schizophrenics was well known in psychiatry. In 1926, Robert Gaupp, a psychiatry professor in Tübingen, mentioned this in passing, as though his readers were already well aware of it: "The surprising rarity of a patient with epilepsy later developing schizophrenia has often been remarked upon, and it is in fact striking when we consider that epilepsy and schizophrenia are both indeed very common diseases. I myself can recall only two cases of such a combination."[55]

As Meduna followed this epidemiological trail, he asked Julius Nyirö at the state asylum in Budapest-Lipotmezö if he knew of evidence linking epilepsy and schizophrenia. Nyirö called Meduna's attention to a paper that he and Albin Jablonszky at the State Office of Social Insurance had published in a German journal in 1929 on epileptics who developed schizophrenia: once a psychotic break occurred, their incidence of subsequent epileptic attacks dropped way off. Of 176 patients either with pure epilepsy or with a combination of epilepsy and schizophrenia, only 1 percent of those with pure epilepsy recovered from the epilepsy, but 16 percent of those with epilepsy-schizophrenia recovered. In contrast to Gaupp, the authors noted that it was not unusual to find epilepsy and schizophrenia coexisting. Yet, "in regard to the epilepsy of these combination patients, relatively often there is a recovery."[56] Meduna asked himself: *Could it go the other way?* Could giving schizophrenics epilepsy help cure their schizophrenia? Other studies found few epileptics among populations of schizophrenics (this is not universally true, however).[57] Unknown apparently to Meduna, in 1931 Georges Heuyer—the originator of child psychiatry in France—had postulated an antagonism between catatonia and epilepsy: "It is very rare to find a patient with catatonic schizophrenia who is simultaneously epileptic."[58]

In 1932, Karl Wilmanns's volume, *Schizophrenia,* had just appeared— part of a massive collection on psychiatry edited by Oswald Bumke at the University of Munich that represented the apex of world knowledge of the subject at the time. Wilmanns was a professor at the University of Heidelberg, and two of his staff doctors, Gabriel Steiner and A. Strauss, had discovered that among six thousand cases of schizophrenia seen in that university hospital there were perhaps twenty who showed convulsive phenomena, either during their stay or in their previous history. And many of those attacks were not considered epilepsy, either. In fact, at that clinic in the years 1910–1931 there had been only one episode of real epilepsy.[59] In 1930, Georg Müller, a staff doctor at an asylum in the Lippe area, reported two young women with apparent schizophrenia who recovered after developing epilepsy.[60]

What impressed Meduna most in the epidemiology of epilepsy and schizophrenia was Alfred Glaus's observation in 1931 that whenever schizophrenia and epilepsy occur together, they seem to alternate—or one excludes the other. Glaus concluded: "Most often [in these patients] schizophrenia develops as acute epileptic phenomena subside or no longer appear."[61] It was an inference so pregnant that Meduna later said it was Glaus, a junior staff doctor at a Swiss asylum in St. Pirminsberg, who should have credit for developing the concept of convulsive therapy.[62]

"Any credit due me," Meduna later said, "is due to the fact that I was raised and trained in the school of Prof. Schaffer, a school in which nothing was sacred unless you could prove it with hard cold facts, and this I proposed to do."[63] First Meduna had to find a substance that would produce epileptic attacks in animals and that could later be used in patients. There are eighteenth-century accounts of psychotic patients given camphor (from the camphor tree, used traditionally as a stimulant and today in mothballs), and Meduna may have come across this obscure tradition in medicine.[64] In any event, he approached a physician at the International League against Epilepsy who recommended monobromide camphor. Meduna used simple camphor, however, because it was less toxic. In research on guinea pigs he determined that camphor did not affect any organ system except the central nervous system, where it did not cause inflammation. He published the results in 1934, without mentioning that human experiments were already in progress.[65]

On the morning of January 23, 1934, Meduna gave the first camphor injection to a patient. It was fortunate for him that the patient's main symptoms were catatonia (in this case stupor), because catatonia responds beautifully to convulsive therapy. "After forty-five minutes of anxious and fearful waiting the patient suddenly had a classic epileptic attack that lasted sixty seconds." Meduna apparently maintained his composure in front of his gathered colleagues, but as the patient recovered consciousness, Meduna's legs gave out. "My body began to tremble, a profuse sweat almost drenched me, and, as I later heard, my face was ash gray." Two male nurses had to support Meduna down the stairs to his family's apartment below (physicians lived in the clinic in those days). "My hands were trembling so I could not put the key into the lock." His wife approached him: "You did it!" she exclaimed.[66]

Meduna went back up to look at the patient. Nothing had changed from his previous symptoms. He lay still catatonic in bed, this patient who for the last four years had "never moved, never ate, never took care of his bodily needs and had to be tube-fed." Four days later Meduna gave him another injection of camphor. Two days after the fifth injection, on February 10, "for the first time in four years he got out of his bed, began to talk, requested breakfast, dressed himself without any help, was interested in everything around him, asked about his disease that he recognized, and asked how long he had been in hospital." When the staff told him "four years," he was unable to believe it.

The patient, who had lain without any signs of life for four years, "with a big smile called me by my name."

"Oh, Dr. Meduna!"

"How do you know my name?"

"Oh, I heard everything while I was sick," he replied. "I heard them talking that you were going to make some crazy experiment? Did you do it?" he asked.

Meduna turned his head away. "I could not lie and it was too early to tell the truth."[67]

The next day the patient did well, then relapsed into his catatonic stupor. Meduna continued the injections, producing another epileptiform attack. The following day the patient's stupor disappeared again. "He talked quite normally and begged us to notify his wife and ask her to come to see him. His wife came in and they had a very lively discussion during which time the wife told him that he had been sick for four years by now and she was living with her cousin." There was another relapse, then another treatment.

The next morning when Meduna came into the ward he asked the nurse: "How is Zoltan?" She grinned and answered: "We had quite a time with him. He escaped last night from the institution, went home and found out that the 'cousin' living with his wife was not a relation at all but a lover of his wife." He beat up the cousin and kicked him out of the house, declaring that he preferred to live in a mental hospital than in this crazy world. From then on Meduna considered the patient cured, and in fact he remained well at the time Meduna emigrated from Hungary in 1939.[68]

Meduna rapidly treated five patients, and every one recovered. He felt elated beyond words, wrote up the findings for a German journal, and took the manuscript to Schaffer, not knowing quite what to expect. "Well, a storm of emotions I got. . . . He called me a swindler, a humbug, a cheat, every bad name he could think of. How did I dare to claim that I cured schizophrenia, an endogenous, hereditary disease?" Schaffer told Meduna that he would disown him if Meduna published the paper. "And if ever anybody asks me whether you were my pupil I will deny it, and your name will never be mentioned in my presence."[69] Meduna collected a few more cases and published the paper anyway in 1935 under the title "Some Experiments on the Biological Influencing of the Course of Schizophrenia: Camphor and Cardiazol Therapy."[70] The initial patients were treated in the department of psychiatry, the later ones at the Lipótmezö State Mental Hospital, where director Rudolf Fabinyi exercised benign surveillance. (Meduna later deposited a copy of his book on Metrazol in "Uncle Rudi's" coffin as it was being lowered into the ground.)[71]

Some of the patients in the 1935 paper had been treated with camphor, while others received a new camphor-style drug introduced in 1926 and named generically pentylenetetrazol, brand-named Cardiazol in Europe and Metrazol in the United States.[72] Meduna came to prefer Metrazol to camphor because it was more soluble and acted more quickly. Neither drug was ideal, because as the patients lay there waiting to convulse, they were often overcome with dreadful feelings of anxiety. Also, the drugs frequently caused cerebral hyperexcitability, triggering distracting spontaneous seizures later in the day, or week. For psychosis, however, there was substantial relief, or indeed the possibility of a cure for a devastating illness that had previously been considered hopeless. The side effects were minor inconveniences.

When Meduna submitted the paper, of the twenty-six patients treated, ten were regarded as "remissions," three showed a temporary improvement, and in thirteen there was no change. A number of the patients in remission had strong catatonic features in their illness, and a different patient population might well have produced less impressive results. Yet not all those who improved had catatonic schizophrenia, and there is no doubt that convulsive therapy has real benefits in schizophrenia for the so-called positive symptoms of delusions and hallucinations.[73] In Meduna's 1937 monograph he reported on 110 patients, of whom 62 were "process schizophrenics," a term for poor-prognosis patients. Of these process schizophrenics, 80 percent experienced a remission.[74] On the basis of these statistics, Metrazol therapy was just as effective in schizophrenia as insulin therapy.

There is probably something about discovering a new technique that leads to assessing its results with the eye of faith. Australian psychiatrist Reginald Ellery, visiting Meduna's service in Budapest in 1937, said that "in 50 percent of unselected cases [ill from one week to ten years] a good remission has been obtained."[75] Although not bad as results go in the treatment of a chronic illness like schizophrenia, this is considerably less than 80 percent. As Lothar Kalinowsky, who fled the Italian racial legislation and was teaching ECT in London, said in 1939: "The methods of Sakel and Meduna have been discredited by many critical physicians because the percentage of remissions they had found in the beginning was not confirmed by any other worker."[76]

Remission statistics aside, Metrazol convulsion therapy was superior to insulin coma therapy (ICT) because it was safer—patients in deep coma were often at the brink of death. The insulin treatment had a death rate of 2 to 10 percent. And Metrazol acted with a shorter course of therapy. With ICT, forty or fifty treatments were typically necessary. Moreover, to Sakel's chagrin, Meduna complimented himself as having developed the treatment on the basis of a theory; insulin coma was, Meduna said, "empirical." The essential factor in Metrazol therapy, he maintained, was the convulsion, whereas in insulin coma the agent was hypoglycemia.[77] The aplomb with which Meduna delivered these judgments stoked Sakel to a rage and helps explain the bitterness of their confrontation at the Paris World Psychiatry Congress in 1950.

There was, however, one chief difference between Meduna and Sakel in terms of personality and character. Whereas Sakel's entire identity was caught up with his insulin treatment, Meduna always maintained a kind of ironical detachment toward Metrazol, regarding it as a *pis aller*, a stopgap solution, until something better came along. There was an almost unduly violent aspect of the procedure, he conceded: "I want to tell you about a surprising conversation I had with the Hungarian pathology professor Herr Balo," Meduna told a group of Dutch psychiatrists in 1938. "It took place in the early days of the Cardiazol treatment, as I was still full of doubts about the wisdom of publishing my method. Prof. Balo observed to me that in all areas of intellectual activity there is a singular parallelism. So it's no surprise that now, parallel to the rather violent tendencies going on in our society [the mid-1930s rise of fascism in Hungary and Nazism in Germany], in medicine as well treatment methods are surfacing that appear to be steadily more violent, so that we are almost forced to drive the Devil out of our patients with Beelzebub."[78] For Meduna to contribute this observation to a conference critically assessing his work was astonishing, evidence of the kind of dispassionate detachment of which Sakel would never have been capable.

Meduna's idea of antagonism between schizophrenia and epilepsy has not been reliably confirmed, and there is some evidence of epilepsy in schizophrenic populations.[79] A diagnosis of schizophrenia itself is a slippery concept and is not verifiable, furthering the confusion about the relationship. At the symptom level there may well be an antagonism between the pathophysiology of seizures and psychosis, rather than between the systemic disorders of schizophrenia and epilepsy.[80]

For Meduna himself, the discovery of the safety and effectiveness of convulsive therapy brought him much disgrace at home and celebrity abroad. His book *The Convulsive Therapy of Schizophrenia* became an international sensation, and a stream of American visitors to Budapest followed. The reception at home, by contrast, was disbelief and scorn. Most Budapest psychiatrists "considered me, giving me the benefit of the doubt, a crack-pot, or lacking that, a humbug." Meduna was asked to leave the university immediately, whereupon he took a post at Budapest-Lipótmező asylum, and later at Budapest-Angyalföld asylum once Nyirö had become director there. Schaffer's successor (whom Meduna does not name but was evidently Ladislaus Benedek) was even more contemptuous and "poured upon my head every possible accusation: the method was no good, it did not cure anybody, it was barbaric, it was non-permissible torture of the patients."[81]

Vindication of sorts came in 1937, when Meduna was invited by Max Müller to a big international conference on the new physical therapies at the Münsingen asylum in Berne. He met Jakob Klaesi, who had popularized deep-sleep therapy in psychiatry in the 1920s. "Professor Klaesi shook my hand in a perfunctory way, looked around and asked me, 'Where is your father?'" Meduna did not quite understand and answered, "Well, he was not invited." "Yes," thundered Klaesi, "I signed the invitation myself." Meduna was perplexed. "But," he said, "my father isn't even a doctor." "What!" shouted Klaesi, "You are the Meduna who discovered the Metrazol treatment?" Klaesi embraced him, in a moment of triumph.[82]

CHAPTER THREE

"Madness Cured with Electricity"

In early April 1938, the Police Commissariat of Rome brought to Ugo Cerletti's psychiatric clinic a mechanic from Milan named Enrico X. A man in his forties, Enrico had been picked up at the Rome railway station trying to board various trains without a ticket. "The subject does not appear to be in full possession of his mental faculties," the conveyance slip noted. Three days later, as Enrico was examined at the clinic, he seemed "lucid and oriented," meaning that he knew where he was. But he "expresses in neologisms delusional ideas about being influenced." In fact, the patient spoke in a strange kind of jargon; he also believed that his thoughts were being transmitted to others. Aside from that he seemed indifferent to his surroundings and showed little emotion; on the ward he lay about mumbling. The diagnosis of the clinicians was schizophrenia[1] (in its generic form recognized at the time, though he also meets the criteria for delirious mania, a disorder that is eminently responsive to induced seizures).[2] Enrico had previously been hospitalized in 1937 at the Mombello asylum in Milan, where he received Metrazol therapy. After his successful treatment at Cerletti's clinic with ECT, starting on April 11 and continuing through May 1938, Enrico's schizophrenic mutterings were replaced by normal speech and his pathological jealousy of his wife lifted. Enrico X was the first patient in history to be treated with electroshock.

An American colleague later wrote to Cerletti: "Electroshock can boast of having liberated humankind of millions of tons of suffering."[3] Historically the procedure ranks among the most effective interventions in mental medicine, for suicidal ideation fades with the second or third treatment, the agitation of mania is subdued almost at once, and the mental pain of melancholia is usually vanquished by the sixth application. The importance of Cerletti's achievement lies not in its conceptual value, as Metrazol had already demonstrated the effectiveness of therapeutic convulsions in treating psychiatric illness. The importance of the convulsive principle was therefore already clear, and no one has ever shown electrically induced seizures to be more effective than Metrazol-induced seizures. The significance of ECT lay in the fact that it acted more quickly than Metrazol and was better tolerated by patients, who hated the feeling of dread they experienced with the drug as the loss of consciousness loomed (with ECT loss of consciousness is instantaneous). ECT therefore quickly replaced Metrazol as the convulsive therapy of choice and stands for a triumph of the principle of convulsive therapy, not for the principle of electricity. To anyone's knowledge, there is yet no better convulsive agent than electricity.

Ugo Cerletti and the Invention of ECT

Ugo Cerletti was born in 1877 in the small town of Conegliano near Venice, the son of an agricultural engineer who had moved there from Lombardy. Cerletti read medicine first in Turin, then after spending a year studying with the German histopathologist Franz Nissl in Heidelberg, he returned to Italy and graduated with a medical degree in Rome in 1901, finishing with a host of academic honors. Interested in biological psychiatry, Cerletti became an assistant (equivalent to a medical residency or postdoctoral position), initially with psychiatry professor Ezio Sciamanna, then with his successor, Augusto Tamburini, two of Italy's most prominent academic psychiatrists before World War I. Cerletti set up a small laboratory for research in neuropathology in the Clinic for Nervous and Mental Diseases at the University of Rome, where he and Gaetano Perusini, later a collaborator with Alois Alzheimer in the study of dementia, would prepare slides from brain tissue taken at autopsy and examine them under the microscope. It is said that when Nissl visited Cerletti's laboratory in Rome, he broke into tears at the primitiveness of the setup and said: "Impossible! Why don't you come work with us!"[4]

In the decade before World War I, Cerletti traveled to study in the world-famous psychiatric institutes of Germany and France, back to Nissl's lab in Heidelberg, and then to Munich to work with Emil Kraepelin—a leader of modern psychiatric diagnostics. In Munich Cerletti also worked with Alzheimer, and in Paris with Pierre Marie, the star

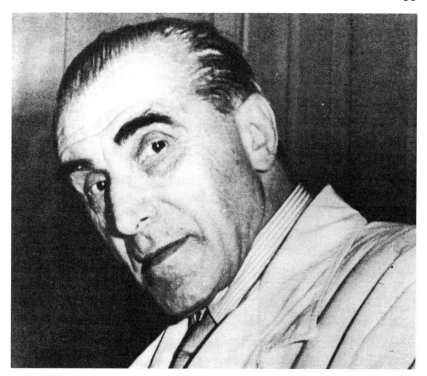

Ugo Cerletti (1877–1963), originator of electroconvulsive therapy, Rome university psychiatric clinic, 1938. The principle of convulsive therapy was already established, but Cerletti used electricity to initiate the seizures. *Settimo Giorno* (July 1951).

figure of French neurology. The clinic in Munich offered postgraduate training courses in biological psychiatry that Cerletti and Perusini attended with physicians from all around the world.[5]

In Rome, Cerletti worked in the outpatient department for "nervous diseases" of the psychiatric clinic. Compared with the research superpowers of France and Germany, Italy in those years was a backwater. Perusini just threw up his hands at even the thought of comparing Italy to Germany, where the classrooms had hot and cold running water and slide projectors! But as a member of the elite group of Italian psychiatrists who spoke German and frequented the fast-lane clinics north of the Alps, Cerletti figured among the stars of Italian psychiatry.

After volunteering as a military physician and serving at the front in northern Italy during the war, around 1919 Cerletti became director of the Institute of Neurobiology, which was the research laboratory of Mombello asylum, a large psychiatric hospital in Milan with 3,500 beds. At this point, Cerletti marched through a series of professorships.

In Italy and Germany in these years, the "professor of psychiatry" was both chair of the department of psychiatry and director of the university psychiatric hospital, or "clinic." Cerletti started this progression at the University of Bari, becoming professor of psychiatry there and founding in 1925 the psychiatric clinic of the university hospital. In 1928, he moved to the University of Genoa, building up its university clinic. Finally, in 1935, at the age of fifty-eight, he was called to the most prestigious chair in the entire system, the professorship of psychiatry in Rome and director of the Clinic for Nervous and Mental Diseases of the University of Rome.[6]

The ECT story began shortly after Cerletti's arrival in Genoa. In line with his interest in tissue changes in the central nervous system, in 1931 he decided to determine whether the hippocampus (or "horn of Ammon," a region of the brain now known to play a role in learning and memory) was involved in epilepsy. How to investigate something like this? Induce epileptic fits in dogs and then examine tissue from the brain area in question. In 1933, the physiologist Gaetano Viale suggested to him that electricity might be a nontoxic way of inducing epilepsy in dogs (so that the tissue would not be changed by the convulsive agent itself),[7] and Cerletti began experiments on dogs, with one electrode in the animal's mouth, the other in the rectum—so as not to pass electricity directly through the brain itself. There was nothing innovative about this as such, and the mortality of the procedure was very high because the current passed through the dog's heart, disrupting its electrical (pacemaker) activity. Several previous physiologists had used electric current as a convulsive agent, and in 1934, in an article in the journal Pathologica, Cerletti's student in Genoa, Angelo Chiauzzi, was able to demonstrate that, using Viale's method, one could induce epileptic fits safely in dogs with a 50-cycle (50-hertz) current of 125 volts at a duration of one-half second.[8]

When Cerletti was called to the professorship in Rome, he wanted to continue his research and asked an assistant professor at the clinic, Lucio Bini, to help him with this work. Bini built a machine that could conveniently cause seizures in dogs with controlled doses of electricity. Born in Rome, Bini was twenty-seven at the time and had graduated in medicine in 1932 with a doctoral dissertation in the area of psychiatry. Bini also had considerable competence in building electrical devices. With the aid of the clinic's electrician, he proceeded to construct a primitive machine that had a stopwatch for controlling the duration of current and a rheostat for adjusting the voltage. It was designed to use alternating current from wall sockets. Cerletti had already determined that a duration of one-tenth to one-fifth of a second was sufficient to provoke a seizure. Because the mortality of the dogs in Genoa had been so high, Bini determined that the best placement for the electrodes in giving dogs convulsions was to put both of them on the cranium, avoiding electrical disruption of the heart.[9]

Meanwhile, in 1935 Meduna had announced his finding that inducing fits with Metrazol could relieve schizophrenia. This news caused gradual awareness in Cerletti and his team that their electrical method of inducing seizures was applicable to schizophrenic treatment. Cerletti knew from his dog experiments with electricity that the loss of consciousness was instantaneous, and that, to spare the Metrazol patients the subjective suffering that occurred prior to the onset of convulsions, they might be switched to electricity.[10] Cerletti needed to determine if electricity could similarly induce therapeutic convulsions. The first step was to establish through animal research that electricity could be applied safely. Public images of electrocutions and capital punishment using an electric chair served to raise concerns, and the whole idea of applying electricity in convulsive doses seemed culturally ill-starred.

The Cerletti team also needed to acquire greater knowledge of insulin treatments (which they were already doing in the Rome clinic) and Metrazol therapies. In 1936, Cerletti, accompanied by two assistants—Bini and a German neuropsychiatrist named Lothar Kalinowsky—traveled to Vienna to have Sakel demonstrate insulin therapy. There they witnessed Metrazol therapy as well. Cerletti returned to Rome, but Bini and Kalinowsky stayed on for several months. When they came back and discussed what they had learned about the Metrazol therapy, Cerletti's first question was related to convulsive, not coma therapy: "Why was Meduna not using the much simpler method of inducing fits with electricity?"[11] In October 1936, Bini called his main assistants together to outline a research agenda and to ask each to assume responsibility for a certain aspect: Bini and Ferdinando ("Nando") Accornero would study insulin coma; Lamberto Longhi would be responsible for Metrazol treatments, which began the following year; and Bini would investigate the electroconvulsive safety question in dogs.

In May 1937, Bini and Accornero traveled to an international conference arranged by Swiss psychiatrist Max Müller at the asylum in Münsingen, also attended by Meduna and Sakel. Its theme was the treatment of schizophrenia, a subject that did not exist five years previously.[12] Here Bini met Meduna and told him of their plans to try

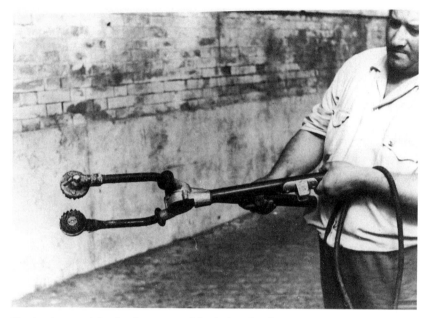

Electrodes used in the Rome municipal slaughterhouse to stun pigs, c. 1938. *Sapere*, no. 154 (May 1941).

electroshock. "Would it work?" Bini asked. "Why not?" answered Meduna. "It is not the camphor or the Metrazol that cures the patients but the convulsion produced by those drugs."[13]

When the two assistants returned to Rome, Accornero reminded Bini that electricity was used to kill pigs at the Rome municipal slaughterhouse, and that they should go there to investigate the safety of such an approach. Bini and Accornero were politely received (although by Cerletti's account it is he who had the idea and went first to the slaughterhouse). They learned that the pigs were not actually killed with electricity but merely stunned into unconsciousness so that their throats could be cut more easily. Yet the stunned pigs, if not immediately dispatched, clearly exhibited the classic symptoms of grand mal epilepsy: a big clonic contraction of the muscles, followed by clonic-tonic (back-and-forth) movements of the limbs. Cerletti apparently asked Bini to undertake systematic studies of the safety threshold: How large a dose of electricity was required to kill a pig? How great was the window of safety between the convulsive dose and the fatal dose? (It was in fact large: 400 volts was fatal, 120 volts convulsive.) And how much time was required for a fatal dose? (About 60–150 seconds.) So there was an ample margin of safety.[14]

Afterward in the slaughterhouse, Cerletti, Bini, and Accornero discussed a course of action. The young assistants were keen to press ahead, but Cerletti's position was more conservative. The Rome clinic already had a controversial reputation for being interventionist. If something went wrong, argued Cerletti: "The reputation of our school would fall into enormous discredit."[15] Nonetheless, by November 1937 Cerletti was resolute enough that he telegraphed his next move at a conference on schizophrenia in Milan: "One might foresee that even the present methods of shock will not be kept in use for long, at least not in their current forms, but will be replaced, perhaps in a little while, with newer, more simpler methods, agents acting directly on the morbid core of illness through mechanisms that are better understood and more easily regulated."[16] Finally, in April 1938, the patient Enrico X was admitted to the clinic. On the evening before April 11, Bini told Accornero: "It's been decided. Tomorrow we're going to try it."

The First Electroshock Treatment

The list is long of those who claimed to have been present at the first electroshock.[17] Accornero remembers only himself, Longhi, Bini, and Cerletti, but admits to being nervous enough at the time that he might have forgotten others. A psychiatrist named Giorgio Alberti, who also worked as a part-time journalist, later claimed that he was present but discredited his account by placing it in the afternoon.[18] Cerletti recalled another assistant, Edoardo Balduzzi (whom he brought with him from Genoa) as being present (a point on which Balduzzi anxiously queried him later, when credit for being among the pioneers was being handed about); Cerletti also recalled Kalinowsky and Giovanni Flescher.[19] This would already be a full house for a small room and a patient who at the beginning was fully conscious, but later applications of ECT would be virtual three-ring circuses, as audiences of curious physicians were summoned—by two blasts of a trumpet no less—from all over the clinic.

Lucio Bini's laboratory notebook stands as documentation for what occurred on that day. On the basis of other evidence, the patient was Enrico X. The notebook records, on April 11, 1938, at 11:15 A.M., "the patient is laid supinely on the bed," arms tied (in contrast to later practice). The electrodes are attached to his temples with a rubber band.[20] For the first dose, the Cerletti team applied 80 volts of electricity for a quarter-second. The patient had a slight spasm of the muscles of the trunk and

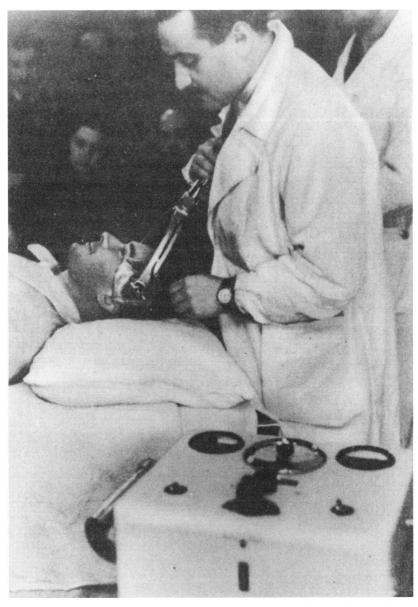

Lucio Bini administering ECT in the Rome university psychiatric clinic, c. 1940. *Sapere*, no. 154 (May 1941).

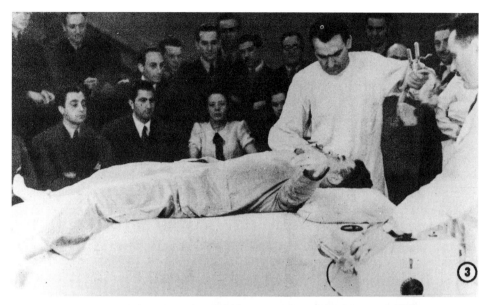

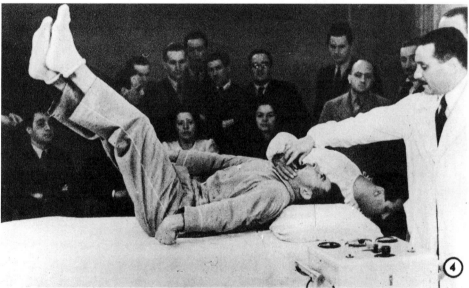

ECT in the Rome university psychiatric clinic, c. 1948: (Top) attendant removes electrodes immediately after inducing seizure while Bini looks on. (Above) Bini checks mouthguard in an unmodified grand mal seizure. *Tempo* (March 1948).

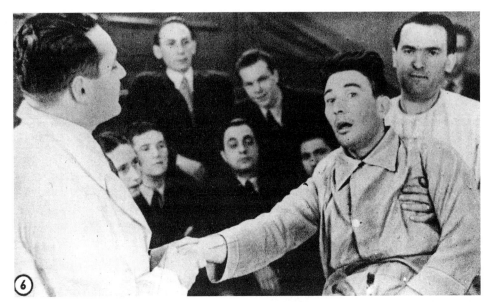

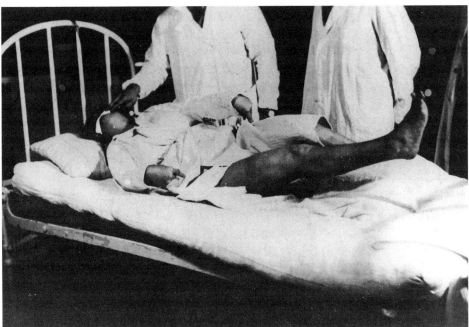

ECT in the Rome university psychiatric clinic, c. 1948: (Top) ECT patient awakens after end of seizure and talks with Bini. (Above) N.B.: characteristic head rotation and extension and outward rotation of limbs before flexion during unmodified seizure in convulsive therapy. *Sapere*, no. 154 (May 1941).

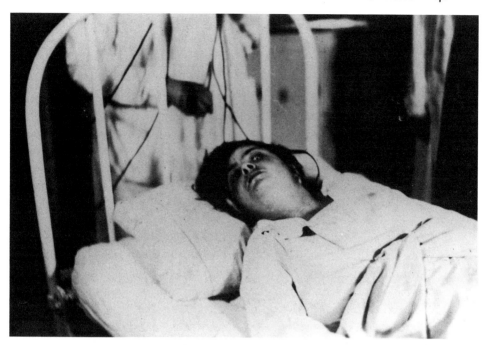

The second patient (first female patient) to receive ECT, April 1938; photograph taken in the Rome university psychiatric clinic and published in an Italian journal in 1940. From Lucio Bini, "La tecnica e le manifestazioni dell'Elettroshock," *Revista Sperimentale di Freniatria* 64 (1940): 363–458.

limbs, became pale, and began singing loudly, but he did not lose consciousness. The treatment had failed: There had been no grand mal convulsion. The second dose occurred ten minutes later; this time 80 volts for a half-second. The results were the same. The worried psychiatrists consulted about whether to press on; the assistants all urged that it be "postponed"; while Cerletti himself was indecisive. The patient, who had been listening to the discussion, cried out, not in his usual jargon but in clear Italian: "Attention! Another time is murderous!"[21] Cerletti decided to forge ahead. Fifteen minutes later, they gave a third dose of 80 volts for three-quarters of a second. Again, no grand mal seizure or loss of consciousness resulted. "The patient is freed," noted Bini, "gets up immediately, walks quietly back to the ward, talking in his usual loose way." The first attempt to induce ECT had failed.

More than a week later, on April 20, 1938, the physicians tried again. After treating a female patient, they readied Enrico S. once more, but this time, instead of progressively increasing the duration of the 80-volt stimulus, they decided to give higher voltages. At 92 volts for a half-second, the patient responded with a general tonic spasm, then clonic contractions of the limbs and trunk that lasted for about 80 seconds, followed by a period of 105 seconds in which he did not breathe. Bini counted out loud the duration of the apnea. The patient ejaculated semen (which is not uncommon in a grand mal convulsion, as is also a spontaneous loss of urine). Enrico's face became "quite cyanotic" (pale), and corneal reflexes were absent, indicating a state of unconsciousness.

After four to five minutes Enrico began to move his head and limbs and to open his eyes. But he did not respond to questions or stimuli. His Babinski reflex was "positive" and abnormal, reflecting a change in brain signals to the limbs (a normal Babinski means turning the big toe downward in response to tickling the sole of the foot). Ten minutes after its induction, the convulsion ceased and "he seems partly to have regained consciousness." About three minutes later, he started to respond to questions and to carry out a few simple instructions. Another two minutes after that he began to speak, stating that he remembered nothing. "When he was shown the electrodes and asked if he wished to repeat the experiment, he was completely indifferent." Enrico S. got out of bed and walked back to the ward.

Six or seven further treatments are recorded in Bini's notebook,[22] and we know from Cerletti's account that Enrico X had perhaps four more beyond these, for a total of eleven. By May 14, 1938, he was able to "write to the physicians of the Clinic a well-composed letter, in which he gave information about his previous illnesses and the attempted treatments and thanked the physicians." On May 28, Cerletti and Bini presented Enrico X to the Royal Academy of Medicine of Rome in a session titled "A New Method of Shock Therapy: Electroshock.'"[23] To make the point that ECT was superior to Metrazol, they gave Enrico ECT before the astonished audience. A second patient received Metrazol. A headline story the following day in a major Italian daily paper announced: "Brilliant New Method of Treating Psychosis"; the session was said to have been greeted with "hot applause."[24] On June 17, Enrico X was discharged from the clinic, "calm, well oriented," as Cerletti later said. As the patient's chart noted: "He takes part eagerly and flawlessly in the routines of the Clinic. Thought and memory unimpaired. He has full awareness of his former hallucinations regarding the ideas of persecution, attributing all of them to his illness. He has been in correspondence with his family." He was sent back to Milan.[25]

The first electroshock treatment produced a positive therapeutic result. Enrico had been rescued from a debilitating illness. Interestingly, Cerletti and Accornero distorted the record a bit, and in their published accounts they conflated the treatments of April 11 and April 20 to sound as though Enrico had received two failed shocks and then a triumphantly successful one in the first day of treatment.[26] Bini's notebook tells a different tale. The creators of electroshock had been so eager to give the public a perfect story that they concealed a few weaknesses to their claims present in the record.

There is another imperfection that they covered up. Almost two years later, on March 4, 1940, Enrico's wife wrote to Bini saying that her husband had been readmitted to Mombello Psychiatric Hospital in Milan.[27] She asked Bini to contact his clinician there. Bini forwarded the note to Cerletti with "Urgent, important" scrawled at the top. Cerletti neither acknowledged nor responded.

Getting Going

After Cerletti and Bini's presentation at the Academy of Medicine, news spread quickly about an effective new treatment for "schizophrenia." Families of patients from all over Italy wrote to the clinic, and patients treated with "electric jolts" began to get better. "The schizophrenics coming out of epileptic convulsions have a visible sense of calm and repose," reported one big daily paper in August 1938. The reporter talked with a young history graduate student who received treatment. "And he discussed with us, in the greatest clarity and precision that one can imagine, the study he was researching of the Emperor Hadrian, which he intends to get back to as soon as he is discharged from the Clinic. Life is regaining all of its profundity and color for this young man, who for an entire year had not been able to leave his bedroom."[28] "Madness Cured with Electricity" was the headline of the story.

Shortly after the first patient had been given ECT, Cerletti convened his assistants and gave them assignments. He wanted to work up a scientific dossier on the mechanism, technique, and side effects of the new treatment and asked each one to undertake an investigation: this one was to study changes in the fundus of the eyeball in ECT, that one to study blood chemistry. For lack of funds, they did not have what would have been the most useful investigative aid of all—an electroencephalograph (EEG) to record patterns of the brain's electrical activity before, during, and after ECT treatments. (Though EEGs were available since Hans Berger first described the procedure in 1929, the Rome clinic did not get one until 1950.) As if the patients were race cars at a pit stop, the assistants would swarm over them as they lay in bed in the ECT suite—reflex hammers, ophthalmoscopes, and syringes in hand. Although, as Accornero conceded, an occasional shoe was thrown at this industrious crew, by and large the patients were not hesitant about the procedure and accepted it readily.[29]

Following the insulin and Metrazol models, clinicians at the Rome clinic gave long courses of ECT, and the number of treatments would later be regarded as "abuses." Of the twenty patients at the clinic whose ECT series started between May 23 and September 14, 1938, the average number of treatments per patient was twenty-one, a rather high number in the wisdom of hindsight. And some of those treatments included multiple stimuli (typically, if the first stimulus failed to elicit a grand mal, a second or third might be given).[30] The clinicians were groping their way in the dark and had only the examples of other somatic treatments to guide them. They developed their own jargon for giving a stimulus (*zapare*) and for describing patients who were "poorly zapped" (*mal zapato*). The results of these early trials were published in 1940 in a special issue of the *Rivista Sperimentale di Freniatria* (Italy's *Journal of Experimental Psychiatry*) that was immediately reissued as a book. Until after the war, this special issue became the standard scientific guide to the administration of ECT.[31] Because of the war, however, few copies of the journal reached readers outside of Europe, and great uncertainty prevailed abroad about exactly how the procedure should be conducted.

One stumbling block to its acceptance outside the Rome clinic was the electrical technology for administering the stimulating voltage. What began with a contraption cobbled together by Bini for dog studies needed to evolve for use in humans in clinical settings. As early as July 1938, Cerletti and Bini had contacted the Arcioni company in Milan, asking it to build a proper device, for which Arcioni would then have an exclusive license. In the meantime, Bini applied for an Italian patent. Asked if he wanted to be listed on the patent as a co-inventor, Cerletti refused, saying that he did not think the machine represented truly new principles.[32] But one wonders if Cerletti's reluctance to get involved with patents did not stem from the traditional physicians' distaste for any kind of exclusivity attached to their discoveries: medicine was supposed to be about advancing the welfare of humankind, not commerce, it was once thought. (It is interesting how today, in such fields as psychopharmacology, any vestige of this high-minded reluctance has been mercilessly obliterated.) By October 1938, Arcioni produced the new device, and it was used in the Rome clinic for the first time on the fifteenth of the month.[33]

With a respectable machine in hand, Cerletti could now assent to the many physicians wanting to come to the clinic for a day or two to observe. Throughout 1939 and 1940 there was extraordinary interest among Italian psychiatrists, both in private nervous clinics and provincial hospitals, in learning ECT and acquiring the new machine. The psychiatric hospital in Naples told Bini it needed to get hold of a machine "urgently."[34] Several neurological centers, on the face of it dedicated to the care of victims of the "lethargic encephalitis" epidemic that swept Europe after World War I (a sign of the euphemisms in which the care of psychiatric illness in those days was often cast), expressed a lively interest in ECT machines.[35] It was also helpful to the cause of ECT that the Italian Ministry of the Interior, in the face of a growing national shortage of insulin, mandated in the summer of 1940 that electroconvulsive therapy be used in all psychiatric hospitals rather than insulin coma therapy.[36]

By the summer of 1940, therefore, Cerletti had every reason to be pleased with himself. He had launched a major new therapy in the treatment of schizophrenia and depression, and indeed had already discovered that it was more suitable to depression than to schizophrenia (in which latter disease it was effective mainly in cases of recent onset).[37] He had scientifically determined, on the basis of five years of animal experiments, the appropriate voltages and duration of current. And he had ensured that it could be administered safely: the reason for the lack of human histopathology studies in the Rome clinic over the years was that they never had any patient deaths.[38] Although fractures and dislocations were theoretically possible—and did in fact occur—they did not happen often, and most patients were physically unscathed from the treatment.

But Cerletti was always bothered that the procedure was known as the Cerletti-Bini technique—indeed sometimes the Bini-Cerletti technique! Cerletti was not intellectually ungenerous and insisted over the years that the credit for the idea of convulsive therapy belonged to Meduna. Yet he felt obliged to include Bini's name on the first publication, the summary of the session at the Rome Academy of Medicine on May 28, 1938, mainly because he needed Bini's help in demonstrating the procedure. For Cerletti, Bini's claim to the development of ECT was not substantial. Bini designed and built the first machine for inducing seizures in dogs and carried out animal studies in which stepping up the voltage was seen as less harmful than increasing the duration of the current.[39] In addition, he contributed several ideas about technique, such as multiple seizures on the same day, a practice rather unfortunately referred to as "annihilation."[40] But the vision of therapeutic epilepsy—of applying electricity to the human brain with the intention of healing—and the courage to carry it out, were Cerletti's. Later, Cerletti also got credit for the view that ECT affected neurohormones controlled by the basal ganglia and the brain stem, rather than conceptualizing shock as solely a cortical phenomenon.[41]

Cerletti seethed in private at the double-barreled "Cerletti-Bini" eponym, and when his widow, Etta Cerletti, donated her husband's papers in 1965 to the Menninger Foundation in Topeka, Kansas, she insisted that they be kept separate from Bini's: "This is because for a period, and particularly in English-speaking countries, the double parenthood of Cerletti and Bini was applied to the E[lectro].S[hock]. In reality this therapy had been conceived and worked out by my husband."[42]

How could the outside world have got it so wrong?

Kalinowsky in Europe

In 1938, when Lothar Kalinowsky and his wife returned to Germany to buy a car so they could tour around Europe, the thirty-nine-year-old already had an important reputation in Germany as a neuropsychiatrist. The son of a lawyer, Kalinowsky was born in Berlin but grew up in suburban Bernau. In 1917, he began medical studies at Berlin University, even though he had a strong philosophical orientation and commitment to social activism. After serving briefly in World War I, he continued with medicine, listening to psychiatrist Hans Gruhle lecture on schizophrenia at Heidelberg (and Karl Jaspers there on philosophy); he also attended Emil Kraepelin's lectures in Munich. After qualifying in 1922, Kalinowsky trained in psychiatry under Wagner-Jauregg (and his assistant Paul Schilder) in Vienna, and—following Schilder's lead—had a strong interest in psychotherapy. Between his return to Berlin in 1925 and his definitive departure from Germany in 1933, Kalinowsky did a series of extended fellowships at the major German psychiatry and neurology centers, for example, in Breslau with the neurologist Otfrid Foerster (who had treated the dying Lenin). Kalinowsky was also involved in community outpatient clinics. He was not just another dispassionate brain researcher, in other words, who saw his patients mainly in terms of the autopsy findings he would soon derive from their brains. As he later noted in his autobiography, "What we were missing at the time was the possibility of active treatment for our patients."[43]

Kalinowsky's mother was Jewish, and after Hitler's seizure of power in 1933, Kalinowsky realized he did not have an academic future in Germany. He decided to emigrate to Italy, "the land of longing for every German," as he later put it. Foerster wrote a letter of recommendation to the professor of psychiatry in Rome, and in May 1933 Kalinowsky arrived there, knocking on doors and looking for work. He wound up in the psychiatry clinic, two years before Cerletti's arrival. To become licensed in Italy, Kalinowsky had to do a year's worth of studies in subjects such as tropical medicine that were not offered in Germany. By 1935, he passed both his licensing exam and the specialty exam in psychiatry in the clinic in Rome.

Kalinowsky, with his background in social activism, philosophy, and community psychiatry, was initially horrified at the idea of electroshock—as Cerletti reminded him when the two clashed at the Paris World Congress of Psychiatry in 1950.[44] But the new procedure offered possibilities of active treatment, and Kalinowsky was soon won over. He became a personal friend of Bini, and the two worked closely together. Then, in 1939, government decrees forbade the practice of medicine in Italy to "foreign non-Aryans," and Kalinowsky was obliged to leave. He often reflected later on the sweetness of life in the Italian capital. He had a small private psychiatric practice in the afternoons at the Porta Pinciana, where he saw mainly foreigners; mornings he was at the clinic; and at noontime they would wander over to the Via Veneto for a leisurely lunch.

In 1939 he, his wife, and their two children piled into their new car and drove to Paris from Germany. Though Kalinowsky acquired an ECT apparatus from Arcioni, he left it behind, taking only the designs with him when he departed Italy. These, however, he somehow failed to produce from his luggage, and he really had very little to show Professor Henri Claude at the Ste. Anne Mental Hospital.[45] He drifted on to Brussels and Amsterdam, where he discussed the new procedure with local clinicians. Finally, in July 1939, the Kalinowskys settled in London.

Throughout this period, what was driving Kalinowsky was not so much the frisson of scientific excitement, being the Johnny Appleseed of a brave new technique, but the question of patents. Bini held the patent for Italy, but being unable to negotiate patents abroad, he had ceded to Kalinowsky the patent rights for England and the United States. Therefore, as long as the foreign patents were not in place (which they never were because Kalinowsky, like Bini, was never successful at securing them), everywhere Kalinowsky went he talked about the Bini-Cerletti technique. He did this to promote his friend's invention over its competitors (Bini received from Arcioni a thousand lire per machine sold.) At the end of 1939, he wrote to Bini that he had an article on ECT forthcoming in an English journal. "And I've succeeded, even before the publication of this article, in having a paper of mine on method published in which I shall point out the name of the company that makes the machine you've licensed to them. . . . In a few weeks your method will be not less known and accepted in England than in Italy." [46]

It is doubtful that Cerletti was aware of all the patent machinations his younger assistants were undertaking. In any event, it was in vain, for neither Bini nor Kalinowsky made any money from their ECT patents.[47] Yet this is where much of the "Cerletti-Bini" (not to mention, the "Bini-Cerletti") talk was originating—from Kalinowsky as he tried to chat up the Bini machine. Cerletti was forced to retire from his professorship in 1948 at the age of seventy. It forms a rather piquant note that an increasingly embittered old man did not realize that his two assistants were involuntarily muddying the credit for his scientific accomplishment.

CHAPTER FOUR

From the University Clinic to the Psychiatric Institute
Shock Therapy Goes Global

On November 30, 1937, a female schoolteacher in her early twenties was admitted to Hillside Hospital in Hastings-on-Hudson, New York (its original location, before it moved to Queens). Mae X's problems started when she was working at a summer camp. "While there, a man kissed her, according to the patient for the first time in her life."[1] She became panicky and imagined that everybody at camp knew about it and was talking about her. She experienced auditory hallucinations, believed that everyone had turned against her, and failed to return to the classroom that fall. She came to Hillside with a diagnosis of schizophrenia; before her admission the family was told that she would be receiving insulin therapy. On December 2, doctors began giving her insulin injections four times a week. By February she was regularly induced into comas with injections of 100 units of insulin at a time (a considerable dose). Erwin Levy, a resident physician recently arrived in the United States from Germany, was her primary physician and administered the insulin. Levy saw that she remained psychotic, and he penned in her chart: "Dr. Osserman [whom she had previously seen] was told to write a new Bible and as a reason for that she states that he treats the three sisters and that she was vomiting every night. The patient does not have any insight into the complete nonsense of this statement and the causal connection."

By January she was hearing voices telling her that "they throw people down the sewer." All the while she was having insulin treatments and was now going easily into comas. But the treatments did not seem that successful. Sometime in early March 1938, she wrote a letter home: "Dear Folks, I have little to write. Feeling low but trying to make the best of it. Take it easy at home. Don't fight with each other. . . . Also do not pay attention to those around you. Learn to get hard yourselves and remember that you are Jews, not Italians." The letter concluded with a P.S. "Don't be fooled by anyone, especially when going home and coming." Because her paranoia continued, she was shortly taken off insulin, as there was no evidence it was having any effect.

Around the middle of April 1938, Metrazol therapy was started, and its effect in reducing her paranoia was at first minimal. Obsessed "about the idea that [she] has never been given a chance, has had to suffer from prejudice because they were Jews, that she cannot stand it anymore," she complained that "in one of the doctor's offices she found some gas, and that the first meal that [she] received in this hospital was poisoned." Banging her fist on the table, she "shout[ed] at the top of her lungs, with the tears running down over her cheeks."

After several trials of Metrazol her condition improved. She appreciated Levy's friendliness and believed him and Dr. Morris D. Epstein to be her allies, whereas Dr. Louis Wender, Hillside's medical director, was her enemy. By June she began to mix with the other patients, and the chart note of July 26 says: "The patient has shown very good improvement since the last note was dictated. The insight is growing deeper, and she is at present quite amazed at the fact that such minor incidents as a kiss at the camp should have been able to throw her off balance." On September 27, 1938, she was discharged and returned to the classroom.

Only seven months before Mae X arrived at Hillside, Erwin Levy had treated the first patient to receive ICT there. Wender had instructed him to begin the treatment, but Levy had been skeptical about it at the time. After his experience with Mae X, Levy noted a therapeutic distinction between the two protocols: "One feels that this patient has responded to Metrazol and not to insulin, for after the cessation of the insulin therapy, the patient continued to be psychotic, delusional and asocial, and the response actually appeared after the injections of Metrazol. One feels that this patient's recovery is due to the chemotherapy she received."

In the late 1930s and early 1940s, the three new physical therapies—ICT, Metrazol, and ECT—left their institutional homelands in Vienna, Budapest, and Rome to become applied all over the world. At hospitals like Hillside, the three therapies were used in conjunction, serially, or even simultaneously on the same patient. Twenty years later, only ECT would remain in practice. Insulin coma came to be seen as a specific treatment for schizophrenia but became therapeutically obsolete in the decade following the advent of the first antipsychotic drugs, beginning with chlorpromazine in 1952. ECT ultimately vanquished Metrazol as the better of the two convulsive therapies. Metrazol typically triggered partial and incomplete seizures, whereas ECT reliably elicited a full response. Metrazol was also accompanied by occasional tardive convulsions—seizures that occurred spontaneously later in the treatment day. And so by the late 1950s, ECT remained alone on the field among the somatic therapies.

This story has been misunderstood by subsequent observers, who have tended to dismiss the various somatic therapies as faddish, brutal, or somehow just embarrassing in view of the simplicity of opening a bottle of pills or the supposition that only psychoanalysis could get to "the roots" of the problem. But these arguments fail to account for the rapid spread of the treatments—ultimately spanning the globe—in late 1930s and 1940s. By the mid-1940s, they had become part of the therapeutic apparatus of nearly every mental hospital, not just in the western world but in Asia and Latin America and many private practices as well—because they were effective. What was forgotten by later generations was just how well they did work.

The Insulin Period

As insulin treatment for schizophrenia burst on the international scene, its initial impact was in Switzerland, a world center of psychiatry known for its clinics in Zurich and Berne. At the Psychiatric Hospital and University Clinic of the Zurich Canton (Burghölzli) in Zurich, Eugen Bleuler coined the term *schizophrenia* in 1908; in Berne, Jakob Klaesi popularized deep-sleep therapy in the 1920s.

In 1919, Bleuler diagnosed Russian ballet star Vaslav Nijinsky with schizophrenia, and soon after Nijinsky was admitted to the Swiss nerve clinic, Bellevue, in the village of Kreuzlingen in Thurgau Canton, a private sanatorium run by the Binswanger family. In 1936, Nijinsky's wife, Romola, learned of Sakel's insulin treatment and contacted him in Vienna, wondering if insulin hypoglycemia could relieve her husband's illness. Sakel came to Kreuzlingen, consulted with various Swiss psychiatrists, and promised to administer the treatment as soon as he was free.

In August 1938, Sakel returned to Kreuzlingen and began to put Nijinsky into insulin comas. The treatment was interrupted when Sakel left permanently for the United States, and Nijinsky was transferred to the state asylum in Münsingen, where staff psychiatrist Max Müller continued the treatment. According to Romola: "The improvement was slow and steady but distinct." Nijinsky progressed so well that he and his wife were able to take a cottage in the Bernese Oberland district; he even resumed dancing. Romola reported: "Vaslav began to act and behave quite normally. The insulin shock had decidedly freed him from hallucinations." (Unfortunately, the story did not have a happy ending. Nijinsky relapsed, and though he wanted to follow Sakel to New York to continue treatment, the U.S. Consulate blocked the visa on a pretext. Nijinsky died in Europe ten years later, again insane, in 1950.)[2]

As Romola and Vaslav waited for the treatment to begin, Müller, excited by the gains he had been making with the insulin cure in other patients at Münsingen, persuaded the Swiss Psychiatric Society to dedicate its 1937 annual meeting to insulin. Although normally only about sixty psychiatrists turned out for such an event, in May 1937 more than two hundred participants from all over the world converged on Münsingen for the first international presentation of the insulin cure.[3] The meeting was crucial to insulin's international launch: "People trust Müller," said one observer. "They don't trust Sakel. People trust Münsingen; they don't trust Vienna."[4] At the conference there were some sixty-eight scientific contributions on insulin therapy, a showcase event that, in the words of Joseph Wortis, truly put insulin coma therapy "on the map."[5]

Müller visited Sakel in Vienna sometime early in 1935 to learn the insulin cure, then in September of that year introduced it to Münsingen, where refugee German psychiatrist Gertrud May took charge of the service. ICT's popularity in Switzerland was not at the conservative state asylums but rather at the market-oriented private nervous clinics such as Bellevue in Kreuzlingen. German patients were said to flock to these private clinics seeking a recovery in order to avoid being sterilized under the Nazi eugenic legislation back home.[6] Even before the conference in 1937, the Swiss psychiatric scene had been heavily infiltrated by insulin therapy. By the time of the conference, the cure had been implemented at André Repond's Maison de Santé Malévoz in Monthey (Valais Canton), at the clinic Les Rives de Prangins (Vaud Canton, run by Oscar Forel, the son of psychiatry professor Auguste Forel), and at Felix Georgi's Bellevue Clinic in Yverdon (also in Vaud Canton).

Elsewhere in Europe, it was well established in university centers such as Budapest in Hungary, and Tübingen and Giessen in Germany. Some of the most progressive figures of the age had begun to take it up, such as Paris psychiatry professor Henri Claude and Rolf Gjessing in Oslo (who in 1932 described "periodic catatonia"). In May 1936, Sakel boasted to Joseph Wortis that insulin treatment had been adopted in seventeen university psychiatry clinics around the world, from Tokyo to Poland.[7]

In Britain, Herbert Pullar-Strecker, born and trained in Germany, initiated insulin coma therapy at the Royal Edinburgh Hospital for Mental Disorders, evidently sometime early in 1936.[8] The crucial moment for British acceptance of insulin was the report of Isabel Wilson, a medical commissioner of the Board of Control of England and Wales, in July 1936. After visits to Sakel in Vienna and Müller in Münsingen, she praised the treatment and urged its adoption in England.[9] In November 1938, psychiatrist Russell Fraser, together with leading somaticist William Sargant, brought insulin to the Maudsley Hospital, a leading psychiatric teaching center in London.[10] Said Sargant later, "Right from the start, one saw patients starting to get better at the Maudsley Hospital with insulin-coma treatment, who might have been treated psychotherapeutically for months before, and on whom every other method of treatment available at that time had been tried, without any success at all."[11]

Another leading insulin center in the United Kingdom was the Crichton Royal Hospital in Dumfries, Scotland, under Willy Mayer-Gross, the émigré German psychiatrist and former member of the "Heidelberg School" who forcefully advocated the somatic therapies in Britain. It was known that schizophrenics treated with insulin were likely to relapse. In a three-year follow-up study, Mayer-Gross established that fresh-onset patients had a much lower relapse rate than did untreated controls: the recovery rate in schizophrenics ill less than one year who had been treated with insulin was 56.9 percent; in those ill one to two years, 43.4 percent recovered. By contrast, the recovery rate in untreated controls who had been ill less than a year was only 34.5 percent.[12]

World War II introduced a major discontinuity into European research on the somatic therapies. Nurses disappeared into army hospitals; many mental hospital beds were given over to military casualties; the physicians were forced to focus on muddling through rather than on scientific work. In the Denbigh Mental Hospital of North Wales, for example, the insulin shock unit was simply abandoned. As the superintendent noted with a stiff upper lip in the *Annual Report* for 1940: "When the War came, the organisation of a Department for the treatment of Dementia Praecox by Insulin Shock was complete and a preliminary trial with six cases had been successfully accomplished, the nursing staff had become familiar with the exacting technique and all was set for commencing on a full scale. It was, therefore, with considerable regret that we abandoned the project." They had had to yield the space and the nurses to other needs.[13]

With war raging in Europe, the psychiatric theater for insulin moved to the United States, and it was there that the treatment enjoyed its greatest success. The American interest in ICT harkens back to 1933, when four eager physicians from the United States separately visited Sakel in Vienna to learn the new technique.[14] One was Henry Brill, then twenty-seven and a junior staff psychiatrist at Pilgrim State Hospital in West Brentwood, Long Island, part of the New York state hospital system. The New York State Department of Mental Health was keen to develop innovative therapies as a way of reducing costs in its exploding patient population. A second American visitor was Bernard Glueck, whom Brill recommended see Sakel. Glueck, then fifty, was the director of Stony Lodge in Ossining, New York, an expensive private nervous clinic similar to those in Switzerland and intent on gaining a competitive edge. Glueck had been born in Poland and presumably spoke German, as Sakel in those days knew little English. Clarence Oberndorf, fifty-one in 1933, who in 1913 had organized a psychiatric service within the neurology division of Mount Sinai Hospital in New York, was the third.[15] Though a founding member of the New York Psychoanalytic Society, Oberndorf—like many analysts in those years— was quite curious about the new somatic therapies and readily referred patients for them. He was also a member of the board of directors of Hillside Hospital, where insulin was introduced in April 1937.[16]

The fourth American to visit Sakel came early in 1934. Joseph Wortis, twenty-seven at the time, held in those years an exclusive fellowship. In July 1933, a privately wealthy Harvard art historian named Kingsley Porter had committed suicide, torn, as were so many gay individuals in those days, between the desire to live as a gay male and the necessity of maintaining the facade of a heterosexual marriage.[17] His widow, Lucy Wallace Porter, intent on learning more about the nature of homosexuality, asked Havelock Ellis (an English sex researcher) and Adolf Meyer (professor of psychiatry at Johns Hopkins University) to nominate a young psychiatrist who might undertake a private research project for her, and Meyer suggested Brooklyn-born Wortis. In addition to being very bright, Wortis was an ideal candidate to do research in Europe because he had received his medical degree in 1932 from the University of Vienna, and had also studied in Paris and Munich. Wortis held this exclusive fellowship from 1933 to 1940, reporting periodically to Mrs. Porter about his activities.[18]

In 1933–1934, Wortis interned at Bellevue Hospital, the city hospital of New York at First Avenue and Thirtieth Street, and late in 1933 spent time with Sigmund Freud in Vienna studying his psychoanalysis. In January 1934, he joined Sakel at the university psychiatric clinic, witnessing there the work with insulin. Later that year Wortis returned to Bellevue as an unpaid research fellow and set up, with the support of staff psychiatrist Paul Schilder, another Viennese, an insulin service, apparently the first in the United States. Bellevue became an important training center for the somatic treatments because the head of psychiatry, Karl Bowman, decided to encourage insulin. Around 1937, at the therapy's height, the insulin service under Wortis boasted twenty-six beds, two assistant physicians, ten nurses, and a secretary.[19] Indeed, in September 1937, Wortis organized a postgraduate course on insulin at the hospital, all the while traveling extensively to introduce it to the medical profession.[20] Yet the therapy was simply too complicated and risky for a municipal psychiatric hospital that was strapped for funds. In 1942, after an insulin patient at Bellevue died, Samuel ("Sam") Bernard Wortis, a cousin of Joseph's who had become head of psychiatry there, forbade further insulin coma treatments.[21]

Sakel himself played perhaps the greatest role in insulin's dissemination in the United States. Around September 1936, Sakel visited New York, lured by the prospect of treating a wealthy member of the Gimbel family of New York's Gimbel's department store (with an honorarium somewhere in the range of three to ten thousand dollars[22]—the equivalent of the annual income of a family doctor in those days). He returned to Europe in May 1937 for the insulin meeting in Münsingen, then in September he moved permanently to New York. He took up residence at the Murray Hill Hotel on Park Avenue, where he also saw patients, sending some of them to expensive private nervous clinics such as Dr. C. Jonathan Slocum's Craig House in Beacon, New York. William Karliner, then recently arrived in New York as a refugee from Vienna, recalls driving up with Sakel in a hired limousine to administer an insulin treatment. Other patients Sakel saw in the hotel, where he gave them small doses of insulin (to induce a subcoma) for such indications as nervousness. He treated a large number of patients for free, yet became himself a wealthy man treating New York's elite at steep prices.

Sakel largely cut himself off from academic affiliations—partly because colleagues at such places as the Payne Whitney Clinic of New York Hospital, where he might otherwise have been welcomed, were offended by his arrogance and rapaciousness.[23] As Lothar Kalinowsky told Lucio Bini in 1940, Sakel had in New York "the worst possible reputation as a money grubber [*un affarista*]."[24] Ladislaus Meduna had plenty of reason to be leery of Sakel for the latter's unremitting attacks on him over priority. As Meduna snidely observed in 1949 in a conversation with Herbert Pullar-Strecker: "I understand that he is among the big money makers of our profession and is doing marvelously in New York. So far as I know, he is not connected with any University; probably, he has found private practice better suited to him than the somewhat sour honey of research."[25] At the time of his death from a heart attack in 1957, Sakel left a well-endowed private foundation on whose board served some of the social eminences of New York, including advertising executive and charity benefactor Emerson Foote.[26] (He also bequeathed two million dollars to his female companion, Marianne Englander.)[27]

Sakel's reputation was so strong that he did not need an academic title to promote insulin therapy. Indeed, he spurned the offer of a professorship in the psychiatry department of Albany Medical College.[28] But under his aegis, insulin coma therapy took wing in the United States. His first major public appearance occurred at a combined meeting of the New York Neurological Society and the psychiatry section of the New York Academy of Medicine on January 12, 1937, which more than a thousand people attended. Also on the program were Joseph Wortis and Karl Bowman of Bellevue Hospital; D. Ewen Cameron, who, in March 1936, introduced insulin coma at Worcester State Hospital in Massachusetts[29] (he later, as head of psychiatry at McGill University, would undertake "depatterning" experiments with intensive ECT); Bernard Glueck, who had come down from Stony Lodge in Ossining;[30] and Adolf Meyer from Johns Hopkins University, who in 1935 launched his department into insulin treatment (without apparently having much idea of what he was doing).[31] The *New York Times* ran a story about insulin coma the day after the meeting and the following day an editorial about insulin treatment: "If the chemist has given us something that makes it possible to explain and therefore to treat mental disease physically, who is to blame us if we prefer mechanism to a mysticism which must be taken on faith."[32] (This latter remark was a swipe at psychoanalysis, unusual in the *Times*.)

Sometime during Sakel's first trip to the United States in 1936, Frederick Parsons, the commissioner of mental health for New York State, asked Sakel to take responsibility for training psychiatrists in the asylums of the huge state system in insulin coma therapy. Beginning on December 8, 1936, Sakel gave a six-week demonstration of the treatment at Harlem Valley State Hospital in Wingdale, New York. The reports then coming out of the New York State system represented the first authoritative confirmation that there was something beneficial in Sakel's treatment: it made schizophrenics better rather than merely operating, as critics charged, via the mechanism of suggestion or attentive care.[33]

Sakel traveled to other centers as well, for the chiefs of service in American psychiatry were avid to learn the new technique, given the previous impossibility of doing anything for their thousands of patients with schizophrenia. Yet there were rustles of hostility from the American psychiatric establishment that even then whiffed danger. This was a physical treatment of illnesses that Freud believed to be psychogenic and treatable exclusively with psychotherapy. When in January 1937 Sakel discussed his treatment at St. Elizabeths Hospital in Washington, D.C., the psychiatric hospital of the Public Health Service, superintendent William Alanson White, a great fan of psychoanalysis, was said to be so apprehensive about the visit that, as Wortis recalled, he "fretted while his staff besieged Sakel with questions. There was a politely hospitable but constrained luncheon, and when White then escorted us to the gate Sakel clicked his heels in Central European style, bowed, put forth his hand and said, in halting English, 'Dr. White, I wish to thank you for your hostility.'"[34]

In retrospect, it is difficult not to see Sakel, despite his blemishes, as among the most important psychiatrists of the twentieth century. The *New York Times* called him "the Pasteur of Psychiatry."[35] His insulin coma treatment had opened the door for the convulsive therapies, making the world receptive to the concept of health-restoring convulsions. Sakel demonstrated the effectiveness of a mixture of convulsions ("dry shock") and comas ("wet shock") for one of the mind's most terrible afflictions. With ICT's introduction to the scene of psychiatric medicine, other, expressly convulsive, therapies might be at least entertained. As Paul Hoch, then commissioner of mental hygiene of New

York State, later put it: "[A major] contribution of Sakel . . . was that he pointed out that schizophrenia is probably not a reaction [as Adolf Meyer believed] but an organic disease, and being an organic disease, it can be approached in the same way as other organic diseases."[36]

If insulin coma had been ineffective, Sakel's achievement would have been comparable to the discovery of the mythical phlogiston. Yet the data on behalf of its effectiveness are impressive. In 1938, Benjamin Malzberg, a statistician with the New York State Department of Mental Hygiene, studied one thousand schizophrenics who had been treated with insulin. "There can be no doubt as to the immediate efficacy of the treatment," he concluded. "Insulin shock therapy raised the recovery rate from approximately 4 percent in untreated cases to 13 percent in treated cases. It brought about a marked improvement in an additional 27 percent," compared with 11 percent in controls. "Do remissions and improvement last? Only with the passage of time can this question be fully answered."[37]

Three years later it was answered. The majority, if left without maintenance treatment, relapsed. Yet aggressive insulin treatment gave them significant periods of wellness. In 1941, T. D. Rivers and Earl D. Bond at Pennsylvania Hospital in Philadelphia followed up eighty-two insulin shock patients who had been treated rather timidly in the period 1936–38, and seventy-one patients who had been treated aggressively in the years 1939–40. Of those treated timidly, only 32 percent remained well two years later; of those treated aggressively, 61 percent. Of the entire sample of 153 patients, only 17 percent were still well at *four* years, about comparable to untreated controls. Still, the authors argued for insulin shock therapy, because "recoveries made under insulin have been prompt: this has given them more years of health in the years in which they have been observed, even though they have relapsed."[38]

Powered by positive results such as these, insulin treatment embarked on what was perhaps a twenty-year reign. Sakel starred in a special symposium on insulin coma at the annual meeting of the American Psychiatric Association in Pittsburgh on May 14, 1937.[39] Given this kind of exposure, the treatment spread rapidly through U.S. psychiatry as a whole. According to a poll conducted in October 1941 by Lawrence Kolb and Victor Vogel of the Public Health Service, insulin shock therapy was being used in 72 percent of the 305 psychiatric hospitals that responded.[40] According to researcher Deborah Doroshow, who looked at the state-by-state use of insulin therapy in the late 1930s, by 1939 the treatment had been adopted across much of the United States, with the exception of the southeastern and western states.[41] (The poorer states often did not acquire it because insulin coma was expensive to administer, requiring one nurse for every two to three patients.)

Yet the reign of insulin coma therapy was to be brief. It died under the hammer blows, first of electroconvulsive therapy, then of psychopharmacology after the introduction of chlorpromazine in 1952. As early as 1941, Kalinowsky wrote to Bini that insulin would soon be abandoned in the psychiatric hospitals of New York State because ECT had been such a big success.[42] By the end of World War II the vast New York State system had largely given it up,[43] with the exception of Creedmoor State Hospital in Queens, where insulin coma therapy lingered on until 1968 (when the shortage of ward attendants caused by a strike ended it).[44] After the success of chlorpromazine in the early 1950s, insulin units worldwide were abandoned by the score.[45] In 1953, Harold Bourne, a young trainee at the Fountain Hospital in London, landed a staggering punch with a widely cited article in the *Lancet* titled "The Insulin Myth." [46] Bourne's review of previous studies that found many of them "fallacious," summoned replies of outrage from such experienced researchers as Pullar-Strecker, William Sargant, Linford Rees, and Willy Mayer-Gross, who knew from years of experience that insulin was effective.[47]

Brian Ackner is remembered for treating the American singer, actor, and activist Paul Robeson with insulin coma. Yet Ackner also played a role in discrediting ICT, for in 1957, he and coworkers at the merged Bethlem Royal and Maudsley Hospitals in London published a randomized controlled trial of insulin against deep-sleep narcosis induced by barbiturates (a weakly effective therapy), and found no difference between them.[48] The fact that there were only twenty-five patients in each group, where the lack of a difference does not necessarily mean equivalency (this is called "type II error," which results when a study is "underpowered," that is, does not have enough patients to show small but important differences) was not sufficient for rescuing ICT from its decline.

Another randomly controlled trial carried out in 1958 by Max Fink and coinvestigators at Hillside Hospital found insulin no more effective than chlorpromazine. This virtually guaranteed the demise of ICT, as chlorpromazine was simpler to administer, safer, and better tolerated by the patients, many of whom felt uneasy about being put into comas daily for weeks at a stretch.[49] The Fink study, too, had only twenty-six patients in each set, suggesting the possibility of a type II error in interpretation. After Fink published his study, Joseph Wortis verbally upbraided him for not understanding insulin coma and for misinterpreting the data. Fink later expressed uneasiness about the conclusions reached in his own study: "The death rate with insulin coma therapy is definitely higher than with chlorpromazine. But whether efficacy is higher is still a moot point."[50] In 2000, Max Fink observed: "Often . . . when my best clinical efforts with severely psychotic patients have failed, I have thought that we put aside an effective treatment before its benefits had been adequately explored."[51]

Concern lingered that ICT, a useful therapy for schizophrenia, had been unfairly sidelined in the findings of these isolated clinical studies. A conference in October 1958 at the New York Academy of Medicine agreed that ICT remained a vital remedy in psychiatry, to little effect.[52] Mathematician John Nash—later a Nobel Prize winner whose story was told in a well-known biography by Sylvia Nasar and the related film titled *A Beautiful Mind*—was treated for schizophrenia with ICT at Trenton State Hospital in New Jersey in 1961, when ICT was virtually obsolete in the United States.[53]

In other parts of the world, insulin coma therapy—and insulin subcoma for anxiety—maintained themselves robustly, almost to the present day. In China, only recently have antipsychotic drug regimens replaced insulin. Insulin coma persisted in Russian mental hospitals through the 1990s, not because the Russians were necessarily backward (the political use of mental hospitals in the Soviet Union is another story) but because they recognized that insulin coma reached a certain population of schizophrenic patients who did not respond to drugs. Russian psychiatrists also were not under pressure from an aggressive pharmaceutical industry promoting pills to cure schizophrenia.

It is striking that each of the three somatic therapies—insulin, Metrazol, and ECT—spread worldwide from its origins in the European heartland. In time, hospitals from Palestine to Argentina would embrace them all, as the powerful logic of modern medicine spun the world from regional collections of medical folklore to an international scientific unity.

The Metrazol Moment

Like insulin coma therapy, Metrazol convulsive therapy gained currency on the world psychiatric stage in the mid twentieth century. Its mainstream use lasted a mere five years, yet it is important as the true beginning of convulsive therapy. For Ladislaus Meduna in Budapest, the diffusion of Metrazol therapy began unpromisingly. As he anxiously awaited international reactions to his 1935 paper in a prestigious German journal,[54] the first to come in was a highly negative report by Salvatore Gullotta of the San Lazzaro psychiatric hospital in Reggio Emilia. Gullotta had already made something of an international name for himself with the experimental production of catatonia and epilepsy in animals using electric current.[55] Of the ten schizophrenic patients whom Gullotta treated with Metrazol, none responded positively, and the four catatonics became worse.

Things looked up with the arrival of a German delegation, headed by Adolf Wahlmann of the Hadamar psychiatric hospital. Both Wahlmann and the town of Hadamar were shortly to become notorious names in the history of Nazi euthanasia and death-camp killing.[56] But at the time of the visit in 1935, Meduna did not yet know he was dealing with "the man who gassed many thousands of Jews, Poles, and Czechs," as Meduna later put it.[57] Yet early in 1936, Wahlmann wrote a positive notice of Metrazol therapy, and the international literature began to pay attention.[58]

Thus the adoption of Metrazol (Cardiazol) began first in Germany, where by 1938 more than half of all psychiatric hospitals surveyed used Cardiazol (twenty-two out of forty-five; thirty were using insulin, and seven were using both). Interestingly, the mortality rate associated with Metrazol in German institutions was only 0.4 percent, compared with insulin at 1.6 percent.[59] In the years of Nazi rule and authoritarian asylum governance, some German psychiatrists valued Metrazol precisely because of the terror it evoked in patients. Anton von Braunmühl, who preached humane treatment and advocated triazol, a convulsive agent that produced less apprehension, said: "To be sure there are authors who believe that Cardiazol convulsions function more or less through the immediate and sudden 'process of discipline'; for this reason these authors do not want to see the 'terror component' eliminated."[60]

Meduna himself turned more to Switzerland than Germany. He was invited as an afterthought to Max Müller's insulin conference in Münsingen in May 1937.[61] Elsewhere as well, prescribing Metrazol not only as a treatment for schizophrenia but for melancholic depression was gaining momentum; by 1938 it was used in at least twenty-three state hospitals from England to Hungary.[62] For patients with recent-onset schizophrenia, Meduna said over half achieved "full remission" with Metrazol.[63]

Just after Sakel had migrated from Vienna to New York in 1938, in 1939 Meduna left Budapest for Chicago. Apparently at the instigation of fellow Hungarian psychiatrist Victor Gonda, who lived in Chicago, Meduna was invited to lecture at Loyola University there. At the time that he accepted the invitation, Meduna did not contemplate emigrating. Yet as one biographer pointed out: "The truth was that the spreading of fascism would have meant a life sentence instead of a scientific career [in Budapest] at that point in time. He knew this, and for this reason he did not return home. This was the real motivation for his staying away."[64] At Loyola, Meduna held a faculty appointment. After 1942, he became an associate professor at the Illinois Neuropsychiatric Institute of the University of Illinois College of Medicine in Chicago and a staff psychiatrist at St. Luke's Hospital.

Unlike Sakel, who fought tenaciously for insulin after his arrival in New York, Meduna lost interest in Metrazol, coming to see it as inferior to electroconvulsive therapy. As he wrote to one correspondent in 1947 who had requested an offprint: "You know this old convulsive therapy is past history for me and I believe for almost every psychiatrist. I do not believe the original publications have much value anymore."[65] He said that he preferred ECT to Metrazol "for its simplicity." Without Meduna as its advocate, Metrazol nonetheless was prescribed in the United States. Joseph R. Blalock and William A. Horwitz, in conjunction with internist Meyer M. Harris, at the New York State Psychiatric Institute at 168th Street on Manhattan's Upper West Side, played a role in instituting its use, sometime late in 1936. By June 1937, "PI," as the Psychiatric Institute is called, had treated four patients with Metrazol who had not responded to insulin (Metrazol failed as well to improve them).[66] Earlier that same year, Hans H. Reese at the Wisconsin Psychiatric Institute and August Sauthoff at the Mendota State Hospital, both institutions in Madison, began treating schizophrenic patients with insulin and Metrazol: the insulin results, they found, were much more impressive.[67] In May 1937, Hungarian-born Emerick Friedman reported Metrazol results at a staff conference of the Buffalo (N.Y.) City Hospital, which counts as the first clinical paper on the subject.[68] And it might have been close to the last, had the focus of Metrazol not shifted from schizophrenia to depression.

Adding to Metrazol's appeal in the United States was its efficacy in mood disorders, first noted by Omaha, Nebraska, psychiatrist Abram E. Bennett in 1938. (Internationally, in October 1938, Leslie Colin Cook at the Bexley Hospital for Nervous and Mental Disorders in England reported Metrazol's efficacy in depression.)[69] Depression was considered unresponsive to insulin, and the convention quickly grew up that insulin coma was to be reserved for what everyone was calling "schizophrenia" and Metrazol should be used for affective disorders. Like many dichotomies in psychiatry, this was probably a false one, given that much "schizophrenia" in those days was probably manic-depressive illness, and that Metrazol and insulin were often simultaneously administered in both schizophrenia and depression. In any event, in 1938 Bennett, who was chief of psychiatry at the Bishop Clarkson Memorial Hospital, published an influential article on Metrazol in "depressive psychoses," and in 1939 followed it up with a second, in which he observed that "90 percent of severe depressive reactions are terminated within two to three weeks," as were two-thirds of the cases of mania.[70] By 1941, Metrazol had become even more popular than insulin in American mental hospitals. As Kolb and Vogel discovered in their 1941 survey, of 305 hospitals, 228 were using Metrazol, 219 insulin.[71]

It was on a Sunday morning late in 1937 that Metrazol was first discussed at one of the monthly case conferences at Hillside, in front of an audience of psychoanalytically oriented physicians; their main reaction was alarm.[72] The patient, Jack X, twenty-five years old and born in Austria, had come into the hospital in October with a diagnosis of manic-depressive illness. On the ward he was withdrawn, hostile, and spoke of harming himself. Morris David Epstein, the attending psychiatrist at Hillside treating Jack X, noted psychoanalytically, "He is apparently releasing his hostilities now on the oral level." On December 3, Epstein, who together with Louis Wender had published on Metrazol earlier that year,[73] decided to try Metrazol on this patient and gave him an initial dose of 3 cc. No response. At 4 cc for the next day or so, "There was a slight reaction which consisted of a feeling of coldness all over the left side and a sensation of trembling inside the body with occasional twitch around the eyelids and mouth." Jack X greatly disliked the treatments and was persuaded to continue only after learning that discharge was the alternative. On January 8, 1938, with the fifteenth treatment of 8 cc, Jack had a major convulsive seizure and went on to have two more.

Epstein noted on January 28: "Since the last note was written the patient has made a most remarkable improvement, and it may be now stated that this patient is almost entirely well. He has become friendly and sociable, very cooperative and active." Epstein added in the "Metrazol report" after Jack was discharged from Hillside some time later: "There was some slight evidence of improvement prior to the institution of Metrazol treatment, but on the other hand there can be absolutely no doubt that the patient's recovery was markedly facilitated and accelerated by the administration of the drug. When the dose reached about 7 cc. the patient began to show a very pronounced improvement, and this improvement increased with remarkable rapidity as soon as he had his first major seizure on January 8th, 1938." He had four more injections, two of which also produced major seizures. "From then until the end of his stay in the hospital the patient showed a remarkably rapid recovery," although Jack X at that point did seem to be swinging into hypomania. When Jack X was again presented to the psychoanalysts at the case conference before his discharge, there was "amazement."

Not all the patients at Hillside responded to Metrazol. Harry X, another young man diagnosed at admission with "dementia praecox," did not do well, despite several major therapeutic convulsions.[74] Epstein interviewed him on January 15, 1938:

> Q. "How is your sex life?"
> A. "That is all taken care of."
> Q. "By whom is that taken care of?"
> A. "By my advisors."
> Harry got onto the subject of being overheard:
> A. "They listen in while people talk sometimes. Sometimes it is business men, sometimes it is writers, sometimes it is stenographers. It could be men, talking about death. Death. Yes, they call on the Jews and people are talking about it all the time. The Jews . . . The Jews . . ."
> Q. "What about the Jews, Harry?" (Harry was Jewish.)
> A. "I told you, I don't know Jewish people."

Harry was discharged some time later "unimproved."

Over the following months, the Hillside staff would start patients on Metrazol at frequent intervals. Epstein became their main somatic therapist, and the results overall were quite encouraging. Of the sixteen Metrazol patients treated between December 1937 and November 1938, only three failed to respond (two who had schizophrenia and one with "manic-depressive psychosis"). There were five who recovered fully, usually from manic-depression; the rest had a variety of diagnoses and were sent home either "improved" or "much improved." Almost all of these patients were in their twenties or early thirties, individuals whom psychiatrists typically try hard to save, especially if the alternative is chronic lifelong illness.

Yet there were problems with Metrazol. One was that patients highly disliked the impending feeling of doom they experienced if there was a latent period between the injection and the onset of unconsciousness or seizure. At Hillside, a private institution with a voluntary admissions policy, staff would solve this problem by threatening to discharge the patient to Bellevue, a public hospital in Manhattan, if he or she did not cooperate. Yet therapies that patients detest, such as chemotherapy for cancer, must have convincing benefits or they will be put aside. Louis X came into Hillside in September 1939, with a diagnosis of "anxiety hysteria." By June 1940, both hospital and patient were ready to try Metrazol. "However, as soon as the actual hour approaches, he becomes very panicky and runs away from it." Yet when his brother had visited, Louis absolutely promised that he would take the Metrazol, just as, on previous occasions, he had made such promises to his wife, "and when the time came for the treatment, he ran downstairs [Hillside at Hastings was situated in an old house], offering all sorts of excuses." Louis X never did screw up his courage for Metrazol and remained in the hospital for almost another year.[75]

Second, Metrazol convulsions were often quite violent, putting patients at risk for fractures of vertebrae and other bones. The early convulsive therapists tried to dismiss fractures as an insignificant side effect. Yet as early as 1937, two asylums in the Netherlands abandoned the procedure after their patients experienced two fractures of the humerus and one of the femur.[76] In a 1939 article in the *Journal of the American Medical Association*, Phillip Polatin and coworkers at the New York State Psychiatric Institute reported that vertebral fractures occurred in 43 percent of the patients, as shown by X-rays taken before and after Metrazol treatment.[77] These were typically hairline compression fractures of the anterior rim of one of the thoracic vertebrae, caused when a patient's back arched forward (flexion) in the initial stages of a seizure. These statistics were so compelling that a number of hospitals abandoned Metrazol treatment soon after the article was published.

In April 1939, Harold Palmer of the Woodside Hospital for Functional Nervous Disorders at Muswell Hill in London visited PI and learned of this high fracture rate. On returning home, he x-rayed the twenty patients at Woodside who had received Metrazol and found fractures in a quarter of them. Because the patients had no radiographs prior to the procedure, Palmer and colleagues were unable to tell if the fractures antedated the treatment.[78] Yet among these five, several were severe crush fractures. Like Polatin, Palmer published his findings, sounding the alarm in England. Fractures of this severity did not commonly accompany insulin therapy when those patients had convulsions.[79] Metrazol's demise was inevitable.

There is always a balancing of risk and benefit in medicine. The great majority of vertebral fractures were innocuous, and patients do recover from fractures of the clavicle or humerus, though they are not innocuous. And whatever the benefits of stopping Metrazol, they might be outweighed by the risk of leaving depressed patients untreated. At Hillside, Joseph X, a twenty-seven-year-old who had been admitted with a diagnosis of "manic-depressive psychosis," began Metrazol therapy on March 11, 1938. He had been ill for about six weeks, unable to get out of bed, and was already contemplating suicide. He had four treatments, which produced only minor seizures. "His fifth treatment given on March 21st, 1938, produced a major seizure with a dose of 6.5 cc. This was the last treatment administered to the patient since he unfortunately suffered a fracture of the left mandible [lower jaw] directly attributable to the violent spasm of the musculature during the convulsion. Because of this, treatment could not be resumed."

Joseph X continued to ruminate about suicide. Yet on May 30, 1938, he appeared "cheerful and alert, ate supper and about 6:15 asked the nurse to let him go downstairs to help with the dishwashing, a job he had been doing for the past several weeks. He never reached the kitchen." Instead he went to the place where his mother, against the hospital's instructions, had left him a car. The hospital notified the police. The record continues on June 1: "Yesterday noon we were informed that the body of a man was found in a car in a garage on route 124, the Pound Ridge–South Salem road. The description tallied with that of the patient." Louis Wender, chief physician at Hillside, went to the spot and identified Joseph's body.[80] The message is that one must be cautious, in dealing with major psychiatric illnesses, about attributing too much importance to side effects. Most adverse effects in the convulsive therapies are less serious than a broken jaw.

The Triumph of Electroconvulsive Therapy

ECT first traces its acceptance as a psychiatric therapy from Cerletti's clinic in Rome to other Italian institutions. Hampered by a shortage of insulin, ECT became widely used along the Italian boot during World War II. Of the forty-six machines the Arcioni company in Milan sold by January 1940 (excluding those to members of the clinic itself), thirty-two went to asylums, private clinics, and university hospitals in Italy.[81] Yet Italy was almost entirely cut off from the outside world during the war. After 1946, Italian clinicians pleaded with foreign colleagues to send offprints of articles published about ECT—and the Italian experience had no international impact.

The first clinic outside of Italy to adopt the procedure was Max Müller's asylum in Münsingen in Switzerland. Sometime late in 1938 or early in 1939, Walter Morgenthaler of the university psychiatric clinic in Berne and Oscar Forel (son of the great Swiss psychiatrist Auguste Forel) heard Ugo Cerletti lecture on ECT in Rome, and on their return suggested that Müller try it. Lothar Kalinowsky visited Münsingen with still further encouragement, and in March 1939 he wrote Müller an enthusiastic letter. So Müller ordered an apparatus himself, the twenty-second sold. In September, Müller traveled to Milan to see his friend Professor Corberi, who had also acquired an Arcioni machine. On November 25, 1939, Müller wrote to Corberi: "We started practicing electroshock immediately after our return. We now have a whole series of patients in treatment, and I can tell you that here everybody is enthusiastic! The therapeutic results are excellent; the side effects of the other convulsive methods have been abolished and I am convinced that in the area of convulsive therapy, Cerletti's method is the method of the future!"[82]

When it became difficult to obtain Arcioni machines after the onset of hostilities throughout Europe, Müller loaned his machine to the Purtschert Company in Lucerne, who reverse-engineered it to sell their own model throughout Europe. Oscar Forel at Prangins, the Zurich university psychiatric hospital in Burghölzli, and Georgi's clinic at Yverdon had Arcioni machines, but the other Swiss facilities ordered from Purtschert.

Müller published his results in the *Swiss Medical Weekly* on April 13, 1940. He had found the Arcioni forceps-style electrodes unsatisfactory (like a scissors, holding an electrode at each temple) and devised rubber bands to hold them in place. Müller detailed his technique: how long the shock should be (a tenth of a second); how much current to use (400–800 milliamps); and the finding that it was unnecessary to shave the patient's temples. At Münsingen they administered oxygen to lessen the cyanosis the patients experienced as they stopped breathing for around half a minute during the convulsion. The big advantages of ECT, Müller noted, were that "the painful subjective side effects" of Metrazol vanished. Rather, patients experienced complete amnesia for the time immediately prior to and during the procedure, and so were willing to return for further treatment. In 413 stimuli administered to thirty-two patients, none had produced fractures. "Thus there is no doubt that electroconvulsive therapy is to be preferred to all previous convulsive therapies." [83] The time for insulin and Metrazol therapies at Münsingen had passed.

The only psychiatrist known to experimentally administer ECT to himself is Henri Bersot of the private psychiatric clinic Bellevue–Le Landeron in Neuenstadt (Berne Canton). He experienced what most ECT patients did: soon after the convulsive phase he sat up but was obviously confused and disoriented. "He is pale and his pulse slowed. He obviously is amnestic for the event; we ask him what has happened to him and he is also disoriented with respect to time." Two hours later he was still quite amnestic and believed, for example, "that he had fainted during a house call. In the course of the day his memories were then restored to him. After three days he noted that he could not remember what had happened ten minutes before the shock." [84]

When the Swiss Psychiatric Society met on November 16, 1941, Bersot headed the program and showed a film about ECT; Ludwig Binswanger, best known for his contributions to "existential" psychotherapy, reported on ECT from Kreuzlingen; and another clinician from Tunis talked about his work with ECT. Eugen Bleuler's son, Manfred Bleuler, then at Basel, discussed "healing" schizophrenics with ECT. [85] Given that Germany was then ensnared by Nazism, Italy under the rule of Mussolini, and half of France lay under German occupation, Switzerland was the first country in which ECT visibly flourished for the international community.

Thanks to Bini's and Kalinowsky's entrepreneurial efforts, after Switzerland, Germany was the next country to which ECT spread. In July 1939, the Arcioni Company sold a machine to the university psychiatric clinic in Munich, for which Kalinowsky received half of the license fee. [86] Whether Munich psychiatry professor Oswald Bumke put the machine immediately into use is unclear. One source says that, having ignored insulin coma and Cardiazol, Bumke waited to try ECT until 1941. [87] Meanwhile, Bini and Kalinowsky both were actively pursuing potential German manufacturers and speculated that they could easily win the German patent, "thanks to the political situation." [88] (But they did not.) Instead, the Siemens-Reiniger Company in Erlangen brought out a machine, evidently late in 1939, and the university clinic in Erlangen undertook the first German trials, publishing its results on February 3, 1940.[89]

The Siemens machine could deliver considerably more current than the Arcioni machine, and for a duration of up to two seconds. Indeed, Max Müller thought that the Germans dosed their patients with far too much electricity.[90] Müller also objected to the "block method" of treating patients, which involved administering Cardiazol during an insulin coma on successive days.[91] First suggested by Anton von Braun-mühl, a staff psychiatrist at the Eglfing-Haar asylum near Munich (an institution later associated with Nazi euthanasia), the block method was administered to their chronic schizophrenic patients in order to "orient" clinicians about the patients' further treatability.[92]

From Germany, ECT spread to France. Henri Claude, the professor of psychiatry in Paris who had also brought insulin and Cardiazol to France, apparently was the first to use it, sometime during 1939. Zigmond Lebensohn, later a noted Washington, D.C., psychiatrist and at the time in postgraduate training at the National Hospital for Nervous Diseases in London, was passing through the Ste. Anne clinic and witnessed it.[93] What machine Claude used is unclear, given that the French had been unable to get an Arcioni model and had been slow to build their own. The German invasion in May 1940 forced Claude to close his Paris clinic and decamp for the provinces.[94]

The first published account of ECT's use in France was on April 28, 1941, when Marcel Lapipe, the "electroradiologist" at Vaugirard Hospital in Paris, and Jean-Jacques Rondepierre, a staff psychiatrist in the Paris asylum system, reported to the French Medical-Psychological Society that, unable to procure a machine from Italy, they had built their own, undertaken some animal experiments in the physiology laboratory of the faculty of medicine to satisfy themselves that it worked and was safe, and then had given a stimulus to a patient, René F., age twenty-five. René, a schizophrenic, had already failed insulin and Metrazol treatments. The authors described inducing the first convulsion at 300 milliamps for one-tenth of a second, although they were silent about its therapeutic effects.[95]

By March 1942, the "Sismothère" machine of Lapipe and Rondepierre, built by the Chillaud Company in Paris, became available to French psychiatrists.[96] ECT then became very popular in France. According to Oscar Forel, it was because the pharmacies were empty of medicines, "but nonetheless one had to look after the patients. Electroshock was for a time the miracle cure. A colleague told me jokingly: even for marital squabbles!"[97] In a discussion of an ECT paper at a Medico-Psychological Society meeting in 1945, Paul Guiraud, soon after the author of a major psychiatric textbook, noted how much French families insisted on ECT for their affected members. And psychotherapist Eugène Minkowski added: "We simply had to give in to the pressure of the families."[98] Much later, the French intellectual class became greatly agitated about supposed abuses of ECT during the war and its aftermath. The writer Antonin Artaud was unhappy about a number of treatments at an asylum in Rodez where he was hospitalized for depression; yet the therapy is credited with restoring his creative capacity.[99] Pablo Picasso's former lover Dora Maar was treated with ECT around 1946 by psychoanalyst Jacques Lacan, and it supposedly destroyed her mind.[100] These doleful accounts are, however, at variance with the majority of French experience.

Most active in French ECT research during the war was Jean Delay, who, after 1946, was a professor of psychiatry at the faculty of medicine in Paris. In that year he published one of the seminal contributions to ECT and its mechanisms, *Electroshock and Psychophysiology,* in which he argued that convulsions emanate more from the diencephalon (midbrain thalamus and hypothalamus) than the cerebral cortex. This view had originally been articulated by Cerletti, but was unknown outside of Italy. Delay bolstered it with a large amount of animal research, explaining that disorders of mood took two forms: hyperthymia (manic and melancholic varieties) and hypothymia (of which the main variant was hebephrenic or disorganized schizophrenia). ECT acted, he said, as a sedative on hyperthymia, and as a stimulant on hypothymia.[101] Although Delay is remembered mainly as an advocate of psychopharmacology, his scientific reputation was based on his ECT research.

By the time of the Paris World Psychiatry Congress in 1950, the French were at the forefront of electroshock work. Paul Delmas-Marsalet of the university psychiatric clinic in Bordeaux noted that the overwhelming majority of French psychiatrists were favorable to it, and that such lone critics as Henri Baruk, superintendent of the national mental hospital in Charenton, a suburb of Paris, were exceptions. (For reasons no one could really figure out, Baruk fiercely opposed all the somatic therapies and referred to ECT as "incomplete electrocution with an epileptic crisis."[102] His colleague Jean Thuillier said: "He never really explained it to me in a way that made sense."[103]) Delmas-Marsalet countered Baruk by claiming that 90 percent of patients with endogenous depressions responded to ECT. He felt that rejecting it for abstract theoretical reasons was comparable to reimposing chains on patients, undoing the reforms of Philippe Pinel, the founder of modern psychiatry, who had removed the chains at the Salpêtrière Hospital a century before.[104]

ECT was practiced in the United Kingdom as well. In July 1939, Lothar Kalinowsky arrived in London from the Netherlands, where he had introduced ECT to the Dutch. He visited each of the great neuropsychiatric institutions of the English capital, including the Maudsley Hospital and the National Hospital for Nervous Diseases at Queen Square. In the course of his travels, he encountered Thomas Percy Rees, superintendent of Warlingham Park Hospital, an asylum in London formerly named Croydon Mental Hospital. Rees was well known for having kicked off the chains, in a manner of speaking, from the classic English asylum. When he became superintendent in 1935, he ordered the gates unlocked, opened the wards, and abolished restraint and isolation almost entirely.[105] It was natural, therefore, that Rees became interested in this progressive new somatic method of treating mental illness. Rees and Kalinowsky, apparently together, asked the Solus Electric Company in London to build an ECT machine. (Kalinowsky had tried to import an Arcioni model from Italy but was impeded by Italian export controls.)[106] On December 9, 1939, Kalinowsky published a paper in the *Lancet* on how ECT was used to treat schizophrenia in Italy.[107]

Independent of Kalinowsky's influence in London, neuropsychiatrist Frederick L. Golla, who in 1939 was a founding director of the Burden Neurological Institute in Bristol, and his research assistant, electrophysiologist Grey Walter, became interested in ECT. Walter, the technical expert of the team, commissioned the Edison Swan Electric Company to build a machine. On December 30, 1939, Golla, Walter, and Gerald W.T.H. Fleming reported in the *Lancet* on the first five psychotic patients from the Barnwood House asylum in Gloucester whom they had treated with ECT.[108] The authors set the machine at 140 volts and higher (Kalinowsky made a catty remark to Bini that the voltage was so high because Golla and company believed the brutish patients at Barnwood House to be unresponsive to lower doses.)[109] For a brief period the authors thought they had written the first English clinical report on ECT (it was only the first paper to study ECT with electroencephalography to chart surface brain activity). On the same day as the Golla *Lancet* article, a paper was published in the *British Medical Journal* in which two junior staff doctors at Warlingham Park said: "We have every reason to believe that [our therapeutic results] will compare favourably with those obtained by other methods, and indeed may be better, as the patients do not live in fear and dread of the next treatment day."[110]

Owing to the great interest in ECT then present in the medical community, on January 9, 1940, the Royal Society of Medicine arranged a meeting bringing all the participants together: Golla and his group from Bristol, the team from Warlingham Park, and Kalinowsky, whose major interest lay in getting the British patent and in stymieing Grey Walter.[111] After the meeting at the Royal Society, interest in ECT rapidly spread within the British Isles. In 1940, psychiatrist Eric Strauss, on staff in psychiatry at St. Bartholomew's Hospital, opened the first outpatient clinic in England for ECT, situated at Riverhead House near Sevenoaks.[112] In 1940, John G. Porter-Phillips, long-standing superintendent of Bethlehem Royal Hospital ("Bedlam"), which had just moved from Lambeth to Beckenham in Kent, installed ECT there.[113]

For this generation of British psychiatrists, ECT was a talisman. A. Spencer Paterson, a staff psychiatrist at Middlesex Hospital in London during the early ECT days, later recalled that in the 1930s, at the psychoanalytically oriented Cassell Hospital near London, he had provided psychotherapy for psychotic patients. "It is almost impossible for younger physicians to imagine the impact which the advent of shock treatments made on the morale and on the outlook of the working psychiatrist. One found that patients for whom psychotherapy given for long periods of time had no effect suddenly became symptom-free."[114] When Leslie Cook took over the female side of Bexley Hospital in Kent in 1935, "there were two wards of 65 to 70 patients each, composed mainly of chronic melancholics, who had been in the hospital for two to over twenty years. They had lost the sharp edge of their depression, but were anergic, almost inaccessible to stimulation, and preoccupied with delusions of unworthiness, hopelessness, and bodily illness which gravely incapacitated them."[115] Years later, Michael Shepherd of the Maudsley, who was the founder of English psychiatric epidemiology and a formidable advocate of psychopharmacology, recalled that description of Cook's, saying: "This corner of mental hospital life has mostly disappeared following the introduction of ECT." He added, speaking in 1959, that "At the present time there is no pharmacological substance whose efficacy can match that of ECT in the treatment of major depressive illnesses."[116] And as Kalinowsky told Meduna in

1947: "In England more work in somatic treatments is done than in any other country."[117] But the enthusiasm for ECT in England was not universal. As English hypnotherapist Cyril Robert Birnie told the psychiatry section of the Royal Society of Medicine at a symposium on ECT in January 1940: "Our patients seem to be in danger of having a very thin time. First we Cardiazolize them, then we insulinate them, and now we are proceeding to electrocute them."[118]

In the late 1930s and early 1940s, ECT spread literally to every corner of the globe. In North Africa, one of Cerletti's assistants, Dr. Felice, was trapped in Tripoli by the outbreak of hostilities. He conducted ECT there with no machine at all, simply putting the electrodes on the patient's head and rapidly pushing the plug in and out of the light socket.[119] In 1940, two Swedish physicians came down to Münsingen to view Max Müller at work.[120] ECT was rapidly establishing itself in Denmark and Sweden (but not in Norway, owing to the influence of psychoanalyst Wilhelm Reich, who emigrated from Germany in 1933 and spent 1934 to 1939 in Norway, preaching his own version of Freud's doctrines).[121] By the Paris Congress of 1950, psychiatrist Snorre Wohlfahrt, of South Hospital in Stockholm, was able to report on a study of one hundred patients treated with convulsive therapy versus the same number of controls during a five-year period between 1944 and 1949. The studies "gave us incontrovertible proof of . . . the saving of lives otherwise resulting in death from suicide and exhaustion in the untreated cases."[122]

In Latin America, ECT came first to the large psychiatric hospital in Buenos Aires, Argentina, toward the end of 1939. In midsummer 1939, Enrico Castelluci, a former resident physician at Cerletti's clinic, had ordered two machines from Arcioni. He told Bini in January 1940 that, together with his colleague Pichon Riviere—and under the benevolent approval of asylum head Gonzalo Bosh—he had successfully treated patients with melancholic stupor.[123] Castelluci's main concern, though, was in getting the Argentinean patent. Yet once obtained, he discovered it to be useless because of all the unauthorized competitors on the market.[124] Close on Castelluci's heels came J. M. Hirsch of the municipal psychiatric hospital in Caracas, Venezuela, who in September 1939 asked Bini about using a machine that Hirsch had already ordered.[125] In the next few years, sales of ECT machines were brisk throughout Latin America, indicating that the treatment diffused rapidly there.

ECT was late to arrive in the United States. On March 1, 1940, Kalinowsky set sail from England to New York, but he is not credited with bringing the therapy to the Americans.[126] Who did so remains unclear, but there are several candidates. According to Walter Barton, the official historian of the American Psychiatric Association, Cincinnati psychiatrist Douglas Goldman first used ECT in the United States, sometime in 1939, and the records are clear that he practiced the procedure by the spring of 1940.[127] Goldman, thirty-three at the time, had trained in Cincinnati, a hotbed in those days of psychoanalysis. When the American Psychiatric Association met there on May 23, 1940, Goldman gave a demonstration of ECT at "a small state hospital here," as Kalinowsky told Bini—evidently Longview State Hospital—to an audience that included Sakel and Meduna among other well-known somatic therapists.[128] Goldman himself was a pioneer of the somatic therapies, and it is a sign of the stigma later to befall ECT that at the time of his death in 1986 his widow diminished the entire accomplishment: "He did a lot of early research with electric shock, years and years ago," she said, and told a reporter that it "isn't used any longer."[129]

In the early winter of 1939–40, New York psychiatrists David J. Impastato and Renato Almansi journeyed to Washington, D.C., with an Arcioni apparatus and "administered the treatment to several of Walter Freeman's patients," as Zigmond Lebensohn recalled. "I was Dr. Freeman's associate at that time and assisted in the treatments," he said.[130] (Freeman had helped to introduce lobotomy to the United States in 1936.) Sometime between February 5 and 8, 1940, Impastato and Almansi treated the twenty-nine-year-old Miss X, who had schizophrenia, with ECT at Columbus Hospital in New York City. She had been referred to Impastato by a Dr. La Bella in 1939; she may have had a first treatment by Impastato in his office on January 7, 1940, but the hospital treatment in February with both Impastato and Almansi is clearly documented.[131] The men used the Arcioni machine that Almansi, a former resident under Cerletti, had brought with him from Italy. Almansi, an Italian Jew, was born in Parma in 1909 and was forced to flee in 1939 because of the fascist racial laws. Impastato was born in Sicily in 1903 and came to the United States in 1910.

When Almansi arrived in New York, he had tried to interest the heads of psychiatry in the "Philadelphia–New York–Boston area, in the method," as Impastato later said. In the fall of 1939, Almansi began working with Impastato, and the two conducted experiments on dogs to determine the proper convulsive voltage. Energetic, young, and scientifically oriented, they opened a large ECT practice in Manhattan, said to have "twenty-six rooms," and did most of their work on an outpatient basis. Their joint article in the *New York State Journal of Medicine* in 1940 is the first publication on ECT in the United States.[132]

It is possible that the first American application of ECT was conducted by Chicago psychiatrist Victor Gonda in 1939. Gonda, one of the American pioneers of Metrazol, had trained in Budapest; in the military hospital in Rózsahegy he had helped develop techniques of treating combat-fatigue patients with mild doses of peripheral electricity.[133] In 1925, Gonda emigrated to Chicago, where he had a staff appointment at the Parkway Sanitarium, and also worked as an attending physician at Cook County Hospital and as a professor at Loyola University. His son recalls his procuring an ECT device from the Genoan firm of Zurli and DeRegibus in midsummer 1939. The son also remembers that Gonda undertook a few animal trials, experimented on his own leg (which jerked so convulsively that he injured it), and then performed the procedure on the first patient in late January 1940 at the sanitarium.[134] Although Gonda was a scientific figure, he apparently contributed to Chicago's reputation of administering excessive amounts of ECT in outpatient "shock shops." Kalinowsky observed to Bini that Gonda gave ECT "in a manner suited to discredit the method."[135] The actual month of Gonda's first treatment of a patient may have been as late as March, and not January as his son recollected. Gonda himself wrote: "Since March 1940, I have treated 40 patients with a total of 612 electrically induced convulsions."[136] He may, though, have been referring to the beginning of a series rather than to the first patient.

Others have claimed the first ECT use in the United States, but only Goldman, Gonda, and the team of Almansi and Impastato are valid contenders. In the summer of 1940, the East Coast must have literally buzzed with electricity. Almansi evidently visited Pennsylvania Hospital in Philadelphia and discussed in November 1939 the design of Bini's machine with Joseph Hughes, a staff psychiatrist. Hughes asked engineer Fritz Schindler to build a machine, and on May 1, 1940, Lauren H. Smith and Donald W. Hastings of the psychiatry department of the hospital (the "Institute"), together with Hughes of the laboratory service, began treating patients.[137] Smith, thirty-nine, had just become head of the Institute; Hastings, junior by nine years, had just finished training there.

In the Boston area, Isadore Green, a community psychiatrist, read in 1939 in an Italian journal about Cerletti's work. He asked Louis Feldman, the director of physical therapy at Boston State Hospital, to help him build an apparatus. Their effort failed, so they enlisted an engineer named Frederick T. Davis to build a machine they called the "Commotor." It was ready by December 1939. Green and Feldman solicited Abraham Myerson, chief of research at Boston State and arguably the most influential scientific figure in New England psychiatry in those years, to help them apply it clinically. Unable to get permission to treat patients at Boston State, the three of them, together with Leo Alexander (Myerson's successor), secured permission from Eliza Lindberg to try it at her private psychiatric hospital, the Bosworth Hospital in Brookline, a close suburb of Boston. Alexander later said that "when the button was pressed, everybody looked the other way."[138] This was apparently in the summer of 1940. Under Myerson's aegis, ECT then spread rapidly in New England.

In New York, Impastato brought ECT to the psychiatric division of Bellevue Hospital, apparently late in 1940.[139] Sam Wortis, mentioned above, worked with Impastato, then in 1942 became chief of the department and further encouraged ECT. Later, it was Seymour ("Sy") Berg who assisted Impastato, taking over the Bellevue ECT service after Impastato retired in the late 1950s.[140] Thus, by the end of 1940, electroconvulsive therapy had been introduced to the main psychiatric teaching centers of the United States. In the tumult that the new somatic therapies such as insulin and Metrazol had whipped up within psychiatry, ECT was clearly gaining the upper hand.

Kalinowsky in New York

Though Renato Almansi, David Impastato, and Sam Wortis were active in New York psychiatry and somatic medicine, the main player was Lothar Kalinowsky. The beginnings of ECT in the United States are indissolubly associated with him. When in the early spring of 1940 Kalinowsky left London for the States, he had in his pocket a recommendation from Zurich psychiatry professor Hans W. Maier that he took to Adolf Meyer, professor of psychiatry at Johns Hopkins University. Kalinowsky lectured at Hopkins, but the only state in which he could become registered was New York, and like so many refugee physicians of Jewish origin, Kalinowsky settled in New York City. Meyer recommended him to Nolan D. C. Lewis, director of the New York State Psychiatric Institute. In New York, Kalinowsky first went to work with Almansi and Impastato at Columbus Hospital. Then in May 1940, Lewis offered him an apparently unpaid post at PI. Around June 17, Kalinowsky conducted the first ECT there under the aegis of S. Eugene

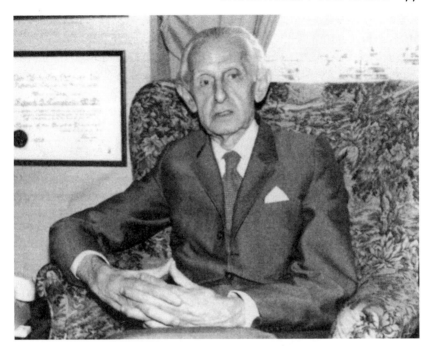

Lothar Kalinowsky (1899–1992) trained with Cerletti in the Rome university psychiatric clinic before World War II, then emigrated to New York and became the premier authority in the United States on ECT. American Psychiatric Association Library and Archives.

Barrera, the New York–born principal research psychiatrist at the Institute. Kalinowsky and Barrera commissioned PI technician Walter E. Rahm to build a machine.[141]

Impastato and Almansi had already approached the Institute, offering to perform ECT with Almansi's machine from Italy. But Barrera had turned them down. This was a source of considerable ill-feeling on all sides.[142] Yet Nolan Lewis was delighted at the arrival of Kalinowsky and with him, ECT. "The method, aside from the great monetary saving, where large groups of patients are to be treated, seems preferable to Metrazol in the sense that no disagreeable sensations or effects are experienced by the patient. . . . As a result, patients show no disinclination to subject themselves to repeated electric shock convulsion treatments."[143]

Animosity between Almansi and Impastato and Kalinowsky further heightened when on July 6, 1940, the first article in the *New York Times* on ECT, "Insanity Treated by Electric Shock," made much of Kalinowsky and Barrera, without mentioning Almansi or Impastato.[144]

Almost a year later, around May 1941, Almansi was still furious about this slight, and he complained to Bini that "in order to create a bit of publicity and can-can around himself," Kalinowsky had arranged the publication of an article that "said they were the first persons to do this work in New York." Almansi, who understood little of American journalism, was sure that Kalinowsky had edited the article and indeed had dictated parts of it himself. "I'm telling you these facts," Almansi said to Bini, "not to make recriminations, but only because I want you to know what is really going on here."[145] Kalinowsky, for his part, complained in his correspondence to Bini (who was a kind of éminence grise) that Almansi and Impastato were trying to monopolize ECT "in the way that Sakel had monopolized insulin in this country."[146]

When Kalinowsky in 1940 initially proposed a demonstration of ECT to the New York Academy of Medicine, he was treated as though he were "insane," as he later told Cerletti: "What? Pass an electric current of 125 volts through the head of an individual!"[147] Yet acceptance of ECT was such that later in 1940 an important medical journal was willing to publish Kalinowsky's and Barrera's findings. The authors commented: "We do not see in the electric convulsion therapy a radically new type of treatment but, rather, technical progress in the method of producing the convulsion. It seems preferable to most other specific methods of therapy because it overcomes most of the objections made against those other methods."[148] So swift was the progress of ECT at PI that Kalinowsky told Bini in July 1940 that they were by then treating most of the patients they admitted with ECT.[149]

Under Kalinowsky, ECT became the main form of somatic treatment at the Psychiatric Institute during World War II. The Institute became a focus of training for the entire New York State asylum system and beyond. By 1942, PI was swamped by the volume of ECT requests. Said the annual report for the year ending March 31, 1943: "As the Psychiatric Institute was one of the first hospitals to utilize electric shock treatments, there has been greater effort on the part of referring agencies and physicians to seek out our treatment facilities. However, it is impossible to provide routine electric shock to meet the general demands of the metropolitan area of New York City, and most of the applications have to be referred to other State institutions."[150] By 1945, almost two-thirds of all admissions to the Institute, the nation's premier psychiatric training center, were receiving ECT.[151]

While continuing to perform ECT at PI, in 1940 Kalinowsky also began an ECT service at Pilgrim State Hospital on Long Island, together

with Henry Brill, a staff psychiatrist at the fifteen thousand–bed institution, the largest in the country. At Pilgrim, Lothar and Hilda Kalinowsky,
together with their two daughters, resided in an apartment. But they
continued to visit New York, spending the night in Kalinowsky's room at
PI to socialize with the "European group" in the research division of PI,
a distinguished circle of émigrés including Hungarian-born Paul Hoch,
the German geneticist Franz Kallmann, the Prague biochemist Heinrich
Waelsch, and the Italian neuropathologist Armando Ferraro.[152]

In 1943, Kalinowsky left Pilgrim to concentrate on the Psychiatric
Institute and a private practice in Manhattan, where he could hospitalize his patients at the Columbia-Presbyterian Medical Center and at
Columbia's Neurological Institute. (The 160-bed PI admitted only patients who met criteria for ongoing research programs.)[153] In the mid-
1940s, Robert B. McGraw, chief of psychiatry at the Vanderbilt Clinic of
Columbia-Presbyterian, asked Kalinowsky to help him set up an ECT
suite in McGraw's private office at 2 East 85th Street. This led Kalinowsky to undertake ECT in his own office, in the same building, where
he worked with anesthetist Salvatore Dell'Aria.[154] Around this office,
and around the special ECT suite at the Psychiatric Institute, the whole
scientific world of ECT in the New York area revolved.

ECT Spreads across the United States

Psychiatrists came from all over to learn the new technique from Kalinowsky. In 1940, rumors of "the miracles that Dr. Kalinowsky was per-
forming with ECT" reached the State Hospital in Trenton. The medical
director sent Dr. John Taylor for an "apprenticeship" with Kalinowsky.
Taylor then returned to Trenton and set up an ECT program.[155] Louis
Linn, later a distinguished psychotherapist and electrotherapist at
Mount Sinai Hospital in New York, was then a junior staffer at Trenton
State. Linn recalled: "Until that time, we had treated our psychotic patients primarily with various forms of hydrotherapy and great quanti-
ties of sedation. ECT changed all that. Before our eyes we saw miracles
unfold. Patients with severe depressive disorders and stuporous states
that had disconnected them from the real world for months and even
years came to life. You can well imagine the impact this had on me as
a beginner in this strange specialty that seemed to offer little help to so
many sufferers."[156]

The striking successes of ECT had an impact on many. Of 305 psychiatric hospitals polled in October 1941 by Kolb and Vogel, 129, or

42 percent, had adopted ECT.[157] Six years later, by 1947, the figure was nine out of ten. Virginia psychiatrist Granville Jones—who was actually not a friend of ECT—summarizing an unpublished survey of the National Committee for Mental Hygiene based on a questionnaire received from 370 public and private institutions, said that "nine-tenths of the mental hospitals in the country are using some form of shock therapy," most of it ECT because it was less expensive than insulin.[158] ECT had thus conquered institutional psychiatry. In office-centered private practice, it became so widespread that psychiatrists responding to a poll in 1950 of the American Psychiatric Association endorsed ECT four to one.[159]

The results, indeed, were impressive. Benjamin Wiesel, who had served as a navy psychiatrist and then established a practice in Hartford, Connecticut, said: "It was a god-send to have electroshock therapy because, compared to nothing, it was an enormous relief." He continued: "It was like a miracle. I always related it to Lazarus risen from the grave. In those days with no treatment and nothing one could do, we used to see severe depressions and suicides. If the patient didn't have enough money for 24-hour nursing coverage until he got over the cycle, the suicide rate was very, very high." Wiesel remembered one woman who was "violently depressed, agitated." "Her dog died. We gave her three or four treatments. She recovered completely, then we asked her about the dog. She said, 'What do you expect; the dog was fourteen years old.' "[160]

In controlled trials, ECT was also shown to be effective. In 1945, Kenneth Tillotson and Wolfgang Sulzbach of McLean Hospital in Belmont, Massachusetts, one of Harvard's teaching hospitals, undertook a controlled follow-up study of seventy depressed ECT patients, comparing them with sixty-eight depressed patients not treated with ECT. Eighty percent of the ECT patients had improved versus 50 percent of the untreated controls. Four patients who had "unrelenting depression for five to fifteen years recovered fully in three weeks to four months after the first shock treatment," and had stayed well at least two years later. One year after discharge from the hospital, 17 percent of the treated patients had relapsed as opposed to 40 percent of the untreated (presumably spontaneously recovered) controls. In the treatment group, the average length of hospitalization was five months, as opposed to twenty-one months in the controls.[161] There were numerous such studies, especially for depression.[162] It was clear that, on a statistical basis, ECT was a highly effective therapy.

Kalinowsky, shunning for once the conservative language of medical description, called the results "amazing": "Everyone who has seen depressive patients mute, stuporous, and tube-fed for years, who after three or four convulsive treatments recover completely, will no more belittle the importance of these treatments. In this group, amazing recoveries are achieved in the majority of all treated cases." The effects on psychiatrists were highly salutary as well. He continued: "To the individual psychiatrist they give a satisfaction that he has missed so long—to become an active therapeutist [*sic*] in, so far, untreatable diseases and, thus, to be a physician in the sense of the word."[163] For psychiatrists, for many years adrift from the mainstream of medicine, isolated either in custodial brick bins or seated silently behind couches in private practices as patients free-associated, these words fell like balm.

Because of the extraordinary success of ECT in medicine, by the late 1940s its curative value was understood in other areas of American society. This was certainly the case in the courts, where malpractice cases were judged and damages awarded on the basis of the likelihood of a patient's responding to ECT. In 1942, one patient, a merchant seaman, "became depressed over ship sinkings and the loss of his comrades." He slashed his wrists one night in a suicide attempt, was committed to Pilgrim State Hospital, and there "was found by an attendant hanging from a ventilator handle in the water section of his ward." His mother sued Pilgrim State for damages on the grounds that the State had been negligent. The Court of Claims of New York found for the mother on the grounds that "with reasonable certainty claimant's intestate [the patient] would have responded to shock therapy and with proper care and treatment would have been restored to usefulness in society."[164]

In 1948, the Pennsylvania Department of Justice gave the opinion that written consent from relatives was not necessary for ECT in state hospitals, on the grounds that "there may be a delay of weeks or months required for relatives to investigate to their own satisfaction before signing such a permit. Furthermore, uninformed lay advice, ignorance and general prejudice, especially from uncooperative families, may deprive a patient of a definite chance for improvement or recovery." In support, the Department of Justice cited statistics on how discharge rates from state hospitals had risen as a result of ECT: Discharges of patients with "involutional" (midlife) depression had risen from 39 percent between 1930 to 1932 to 75 percent in the period around 1944 to 1945.[165] For the legal minds of Pennsylvania, it was clear that the benefits of ECT for the patient outweighed the family's right to be consulted.

All this goes to show that at the beginning of ECT's historic launch in American medicine, there were no anguished worries about memory loss, no antipsychiatry groups protesting permanent brain damage, and no squeamish psychologists and social workers shying aware from a "brutal" therapy. That would come later.

CHAPTER FIVE

The Couch or the Treatment Table?

Back in the 1960s, Joe Schildkraut was a resident physician at the Massachusetts Mental Health Center in Boston. It was a fortress of psychoanalysis where Elvin Semrad, the charismatic chief psychiatrist, referred disparagingly to drugs as "taking a patient to a cocktail party." But it had an ECT service, and Schildkraut, as a first-year resident, was obliged to serve a couple of months on this rotation. At Mass Mental, as it is commonly known, there were many agitated and depressed patients who would pace the halls wringing their hands, saying: "Oh my God. Oh my God. Oh my God. What have I done? Oh my God. Oh my God. Oh my God. Why did I do it? Oh my God. Oh my God. Why did I do it? Oh my God." "This just went on ceaselessly," said Schildkraut, "patients exhausting themselves, grossly psychotic." These patients would receive ECT. Schildkraut thought being assigned to the service was a nuisance requirement, as he wanted to become an analyst. "But the ECT rotation gave me the opportunity to see these depressed, starving, near-dead, vegetating human beings, given a course of ECT, turn into vital, engaging people with charm and dignity and a personality that came alive. It was the most amazing therapeutic transformation that I'd seen in all of my experiences in medicine."[1] Schildkraut kept his thoughts to himself at the time. Ten years passed.

In the early 1970s, Fred Frankel, a psychiatrist at Beth Israel Hospital in Boston, spearheaded a task force on ECT in the state of Massachusetts (see chapter 9). The experience was emotionally exhausting. After it was over Frankel reflected on "the righteous indignation of those who virtually never recommend it, offset by a vehement defense by many of those who do." The battle, he said, "captures the essence of the struggle for identity within the psychiatric profession."[2] Frankel found himself in the middle of this struggle. The early successes of the shock therapies were so dramatic that they precipitated a furious reaction from the psychoanalysts who then were dominant in psychiatry. The shock therapists, pursuing a biological model of illness, argued that jolting the brain itself had somehow produced a therapeutic rewiring. The analysts argued that only deep psychotherapy could get at the "real causes" of psychiatric illness within the intricacies of the unconscious mind. The conflict touched off a forty-year clash. As waged in public, it was no-holds-barred: for the analysts, ECT was a brutal, primitive treatment, sadistically inflicted, and masochistically accepted as an expiation for guilt. Yet behind the scenes many analysts were warmer toward ECT, because they needed it to make their patients better. Without that therapeutic stimulus, they privately acknowledged that some of their mute and unresponsive patients would never reach a state where psychoanalysis could have an effect. Few who were not insiders knew of this backstairs accommodation—an unfortunate circumstance, because it was the public confrontation that helped brand ECT, in the eyes of patients contemplating referral to an ECT-specialist, as a dangerous treatment best to avoid. This chapter tells the story of the conflicted relationship between ECT and analysis—and how ECT triumphed because it ultimately was able to deliver the goods.

Psychoanalysis and ECT: A Love and Hate Relationship

Right up front it must be said that not all psychoanalysts were hostile to the administration of ECT. English analyst Ernest Jones, one of Freud's closest collaborators, kept a separate register of ECT patients and believed that the reason "why the treatment had proved so useful" lay in its impact on levels of "repression" in his depressed patients.[3] But most analysts did not keep records of their ECT patients. Being adamantly opposed to ECT, the analysts, says Copenhagen psychiatrist Tom G. Bolwig, assume "that the underlying problems of all forms of psychopathology are interpersonal conflicts in the early stage of a human being's life." Using Freud as their model, they look for circumstances unknown to the patient and submerged in the unconscious realm. "Therefore, the task for the therapist is to reveal these secrets. This of course is very appealing to psychotherapists." Bolwig then notes that into the midst of this entrenched psychoanalytic tradition that reigned in both Europe and the United States came the biological psychiatrists with their view that sometimes "the brain, the synapses and all the wiring may per se go wrong and create a psychologically complicated situation. That doesn't appeal to them. . . . For some of them, treating a patient with a depression dominated by feelings of guilt, ECT is like throwing a hand grenade in a kindergarten and closing the door from outside. They simply hate it."[4] Electrotherapist William Karliner summed it up succinctly: "The analysts denigrate me, but when their mothers get depressed, they send them to me."[5] When ECT use surged in the 1940s and 1950s, so did the analytic counterattack, setting the stage for the stigmatization that would follow.

At a basic level, the analysts were unable to accept that a jolt of electricity lasting one-fifth of a second might achieve a better result than months of drawn-out talk therapy. It was not so much that they feared the economic competition, for the schizophrenic and melancholic patients receiving convulsive therapy were not part of the elective terrain of psychoanalysis. Rather it was that the whole biological logic of the shock therapies starkly contradicted the psychogenic thinking of psychoanalysis. In 1947, English psychoanalyst Donald Woods ("D. W.") Winnicott explained that there were good theoretical reasons for withholding ECT from needy patients: "My main objection to convulsion therapy is that it comes as an escape from the acceptance of the psychology of the unconscious."[6] It was much healthier, he said, to compel patients to cope with their unconscious minds in psychotherapy sessions than to lift symptoms with mechanical procedures. Aubrey Lewis, head of the Maudsley Hospital, later commented scathingly of this proposal: "The miseries of depression are such that no theoretical argument of this kind warrants the withholding of treatment that can terminate the misery." Lewis contrasted "the theoretical argument put forward by Dr. Winnicott and the appeal *ad misericordiam* which operates for most psychiatrists who see the utter unhappiness of a depressed person."[7]

Although the analysts did not normally deny the effectiveness of shock therapy, they found in it an expression of almost primitive savagery. Edith Weigert, a refugee analyst from Hitler's Germany then practicing in Washington, D.C., called it in 1940 "a desperate attempt to overcome the patient's inward conflicts by catering to his need for punishment and self destruction." "Shock and convulsion therapy," she continued, "is opposed to the main striving of psychoanalytic therapy: to mitigate the cruelty of an archaic superego and to help the patient to endure the necessary, but not the unnecessary hardships of reality."[8] These are not ignoble sentiments, but they would discourage a physician from referring a patient for shock therapy, or a patient from seeking appropriate help.

The analysts interpreted the ECT specialists themselves in Freudian terms: they claimed that some clinicians relished the infliction of this sadistic punition on masochistic patients seeking punishment to relieve guilt. Otto Fenichel, the New York analyst who in those days was probably the lead figure in Freudian psychiatry, said in 1945 that ECT represented a kind of death and rebirth for the patients, but also for the physicians who gave it (he had analyzed a number of them). "Killing the sick person and creating the patient anew as a healthy person is an ancient form of magical treatment," Fenichel theorized.[9] But physicians dislike the notion of engaging in magic. They prefer to think of themselves as scientific, and the arguments of Fenichel and other Freudians represented a large caution light for psychiatry and the educated public.

In September 1947, it came to blows between the somatic therapists and the analysts. The previous year, at a meeting of the American Psychiatric Association in Chicago at the Palmer House, William Menninger of the Menninger Clinic in Topeka, Kansas, one of the central figures of American psychoanalysis, founded a small organization of like-minded psychiatrists called the Group for the Advancement of Psychiatry, or GAP. The GAP was not publicly committed to psychoanalysis but rather to vague reforms that it wished to see carried out in American psychiatry as a whole. Yet many of its members were psychoanalysts who wished to push a Freudian agenda.

The GAP did have members more committed to biological approaches than to psychotherapy, such as Lauretta Bender, who in the 1940s at Bellevue Hospital introduced ECT for preadolescent children with schizophrenia.[10] But the real power at GAP lay in pushing forward psychoanalysis, and it was no accident that the first GAP public bulletin, published in September 1947, was a frontal attack on "shock therapy." The various GAP committees had substantial autonomy, although they were obliged to run their reports by a referee committee consisting of the various committee leaders. The GAP Committee on Therapy was chaired by psychoanalyst M. Ralph ("Moe") Kaufman, head of psychiatry at Mount Sinai Hospital in New York. Of the therapy committee's ten other members, eight were analysts.[11] On January 22, 1947, they issued a preliminary report on ECT to the membership, approved by the referee committee of five members (of whom four were psychoanalysts).[12] Then nine months later, on September 15, 1947, they brought out GAP's published *Report No. 1* on shock therapy. It stated that ECT was the object of "promiscuous and indiscriminate use." It allowed that ECT might have some efficacy in shortening depressive episodes, but that it had no impact on manic-depressive illness or schizophrenia (except on those aspects of schizophrenia that also could be treated with psychotherapy). The complications and hazards of ECT, claimed the committee, could not be overemphasized; its use in office practice was totally wrong; and brain damage from ECT was an inevitable consequence. The committee concluded: "Abuses in the use of electro-shock therapy are sufficiently widespread and dangerous to justify consideration of a campaign of professional education in the limitations of this technique, and perhaps even to justify instituting certain measures of control."[13] American psychoanalysis had given its verdict on ECT, and the verdict was clearly no.

The GAP leadership, for the most part, was initially pleased with this report and sought to promote its message to the public. Leland Hinsie, second in command at the New York State Psychiatric Institute, wanted it published in *Reader's Digest*.[14] Yet the initial distribution was more modest, with the report circulated among the American Psychiatric Association's 4,400 members.[15] The paper evoked a firestorm among the GAP membership and the psychiatric public, however. Kaufman resigned as head of the Therapy Committee, replaced by Robert Knight of the Austen Riggs Foundation, a private psychiatric hospital with the specialty of psychotherapy. The back-peddling began immediately. By autumn of 1948, Menninger convoked a group of consultant electrotherapists, including Kalinowsky and later Paul Hoch, to revise the document. At the GAP meeting at Asbury Park, New Jersey, in November 1948, GAP secretary Henry W. (Hank) Brosin thanked the consultants "for helping us out in this very tense field."[16]

In February 1949, the Therapy Committee met and found that it was completely divided. "The Therapy Committee members do not feel that they can reconcile the differences," Menninger told the GAP membership, and sent out a ballot asking which of several draft "supplementary reports" now circulating the members approved.[17] Menninger himself was forced to participate in some kind of public reconciliation with the ECT specialists. At the annual meeting of the American Psychiatric Association in Montreal in May 1949, Menninger—in his capacity as president of the APA—signed a joint statement with Nathan Rickles, president of the Electro-Shock Research Association, that read: "Electro-shock therapy is accepted today as the most effective physical agent in the successful treatment of the majority of the affective psychoses when given by properly qualified psychiatrists."[18] (In those days serious depression was referred to as a "psychosis.")

Meanwhile, the Therapy Committee and its consultants were struggling with such issues as the legitimacy of outpatient ECT.[19] In September 1949, Knight resigned as head of the committee, telling Menninger: "Unfortunately during almost my entire association with GAP I have been involved with this God-damned electroshock business, a procedure in which I am less than feebly interested. I can't seem to get rid of the damned thing."[20] Maxwell Gitelson, a Chicago analyst in private practice, became the new leader, "somewhat against my will and with grave doubt," he later said.[21] As the new year dawned in 1950, the members of the Therapy Committee were still arguing about the ECT report. Menninger, now completely exasperated, told Max Gitelson: "I confess I think we made an unfortunate statement in the first report. If we are going to have differences of opinion I would rather they would be about something of much more vital importance than this damned Shock Report and I am quite sure you feel the same way."[22] Finally, GAP members Paul Huston and Jacques Gottlieb of the University of Iowa—even then a fortress of biological thinking—were tasked with drafting a final revision of GAP *Report No. 1.* Their draft has not survived, but we know that it was further massaged by psychoanalyst Max Gitelson, the new head of the Therapy Committee. Menninger at this point was exploding with impatience: "Where is that damn Shock Therapy Report?" he stormed at Gitelson.[23]

In July 1950, Menninger, heavy of heart about the whole affair, sighed to Hank Brosin: "Enclosed is a 'Final Revision By the Committee on Therapy of The Electric Shock Report.' . . . It is Max Gitelson's feeling that they [the Committee] have done everything they can to this." Huston and Gottlieb consulted Kalinowsky and the other ECT people in drafting the revision, and Menninger wanted to know if it was worth running the draft past them before publishing it. He decided: "That is not terribly important."[24] The "Revised Electro-Shock Therapy Report" of GAP, published in August 1950, addressed the whole issue in much more positive language. It acknowledged numerous indications for ECT, stating that it was quite safe and effective; office-practice ECT for outpatients was perfectly acceptable given appropriate precautions, and special government controls were not necessary after all.

Both sets of antagonists published minority opinions at the end of the revised report. Some members of the Committee on Therapy, their noses very much out of joint, said that "familiarity with a wide range of psychiatric theory and practice reduces the need for its [ECT] use in general," and that patients' depression would be successfully treated only when "the real situational factors and their attendant emotional problems" were addressed in psychotherapy. These objections were both psychoanalytic mantras, although the analysts almost never mentioned the term *psychoanalysis* in any of GAP's public communications. The somatic consultants also filed their own objections: it was not, in fact, necessary for electrotherapy to be limited to psychiatrists; neurologists and internists with suitable training might also perform it very well. And "psychosomatic indications" might be more appropriate for ECT than the report granted, they said.[25]

The GAP leadership never really got over the slap in the face of this revised report. At a celebratory GAP meeting at the Berkeley-Carteret Hotel in Asbury Park in April 1951, Brosin justified the original report as completely on target: "Whatever your feelings about the language, the logic or the tone in which it was written, it represents a sound and considered opinion," he said.[26] This note of belligerence was much closer to the true feeling of GAP members than the reconciliatory noises of the revised report.

In retrospect, Sydney Margolin, a New York analyst with a Park Avenue address, saw the whole ECT struggle of the Therapy Committee as a classic set-piece battle between two paradigms, the physical treatment approach that ECT represented and psychoanalysis. He said in a letter to Menninger that it was unfortunate that the Therapy Committee ended up composed entirely of analysts: "Those members who were not analysts saw fit to withdraw and their replacements tended to be analysts." Margolin continued: "The Shock Therapy report and the atmosphere of contentiousness which it provoked caused the committee both individually and collectively no end of disappointment and frustration. . . . By accepting the protests and challenges of vested interests in E.S.T., we lost one of our most potent effects. We stopped being energetic catalysts, hard-headed, hard-hitting realists, and found ourselves skirmishing in a battle of attrition. It was the committee that was finally worn out."[27]

The struggle for the heart of psychiatry had now been joined in earnest. The analysts' denunciations of ECT became increasingly strident in the years to come. In 1953, in a letter to the Sunday Magazine of the *New York Times*, analyst Irving Harrison sympathized with the nonpsychotic patients who had been "subjected" to electroshock.[28] The message: anything other than stark, raving madness belongs on the couch, not the treatment table. In private too, analysts tended increasingly to deny any role for ECT. In August 1951, a family doctor in California asked Meduna about his new "carbon dioxide" therapy, saying: "Two psychiatrists have told me they think it's a 'shock' method and as one said, 'after all you can't help someone with this method when his trouble is that his mother never loved him.'"[29]

Robert Cancro, later head of psychiatry at New York University, remembered the battle between the somaticists and the analysts when he trained at Kings County Hospital in New York in the late 1950s: "The use of electroconvulsive therapy for depression and severe agitation was standard. The striking results of ECT in these conditions influenced many residents to think that more than unconscious conflict was involved in pathogenesis. Nevertheless, there were dynamic supervisors who explained that depression was rage turned inward and that use of ECT was dehumanizing." The residents therefore "began to speak two languages depending on the belief system of the supervisor." It was, said Cancro, like a "religious war."[30]

Fred Frankel had endured the ECT wars in Massachusetts in the 1970s. He said that analysts and ECT specialists inhabited two different worlds and the treatment you got depended on the office you walked into, whatever your symptoms: "If that office was an ECT office, you would be given ECT. If you pressed on the button of an analyst, no matter how bad your depression or your schizophrenia was, he would want to sit and talk with you. It was the most schizophrenic way of approaching a problem that I've ever seen! You simply got what the guy did."[31]

Yet beyond these stories of two worlds, there was another level at which psychoanalysis needed electroconvulsive therapy. The analytic method did not have a great track record of success in patients who were melancholic or psychotic, and the analysts needed something on offer that, unlike pharmacotherapy, would not be in direct competition with them. As we have seen, Moe Kaufman at Mount Sinai Hospital was opposed to ECT on theoretical grounds, yet he retained an ECT service in his department. Arthur Gabriel ran it for several decades, beginning in 1958. "The analysts pooh-poohed it," said Gabriel, "but when their patients were suicidal they sent them for ECT." The analysts at Mount Sinai said to Gabriel: "What are you doing with Kalinowsky!" Their theory was that depression represented "repressed anger." Gabriel replied: "That's bullshit."[32] He continued to work there, almost entirely without contact with medical resident training.

Louis Linn, a psychoanalyst, also worked in the ECT service at Mount Sinai. He recalled: "I was sitting in my office, the phone rings. It's Moe Kaufman. He says: 'Lou, come down as fast as you can with your little black box.'" "I come down there," continued Linn, "and they said: 'We have a VIP in the hospital. And we mustn't let anyone know about it. We can't even tell you his name, because if it gets out it could be catastrophic. Just see the patient, and on the basis of your examination, decide if he may be a candidate for ECT, and treat him if you think so.'" So Linn was ushered into the private room, "with people standing at the door so no one could come in. And I said: 'Look, I think this is the kind of case that I can interrupt very dependably with ECT.' And they said: 'For God's sake, do it!' So I gave him the treatment, and five minutes later I gave the second treatment. An hour later I gave him the third treatment. And within twenty-four, forty-eight hours he was sitting up and started to see people."[33] Mount Sinai treated many celebrity clients. And many of them recovered in the ECT service. Arthur Gabriel even remembered taking a portable ECT device into hotels. He once treated a terribly depressed actress in her room who was supposed to perform on television that night. This was in a milieu that ostensibly worshiped psychoanalysis.

When Max Fink came to Hillside Hospital in 1952, it was because he wanted to study psychoanalysis, and neurologist Morris Bender had suggested Hillside as the best place. Yet when Fink arrived, the hospital assigned him to run the ECT service, simply because Fink was already familiar with it from his sojourn in the army (see chapter 10). One of Fink's first scientific papers was on "Homosexuality with Panic and Paranoid States." Fink concluded of the patient: "Sexuality to this boy represents a hostile aggressive act because his relation to women is colored by his intense hostility to his mother. He is fearful that they will reject him when they recognize his hostility, the same fear he felt with his mother."[34] Thus, as Fink gave ECT, he was musing in classic Freudian style about homosexual panic as a defense against castration anxiety.

At Hillside, psychoanalysis and ECT flowed smoothly back and forth, with world-famous analysts such as Sandor Lorand easily referring patients for ECT, yet offering psychoanalytic formulations of their problems. Of one patient recommended for ECT, chief physician Louis Wender commented: "She then failed to marry her father image and therefore is not happy in the marriage. . . . While her super-ego forced her to be a good wife and mother . . . eventually these trends [began to] revolt, and her conscience clashed openly, this resulting in a confused paranoid reaction."[35]

The staff at the New York State Psychiatric Institute prided themselves on psychoanalysis. As Director Nolan Lewis told the press in 1949: "All patients are treated in a psychodynamic framework. Our principal clinical physicians are all psychoanalytically trained."[36] Indeed, as the years passed, psychoanalysis became even more firmly embedded at PI. In 1952, the *Annual Report* noted: "The general trend of therapy on the male service was in the direction of psychoanalytic and psychodynamic approaches. . . . There was a tendency for the residents to prefer to delay all forms of organic treatment until extensive trials of psychotherapy were exhausted." Yet in fiscal year 1951–52, researchers at PI did extensive work on shock therapies, investigating barbiturate anesthetics, looking at "ketogenic diets" in ECT, and studying the effect of shock treatments on memory.[37] Significantly, it was from PI that the first authoritative textbook for conducting ECT and the other somatic therapies emerged: *Shock Treatments and Other Somatic Procedures in Psychiatry*, which Kalinowsky wrote with Paul Hoch in 1946.[38]

At all of these important institutions—all bastions of psychoanalysis—there clearly was no rivalry between ECT and psychoanalysis, no competing of one against another for patients. And despite all the vitriolic fervor in public discourse, ECT, it could be said, was the secret love of psychoanalysis.

An Achilles Heel

ECT had an Achilles heel. Its application was so straightforward and inexpensive that it could be used on large numbers of patients within a relatively short period of time. Given its effectiveness in serious depression, catatonia, and schizophrenia, widespread use was not necessarily inappropriate for a hospital population. As an image, though, it looked awful: as if the psychiatrists were putting patients on an impersonal assembly line without regard to their individualities and "zapping" them. This was completely at odds with the picture of a profession that prided itself on hour-long sessions of individual psychotherapy. As such, opponents of ECT charged it was used indiscriminately, as a tool for the masses of psychiatric patients. Was there truth to this allegation?

In the days of Jim Crow laws and systematic segregation of African Americans, Central State Hospital in Petersburg, Virginia, served exclusively black patients. Conditions there were so dreadful that it was a public embarrassment to the state. Joseph Barrett, the commissioner of mental hygiene in Virginia, said in court that it was "not one to brag about." And in 1955, Judge Hoffman of the United States District Court for the Eastern District of Virginia considered a lawsuit arising out of care at Central, stating: "Virginia has completely failed in its obligations to the mentally ill, both white and colored." He continued: "Other than electric shock treatments occasionally administered, there is no treatment afforded to the patients. They eat, sleep and sit—this is the routine day. In brief, if the shock treatments do not bring forth favorable results, the patients wait to die."[39]

On the surface, this sounds like indiscriminate use of ECT and assembly-line medicine. The alternative was simply no treatment of any kind for these patients. Electrotherapy must have helped many of them, permitting recoveries and discharges that otherwise would not have occurred. As with many aspects of ECT, the social portrait here seems appalling. It highlights the shattering ignorance of the public about the tough realities of psychiatric care. Viewed another way, electrotherapists delivered effective treatments in desperate situations.

In these underfunded institutions with male attendants who drifted back and forth between jobs in the state hospitals and the state prisons, there were abuses. Rockland State, in Orangeburg, New York, was the original "snake pit" (see chapter 7), where Mary Jane Ward, author of a book of that title, was hospitalized. George Simpson, later an important psychopharmacologist, recalled: "When I came to Rockland [in 1957], I couldn't believe that they gave ECT without anything. And, not only that, but the man who gave it wasn't very smart. When I talked to him about using muscle relaxants and so on he thought that was a bit silly. They simply had tongs and they went around just buzzing people. So there was a huge need for something to happen."[40] The kinds of muscle relaxants and anesthesia that Central Hospital in Virginia could not afford the New York State mental hospital system could.

The charge that ECT was used in a punitive manner in these asylums is not fiction. Indeed, it was sometimes administered in totally untherapeutic ways to keep patients in line and passive. ECT came to the Milledgeville State Hospital in Georgia around 1942, a huge asylum of about seven thousand beds, second in size only to Pilgrim State on Long Island. ECT quickly became known to patients and attendants as "the Georgia power cocktail." As Peter Cranford, a staff psychologist at the time, recalled: "The words 'punish' and 'shock treatment' were often synonymous to the disturbed. Which electric shocks were given for treatment, which for punishment, and which for both presented confusing problems to patients, many of whom were paranoid to begin with and felt they were being punished for their 'guilty' deeds performed prior to their illness." The attendants, not the physicians, often decided who was to be shocked. Nonetheless, Cranford said that ECT had a positive influence on many patients at Milledgeville. On November 6, 1951, he noted in his diary: "On the basis of private practice, I was opposed to shock treatment except for the worst cases. But I have seen some spectacular recoveries here. Catatonic stupor one day, playing basketball the next. Myra Bonner, director of nurses, states that the nurses were lukewarm on shock treatment but she, too, had seen some remarkable recoveries."[41]

At Milledgeville, ECT was abused by the attendants from sheer vengefulness and petty-mindedness.[42] At other large hospitals the abuses seem to have been more a matter of neglect and bureaucratic indifference. Kalinowsky, of course, had done pioneer work at Pilgrim State in the early 1940s. Yet when Michael Alan Taylor visited there in the early 1960s, wanting to know how to set up an ECT service for Stony Brook, he found a changed scene: "If that had been your only exposure to ECT, you would never want anything to do with it. It was totally inadequate. It was so bad that I had to look to see whether the machines were plugged in."[43]

There is no point in trying to sanitize the history of ECT, because there are abuses and horror stories enough. Yet ECT has a long history of underuse, not overuse. It does not lend itself well to abuse because it is painless: the patient is immediately unconscious. Each of the major therapies of the twentieth century has its own saga of abuses: the sexual abuse of patients in psychoanalysis and the scandalously high doses of antipsychotic drugs that were often dispensed in psychopharmacology, doses that indeed caused permanent brain damage. Dwelling on abuses, as many writers have done—while mentioning only in passing that ECT is the treatment of "last resort" in depression—has the effect of scaring doctors and patients away from a therapy with remarkably effective results in terms of successful discharges—even at Milledgeville.

Overcoming Disbelief

ECT specialists responded to the intrinsic doubts about the wisdom of passing 120 volts of electricity through somebody's head with statistics on therapeutic results. The adage among its practitioners was that you were doing something wrong if any fewer than 80 percent of your patients showed improvement.[44] It was the numbers that emboldened the electrotherapists in their push for psychiatry's heart.

From the very beginning, it was clear that ECT had a singular effectiveness in depression and catatonia. Of the seventy-three schizophrenic patients whom Giorgio Sogliani treated with ECT at the provincial psychiatric hospital in Sondrio, Italy, in 1939, only 25 percent improved or recovered (patients with the catatonic form of schizophrenia responding best). Of the twenty-seven patients in the depressed phase of manic-depressive illness, 89 percent recovered or improved. (He achieved similar results with Metrazol.)[45] Sogliani concluded that convulsive therapy "is the therapy of choice for depression and stupor in general, and that it always must be attempted even if the illness has been chronic for several years."[46] In 1940, Cerletti also concluded that the results in the depressed phase of manic-depressive illness were better than the results in schizophrenia.[47]

Few Americans had access to Sogliani's or Cerletti's articles on ECT, appearing as they did in German and Italian journals at the onset of world war. But in 1939, Abram Bennett in Omaha, Nebraska, pointed out in the *American Journal of Medical Sciences* the benefits of Metrazol therapy in alleviating depression.[48] As war enveloped clinical psychiatry on the Continent, the next convincing data on the efficacy of ECT came from the United States and England. In 1941, Abraham Myerson conducted a trial of ECT at Boston State Hospital. As he said in the *New England Journal of Medicine,* of twenty-four patients with depression, "all but three showed moderate to marked improvement or had remissions following electric-shock therapy." Of nine patients with schizophrenia, none showed any essential improvement.[49] A year later, a group at Pennsylvania Hospital had studied 156 patients. The results: of those with involutional melancholia (severe depression in middle age), 85 percent had recovered; manic-depressive illness in the manic phase, 70 percent; in the depressed phase, 72 percent; schizophrenia, none.[50] This pointed powerfully toward ECT in treating mood or affective disorders.

By contrast, Kalinowsky confirmed Meduna's good results with "schizophrenia." At Pilgrim State Hospital, Kalinowsky found that, as long as the patients had not been ill for long, ECT was quite effective: 68 percent of 275 schizophrenics treated with ECT recovered or were much improved if they had been ill less than six months. If they had been ill more than two years, only 8 percent did well. (Kalinowsky's results at Pilgrim State with depression were consistent with what others found: 87 percent of those with manic-depressive illness, depressed phase, recovered or were much improved; 84 percent of those in the manic phase; and 87 percent of those with involutional melancholia.)[51]

In 1945, the first controlled studies of ECT for depression appeared. Such analysis was the only way to rule out influences such as therapeutic suggestion and hope in treatment responses. At McLean Hospital in Belmont, Massachusetts, Kenneth Tillotson and Wolfang Sulzbach examined outcomes of fifty-six depressed patients treated with ECT versus thirty-four untreated controls. Eighty percent of the shock therapy patients improved as opposed to 50 percent of the controls—a difference that is both intuitively and statistically significant. Among the patients in both groups who got better, one year after discharge only 17 percent of the treated group had relapsed as opposed to 40 percent of the untreated group—a result that is perhaps even more interesting. In the treated group the average length of hospitalization was five months versus twenty-one months for the controls.[52] Many other such controlled studies of ECT were to follow, and it would be fair to say that ECT has been better analyzed with controlled studies than almost any other procedure in American medicine.

The greatest specter haunting psychiatric practice is a patient's suicide. In the 1940s and early 1950s, at least fifteen thousand Americans died of suicide yearly, so antisuicidal remedies possessed then—and they do now—great desirability.[53] For the early generation of ECT specialists there was simply no question: ECT reduced suicide and suicidal ideation in their practices and their hospitals. "If you want to know the practical consequences of the method," Cerletti told the Paris World Psychiatric Congress in 1950, "it suffices to see the transformation that has occurred in the psychiatric hospitals where the agitated wards have been closed and the important sections where the patients at suicide risk were closely watched."[54] On another occasion he noted: "When a patient expresses a suicidal idea, it becomes absolutely imperative to proceed to ECT." The idea recedes after two or three treatments, he said, even if the depression as such is not yet relieved.[55]

Neurologist Nathan Savitsky and psychiatrist William Karliner— both major figures in the New York electrotherapy community—often collaborated in ECT, either in Morrisania City Hospital in the Bronx, where they were attending or visiting neuropsychiatrists, or in Karliner's extensive private practice, where Savitsky consulted. In 1949, they wrote: "The incidence of suicides in our experience has been strikingly reduced, compared with their frequency before the introduction of shock therapy." Yet one had to be vigilant after treatment began, they warned, because "attempts at suicide are not infrequent during the period of recovery, perhaps because of the absence of severe retardation."[56] Among outpatients results were equally impressive. Theodore Robie, who had a private practice in East Orange, New Jersey, said in 1950 that "the rate of suicide in our practice has declined 80% to 90%. . . . The use of electroshock therapy on an ambulatory basis is a distinct advance in the private practice of psychiatry and, in the hands of competent, adequately trained psychiatrists, should be encouraged."[57]

There were more formal statistics to support the contention that ECT reduced suicides. In a follow-up study of their depressed patients between 1938 and 1943, the Ziskinds discovered that in 109 patients untreated with convulsive therapy, there had been 9 suicides, in 88 treated patients, 1 suicide.[58] Paul Huston at the University of Iowa compared patients with manic-depressive psychosis treated with ECT in the years 1941–43 to a matched, untreated group in the years 1930–38. He found that of the seventy-four patients of the treated group, only 1 percent had committed suicide within three years following the procedure; in the eighty patients of the control group, 7 percent died by suicide, and five of these six patients died within fourteen months of discharge.[59] Huston's findings came on the heels of the antagonistic GAP report of 1947, but there is no doubt that ECT was effective in the prevention of suicide. (This was confirmed in 2005 in a large multicenter study led by Charles Kellner at the University of Medicine and Dentistry of New Jersey: suicidal ideation dropped so quickly after ECT that the authors said it was irresponsible to offer ECT as "the last resort." ECT, they said, should be moved further up the "algorithm," or sequence of treatments.)[60]

Those who respond most favorably to the treatment are often the most depressed, a correlation that seems counterintuitive, for the opposite is true in psychotherapy. But some types of mental illness do not show significant beneficial results. Kalinowsky warned against treating the psychoneurotics, the obsessive-compulsives, and the patients with "anxiety hysteria." As he explained at the annual meeting of the American Medical Association in 1944: "Anxiety is probably the most frequent symptom encountered in neurotic patients, and it is also the symptom least amenable to electric convulsive therapy." It was precisely these patients who "benefited least from the treatment," he said. Some got worse, and "the few who improved slightly under treatment had a relapse after a short time." By contrast, the sickest and most floridly ill often did beautifully. In the discussion of his paper at the meeting, Kalinowsky said: "We get the best results from shock therapy in patients with dramatic symptoms."[61] As he added elsewhere of manic-depressive illness: "The greater the loss of contact with reality, the better the treatment prognosis."[62]

The utility of ECT was not limited to major psychiatric illness such as recent-onset schizophrenia, depression, suicidal ideation, and mania. There were reports of its curing chronic sneezers and stammerers. Doctors claimed that a twelve-day, and quite debilitating, episode of chronic sneezing by Mrs. Albert Sanders in Jonesboro, Arkansas, was caused by a "nervous illness" and relieved by ECT. The report is not as bizarre as it seems, given the effectiveness of ECT in nonconvulsive status epilepticus or catatonic repetitions, two clinical conditions that may be signaled by such episodes of sneezing.[63] In addition to the flood of other reports about chronic headache and the like, one side-note is of interest, given the intractability of Parkinson's disease to this day. In 1938, Eugene Ziskind and Esther Somerfeld-Ziskind, who together had a neuropsychiatric practice in Los Angeles on Wilshire Boulevard and were pioneers of convulsive therapy on the West Coast, reported that five treatments with Metrazol in a thirty-four-year-old woman with encephalitic Parkinsonism resulted in reducing the oculogyric crises—a marked deviation of the eyeballs upward—to which she had been subject. Twice, she was in the middle of an attack as the Metrazol was given. The convulsions had no effect on her Parkinsonian rigidity, but nonetheless, affected a significant manifestation of the condition; the report stands as an initial advance in a disease that has been notably resistant to treatment.[64]

In later years, other scattered efforts were made to treat Parkinsonism with convulsive therapy. The outcomes were inconclusive. In 1950, at the Paris World Psychiatric Congress, Osvaldo Meco, a neurologist in Florence, Italy, reported durable remissions of muscular rigidity in some of the Parkinsonians he had treated with electroshock. Not all of his eight patients responded with enduring remissions—some lasted only a few minutes to half an hour following ECT. Yet the patients who benefited from relief of their psychiatric symptoms were also those who experienced a durable reprieve of their neurological symptoms, especially the rigidity. "In some cases," said Meco, "particularly in the milder ones . . . in giving 5–8–10 shocks, sometimes after a few

minutes, one observes a lasting diminution of the muscular rigidity."
Meco thought it possible that the psychiatric ailments of Parkinsonians
and their physical symptoms might share the same cause.[65] Meco's paper caused a flurry of interest in the possibility of using a psychiatric
technique to relieve a neurological illness, but was forgotten as ECT
fell increasingly into disuse.[66]

ECT for Outpatients

Louis Linn once recalled of his service as an army psychiatrist during World War II: "I carried my Rahm ECT machine with me through
North Africa, Italy, and France. In tent hospitals and without the use
of restraints in North Africa, I was able to treat psychotic patients with
severe excited states, manic and catatonic, thanks to ECT. In the process I saved lives and spared patients much suffering."[67]

ECT does not require admission to a hospital. It can be done safely
and effectively on an outpatient basis, and in the years from 1938 to
about 1970, a majority of treatments took place in the offices of psychiatrists, neurologists, and family doctors, rather than in mental hospitals. Most commonly, it was for "maintenance" treatment, giving it on
Saturday morning to, let us say, a middle-aged man with chronic depression so that he could continue to hold a job and not have to enter a
mental hospital. A person with chronic schizophrenia might be treated
on a weekly basis so that he or she could remain in a halfway house
instead of a hospital ward. On Saturday mornings, William Karliner
might have a line of patients waiting outside his office in the Grand
Concourse of the Bronx, awaiting maintenance ECT so that they could
go to work on Monday morning.[68]

Today, such outpatient treatments are represented as abuses, and
ECT in the United States and Europe is for the most part no longer
done in doctors' offices. But from the beginning, ECT was performed
in nonhospital settings. An advertisement for the Arcioni machine
around 1939 claimed: "In case of use at home, the device may immediately be removed from the cart."[69] In England it was said that "the vast
majority of depressed patients have ECT on an out-patient basis."[70]
Abraham Myerson was the first to introduce outpatient ECT in the
United States, and Myerson discussed it at the May 1941 meeting of the
American Psychiatric Association.[71] Around the same time, Almansi
and Impastato opened a large ECT suite with, as Kalinowsky told Bini,
twenty-four rooms.[72]

The great advocate of outpatient ECT in the United States was Kalinowsky himself. In 1944, he described maintenance therapy of patients with chronic schizophrenia: "short, purely symptomatic treatment in chronic cases where no final remissions can be obtained. A maintenance treatment of one or two weekly, bi-weekly or even monthly treatments will keep the patient on a higher level. This appears to be one of the main tasks for ambulatory electric convulsive therapy. Many patients could be kept outside the institutions if psychiatrists would limit themselves in such cases to occasional symptomatic applications."[73] In Manhattan, David Impastato was sought after for outpatient ECT, and Karliner, in addition to his office on the Grand Concourse, did outpatient ECT at the private hospitals where he consulted over the years, particularly West Hill Sanitarium in the Riverdale district, Lenox Hill Hospital on Manhattan's Upper East Side, Hillside Hospital in Queens, and Gracie Square in midtown Manhattan after it opened in 1959.

Karliner's story is instructive. In 1938, shortly after arriving in New York as a refugee from Hitler's Vienna, he began by helping Sakel, whom he despised although they were distant cousins. In a relatively short time, Karliner opened his own office and began a large ECT practice, but did general psychiatry and prescribed medication as well. Most of Karliner's patients came in for maintenance treatments. "I take a patient who had a first episode of a schizophrenic illness. . . . I treated them with as few treatments as possible and then stopped. Some patients never had a recurrence. But when a patient came . . . because they had recurrences twice a year or more, after ending the course [of regular treatments] I recommended maintenance treatment. I was one of the first to publish and encourage maintenance ECT. I was very successful and many of my patients who had maintenance treatment did not have recurrences." For what he termed "plain" manic-depressives, Karliner would give only a small number of treatments. "If the patient improved after the sixth treatment I just saw them in the office a week later. In seriously ill cases I kept an eye on them for a number of weeks. If they showed any sign of depression, I would give antidepressants [after they became available in 1959]. If this didn't help, I again gave them ECT and then I would put them on maintenance ECT."[74]

In 1949, Karliner began publishing his techniques, and his papers from the early 1950s were widely read as practical guides for outpatient ECT.[75] Kalinowsky and the academic psychiatrists often spoke scornfully of him because he saw so many patients. Yet over the years his patients experienced few side effects; he had only one death in almost

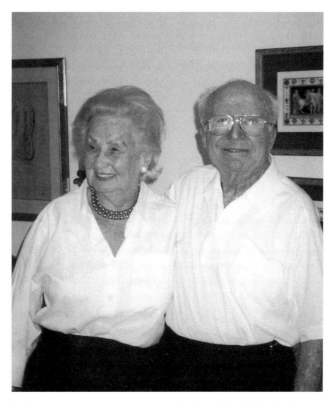

William Karliner (1910–2005), together with his wife, Edith. Karliner emigrated from Austria to the United States in 1938, settled in New York, and tried new approaches to convulsive therapy. Courtesy of Max Fink.

fifty years of practice; and there is no doubt that he made life more tolerable for many families with afflicted relatives who preferred the outpatient clinic to the hospital ward.

In 1953, the American Psychiatric Association ratified the legitimacy of outpatient ECT. Its Committee on Therapy, chaired by Paul Hoch, and including Heinz Lehmann and Joseph Wortis, concluded that "a patient in good health may be treated as ambulatory," provided that the therapist took special precautions in using intravenous sedation or a muscle relaxant such as curare. For the first ten treatments a family member might accompany the patient to and from the therapist's office. After that, the patient might travel alone.[76]

Much of this discussion took place in the days of "unmodified" ECT, which is to say, before the introduction of reliable muscle relaxants (which curare was not), oxygen supplementation, and a short-acting barbiturate anesthetic. That thousands of patients were relieved and grateful to practitioners such as Karliner suggests that these early days of ECT could not possibly have been quite as barbarous as later observers made them out to be.

Thus, by the mid-1950s, two camps clashed directly in their struggle for the core of psychiatry's interests. Was psychiatry a profession more biological in its theories and orientation, or was it psychotherapeutic, theorizing that the mind was somehow different from the substance of the brain? The great success of the somatic treatments, crowned by convulsive therapy, gave strength to the biologists. The concurrent explosive growth of psychoanalysis fortified the approach to psychiatric disorder as an illness of mind, and not of brain, and it ratified in-depth psychotherapy as the superior remedy. Meanwhile, as these two gladiators vied for the prize, a third contestant had quietly appeared, on a sure course for ultimate victory: psychopharmacology. As the result of events beginning with the discovery in 1952 of the effectiveness of chlorpromazine in treating psychotic illness, psychoanalysis and somatic therapy alike would be set aside.

CHAPTER SIX

"ECT Does Not Create Zombies"

n 1965, a practicing psychiatrist in England, depressed and psychotic for some time, received a series of ECT treatments on an outpatient basis. "The way in which memory returns is very interesting," he said. "I have always had a good topographical sense and have been able to memorize maps and, for example, find my way with ease around the Underground system of London." After his ECT he found that he had "forgotten completely the patterns that previously have been almost second nature to me. It is with considerable effort that I am learning again." He discovered his office filing system to be similarly bewildering. He had been depressed and treated with ECT previously. On that occasion, "the defects of memory became gradually fewer and less marked, and at the end of about two months the gaps in my memory had been completely closed." With one conspicuous exception: at a scientific meeting he met a psychiatrist "whose face seemed very familiar, though I could not remember his name nor where I had met him before. I remarked on this to a friend, saying, 'It must be a result of the ECT.' The friend replied, 'I'm not surprised: it was he who gave you the treatment!'" Five days after his most recent treatment, the psychiatrist wrote: "There are still many gaps in my memory, though I am confident that these will close." In the meantime, there was a more positive side, "Every day I am feeling more energetic and I look forward hopefully to a marked positive improvement in spirits in a few weeks' time if events follow the same course as last time." Writing in a psychiatry journal, he said: "I hope that this account will help to dispel the erroneous belief that ECT is a terrifying form of treatment, crippling in its effects on the memory."[1]

Electroconvulsive therapy, like all medical treatments, had side effects. Given the risks entailed in the illnesses for which ECT was indicated, these effects were relatively minor. Patients experienced memory loss of varying degrees, together with, in the early days, a risk of fractured bones. An imagined additional danger was the specter of "brain damage," which turns out to have been false; there is no known occurrence of brain damage associated with ECT. The other risks are small but real. Unfortunately, over the years their significance has mushroomed out of proportion so that today they loom large in the minds of many. The National Institute of Mental Health (NIMH), for example, once refused a grant application for ECT research on the grounds that the patients would never consent to participate in the study "once the risks had been explained to them."[2]

The physical side effects were surmounted relatively early in ECT's history, so that by the mid-1950s, fractured vertebrae and other bones became a phenomenon of the past. Yet memory loss has dogged ECT throughout, its menace indeed rising over the years in the minds of patients and of many practitioners, so that by the 1970s it had become a great black beast, an inducement to many patients and their families to eschew convulsive therapy at all costs. A personal story related this well: I (Edward Shorter) recall a colleague who had endured bouts of chronic depression. One day in the coffee room of the history department, someone asked him: "Have you ever thought about ECT?" "Oh no," he replied. "I'm a historian. I couldn't take any chances with my memory." Several months later the man committed suicide. There are serious issues in the subject of memory loss, yet overemphasizing them has led to tragedies as patients are discouraged from seeking appropriate help by the unnecessary magnification of a minor and mostly temporary effect. As Kalinowsky said in 1942: "In severe mental disorders social death [social stigma] is the outcome in such a high percentage that we are justified in taking a risk."[3]

As for the notion that ECT causes permanent brain damage, it has been even harder to convince the public and many physicians that there is simply no evidence to support this. Arthur Cherkin at the Veterans Administration Medical Center in Sepulveda, California, noted with some exasperation in 1984: "The reality is that ECT of acute endogenous depression [major depression] is the most effective and most rapid therapy in the entire armamentarium of psychiatry. The typical public view, however, is that ECT is a bad procedure which should be constrained by legislation because it 'messes with the brain,' alters personality, is painful, [and] converts defenseless patients into zombies." None of these perceptions is true, Cherkin said. "Today's evidence is already overwhelming that ECT does *not* mess up the brain, is *not* painful, and does *not* create zombies."[4]

Broken bones and memory impairment as side effects were apparent even in the earliest days. Dealing with them led to considerable technical changes in the administration of ECT, so that original ("unmodified") ECT became safer and more memory-sparing as a result of a series of modifications. Ironically, attenuating the convulsive jolt may protect memory, but it is less effective for treating the depression.[5] Even today the full dose of alternating current—Cerletti's original "unmodified" version—may well be the treatment of choice for patients who have high seizure thresholds and are unresponsive to less powerful forms of ECT.

It was, after all, the very effectiveness of unmodified ECT that aroused the curiosity of Tom Bolwig, currently a professor of psychiatry in Copenhagen and a major international figure in neuroscience. In 1962, as a Danish medical student, he interned at a large mental hospital in Sweden. It lacked an anesthetist and so administered ECT "unmodified." "The first ECT I gave was to a young woman whom I shall not easily forget. I had examined her when she was admitted while I was on duty. She had all the features of melancholia. She was a mother of two, about my own age at that time, about 23 or so, and she was almost in a stupor. I decided she had depression and the boss of the ward where I worked looked at her and said, 'You are right; she has severe depression so you give electric shock tomorrow.'"[6]

A senior consultant in the hospital told Bolwig how to do it. "The patient was placed on a bench and assistants held her arms and kept her knees down. I put the rubber bit in her mouth so she wouldn't bite her tongue." They placed the electrodes on her temples. Bolwig pressed the button. "She started to scream leaving me very very weak. I wasn't about to faint but I was very weak. I repeated it because they ordered me to and she had an unmodified grand mal seizure. I had to sit down because it was probably the worst thing I'd done and I was convinced that I could have killed her." Later that day Bolwig saw the woman at the mini-golf course of the hospital, already substantially better. "She didn't recognize me but she said hello and she looked as if she was in a good mood." He gave her five more treatments "and she was completely cured, although of course there was some memory disturbance. I decided, I almost swore at this time, that this thing would never happen again to me. That if I were to be something in the medical profession it should be as far away from torturing people like that as possible."

Yet Bolwig remained intrigued by the therapy. He trained in psychiatry in Copenhagen, by which time modified ECT with anesthesia and muscle relaxation were used. The optics of the scene were very different. For Bolwig, ECT now stood as an effective, humane treatment, despite everything that he had witnessed at the Swedish mental hospital. He decided to go into research to "find out why this crude treatment was so efficient and how it was that some patients—especially depressed patients—got so well and not other types of psychiatric patients."

In its most primitive form, unmodified ECT involves putting electrodes on a patient and delivering a jolt of alternating current. For years and across Europe and North America, this was how it was practiced. But just what were the problems associated with ECT in this form?

Patient Anxieties

Anticipatory anxiety is not, strictly speaking, a side effect. Yet if it builds, it keeps patients from returning for repeated treatments and represents a barrier to effective therapy. Metrazol, the convulsive therapy adopted a few years before ECT, produced acute and foreboding anxiety in patients, and this was one of the reasons for its clinical demise. ECT, on the other hand, did not evoke this level of pretreatment panic. Patients in the early years mostly feared losing consciousness, learning only later from the media that they should experience a sense of doom, memory loss, and other side effects. On the whole, they accepted the treatments they were given and did not fret later about being damaged by them. This is not surprising, as most ECT patients indeed felt much better afterward.

For most of the early generation of electrotherapists, negative patient reactions were unusual. Lothar Kalinowsky and Eugene Barrera described in 1940 the procedure at the New York State Psychiatric Institute: "No patients maintained any unfavorable attitudes toward subsequent [ECTs]. This is considered an inestimable advantage in this method [compared with Metrazol]."[7] In 1941, Victor Gonda described his electrotherapy practice in Chicago: "Not one patient thus far objected to the continuation of the [ECT] treatment."[8] Max Müller in Switzerland recalled in his memoirs that the patients readily accepted ECT, unlike Metrazol, some becoming indeed "addicted to the fits" (*krampfsüchtig*).[9] Said Oscar Forel of the private clinic in Prangins,

Switzerland, where he was working in 1941: "Most of the patients wake up relaxed and smiling."[10]

Early in 1941, Hillside Hospital in Hastings-on-Hudson, New York (later that year the hospital moved to Queens), treated its first patient, a thirty-nine-year-old Russian woman with schizophrenia, using a machine purchased with donations from former patients.[11] She did not respond well and after the eighth treatment "lost her recent memory, became disoriented, believed the hospital to be a hotel, could not remember the names of her room-mates." Her orientation returned quickly, and she did not complain further about the therapy, although it had not greatly helped her.[12]

Also early in 1941, John X, an accountant in his forties with depression, was said to be "somewhat impatient at the fact that [electric] treatment has not yet started." He received twenty-two treatments and was discharged "recovered," despite having had only petit mal responses (a loss of consciousness but no convulsion). Was he uneasy about ECT? We know only that after a few days' discharge, he returned readily to Hillside for further treatments.[13] Charles X asked for the treatments of his own accord but was discharged from the hospital after three sessions because the family were "indignant."[14] Jean X's ECT treatments were started "at her urgent request."[15] These were not reluctant patients.

In other patients, uncertainties and anxieties about ECT did come to the fore. A previously successful dentist, struck by depression, was said to be "somewhat dazed and groggy" after treatment; he had "been complaining of loss of memory." Yet the complaints did not surface again, and after thirty treatments he had shed his depression and resumed his practice.[16] The most negative reaction in the early days at Hillside came from a patient for whom ECT was probably least appropriate, a forty-two-year-old woman who had some kind of personality disorder characterized by histrionic behavior and hysteria. She also had difficulty walking (a psychoneurological gait disorder called astasia-abasia), especially when staff were around, combined with a highly irritable relationship with all of her fellow patients. Her chief complaint was "pressure on top of her head." At a loss for what to do, the staff sent her for ECT. After her first treatment she "reacted . . . with an hysterical outburst. She cried in a loud voice, yelled repeatedly, 'What are they doing to me,' called upon her mother for help and later moaned and groaned. This spell lasted for about an hour." Yet the electric treatments had no therapeutic effect; she was totally disruptive in group psychotherapy (a technique that Hillside pioneered in the United States), and it was finally "felt that this hospital could be of no more service to this patient," as chief psychiatrist Louis Wender put it.[17]

Another patient, a forty-four-year-old male with symptoms of a personality disorder was plagued by a hysterical cough. After being hospitalized for ten months and every approach failing to alleviate his cough, the staff decided to try ECT, which he endured rather sullenly. When his wife came to visit, he had a noisy outburst in Dr. Ernest Lewy's office: "He stated that he would not consent to any more electric shock treatment and that he felt that the hospital was fundamentally obliged to him for having taken those treatments since he had voluntarily become a victim of science. . . ." His wife then broke into tears because of his behavior and told him he did not know what he was talking about.[18]

On balance, among the first twenty or so patients to receive ECT at Hillside, there were none who complained of lasting after-effects.[19] The majority responded well and left the hospital "much improved" or "recovered," and seemingly content with their care. Even those who did not respond, such as a schizophrenic man who, despite eighteen major ECT-induced seizures, "has . . . been listening to his own abdomen a voice from there telling him, 'you ought to have sexual relations,'" had no particular grievance about the ECT."[20]

Despite the general willingness to accept medical authority and to look forward to a rapid recovery from illness, there were anxieties. And these anxieties would swell into a mighty torrent in the decades ahead, overwhelming reason and hope. Abraham Myerson noted some of this sentiment at Boston State Hospital: "It is not quite true that patients have no dread of the electric-shock method," he said in 1941. "There is some dread, probably due to the general fear that is associated with being knocked unconscious." It was much less than with Metrazol, he noted, but nonetheless present.[21] Interestingly, while Cerletti insisted that there were no significant problems with the treatment he had originated, many of his assistants, laboring closer to the patients, detected considerable unease. In 1941, Giovanni Flescher, an assistant at the Rome university clinic, conducted the first study of memory loss in ECT. "Asked about their attitudes, the patients look on with more or less manifestly anxious preoccupation at the preparations for electroshock, because the extraordinary state in which people wake up after electroshock does not escape them, and gives them the sensation of having undergone some grave and dangerous trauma."[22]

Louis Wender, chief psychiatrist at Hillside Hospital, also had a private practice. When in 1943 he and two other physicians reported on the mix of outpatients at Hillside and in Wender's practice, they found that "on the whole, there was no difficulty in getting the cooperation of the patient. Although all patients developed a fear of the treatment to some extent, this was never sufficient to keep them from returning for further treatments."[23] Thus, fears existed, to be sure, but not such as to be a barrier to treatment.

In later years, it dawned on physicians that patients' fears seemed to increase in the course of the treatment, rather than to diminish. Among the first to describe these rising fears during treatment was Alfred Gallinek at the Neurological Institute of Columbia-Presbyterian Hospital. Of the awakening phase, he said: "A temporary annihilation of the sense of familiarity after electroshock provokes basic anxiety, and results in a strong, progressively increasing fear of the treatment."[24] Meduna wrote to his colleague Hirsch Loeb Gordon in 1947: "I read your paper about fear influencing the results of the electric shock treatment. I am positive that you [have] got something here. I do not know whether you noticed in some depressive cases that the patient is not afraid of the treatment at all while he is depressed but his fear increases at the rate of improvement." Meduna said he had quite a job convincing patients to stay the course.[25]

By the mid-1950s, Cerletti too noted this rising fear in the course of treatment, calling it "tardive anxiety." He said: "The patient is not able to explain but it disturbs him at times to the point of refusing to continue the treatment."[26] To diminish this unspeakable fear, Cerletti prescribed barbiturates. Later, other clinicians prescribed the new antipsychotic drugs to help alleviate patient fears. As the ECT manual at the Veterans Administration Neuropsychiatric Hospital in Los Angeles noted in 1956 of the simultaneous administration of reserpine or chlorpromazine with ECT: "The apprehension which develops in a few individuals when ECT alone is used may be controlled."[27]

Memory Loss

When an internationally celebrated actress had an episode of mania in Manhattan, her agent sought out Sidney Malitz of the New York State Psychiatric Institute. Malitz agreed to treat her with ECT, not at the Institute but at his Upper East Side office, and agreed to keep it very hush-hush. The star did well after a course of treatments. "However I had trepidation," said Malitz, "about the fact that she was going to be start-ing a play on Broadway with all kinds of memorizations and things. By sheer coincidence, I had bought tickets to that play before I gave her the ECT. So here we go, the curtain goes up, and I'm dying wondering is she going to forget her lines. But it went well. It worked out."[28]

Yet things did not always work out. "Dear Professor Cerletti," wrote one of his patients on March 4, 1948: "You may remember me. You treated me with electroshock for a nervous depression that I have had for a year and a half. I had six treatments at your clinic . . . and then had to travel back to Egypt." (She was an upper-middle-class Egyptian woman, writing to him from Cairo in French.) Now, twenty days since her most recent ECT session, things were not going well. "Unfortu-nately, I feel bad, very bad. Apparently I'm suffering from amnesia. I feel quite confused, above all when I get up in the morning. And I am very irritable. Above all, I cannot tolerate either noise or music. . . . Movies and night clubs bore me and there are entire days when I have no appetite, then on other days I eat too much and suffer from my stomach."[29] The list of complaints was quite lengthy, but of interest here is the woman's loss of memory.

Disturbances of memory are a real issue in ECT, though not an in-surmountable one. As Fred Frankel, a psychiatrist in South Africa in the 1950s put it: "I had in Johannesburg big business executives, I had the conductor of an orchestra, I had academicians, people who had ECT, came for it, weren't dragged to it, and were delighted with the re-sponse and went out. And they said, you know I don't remember very much of what happened during the period of ECT, and we all said yes you won't, but you will remember stuff afterwards and what happened before will come back slowly."[30] In discussing memory effects with ECT, it was seen as no big deal.

When two psychiatrists interviewed 166 inpatients in 1976, a year af-ter they had received ECT at the Royal Edinburgh Hospital, 50 percent of the sample reported memory loss as the worst side effect, two-thirds mentioned some memory impairment, and a quarter of the entire sam-ple believed it was "severe." Yet on the whole the perceived side effects were not vastly discouraging: 50 percent said that "going to the dentist was more upsetting or frightening" than ECT.[31] These statistics have been widely cited, both by the opponents of ECT (two-thirds lost some memories!) and the supporters (better than a trip to the dentist!). Sta-tistics on memory loss have proven something of a quagmire because they are so subjective. Who among us can remember exactly what we did some months or years ago—and if we are told this is pathological, we dwell on it. (See chapter 9 for a detailed discussion of the components of memory loss.)

In informed circles, serious memory loss has seldom been considered real. The courts have always looked dubiously on the claim of ECT as an exculpation for criminal activity (the defendant alleging he cannot recall the crime). In 1972, a New Jersey appeals court rejected the plea that the defendant's amnesia (he received ECT following committal to a mental hospital) extended back a year and a half, covering the period of the crime: "Retrograde amnesia, as a passing phenomenon, is well known, but respondent's claim that his loss of memory was total a year and a half after the treatment seems extraordinary. . . . Respondent's claim is subjective and we do not credit it."[32]

The pioneer generation of convulsive therapists was for the most part oblivious to the issue of possible impairments of patients' memories. Meduna dismissed cases of amnesia in Metrazol therapy as largely feigned, or a demonstration of patient resistance to the aggressive Germanic interrogative style of the day. He conceded that perhaps one patient had experienced genuine amnesia: after recovering the fellow had chuckled about some embarrassing and now forgotten utterances during his illness.[33] Later, Meduna waved aside the entire issue of side effects in convulsive therapy. His chief at the neuropsychiatric institute in Chicago, Francis Gerty, had forwarded to him a questionnaire from the National Committee for Mental Hygiene about "persistent side effects." "The developing fear of patients toward convulsive treatment is most certainly unfavorable," Meduna allowed. But were the aftereffects enduring? Not really. "I don't know whether the transient impairment of memory, or occasional bone fracture in convulsive treatments should be considered as 'permanent' after effects."[34]

In 1940, Ugo Cerletti stated there was consensus that ECT produced no complications that "could damage the nervous system."[35] And Jean Delay, who had pioneered ECT in France during World War II, dismissed memory loss as a significant side effect on the basis of 1,200 treatments to date: "The prognosis of these amnesias is benign. They clear up in a few weeks."[36] Indeed, the tenor of the discussion of Metrazol therapy and ECT in the late 1930s and 1940s was to play down memory loss and disorientation as transitory phenomena that merited little concern. In retrospect, these observers were largely correct that most patients recovered their recollections of past events. Yet they made the mistake of ignoring the subjectivity of their patients' feelings.

Some members of the first generation of ECT-specialists did look more closely at what the patients were saying and feeling, and for these clinicians, the memory loss and disorientation issues were a red flag for future criticism. As early as 1940, Los Angeles psychiatrist Eugene Ziskind and his coworkers called attention to the harmful effects of Metrazol convulsion therapy on learning and memory. Using six patients and six controls, he found that the Metrazol patients had a 28 percent lower score in learning tests than did the controls. "The impairment in learning with Metrazol would appear to be due to impaired memory," Ziskind concluded.[37]

The following year, in 1941, Ziskind reported on memory defects in a series of thirty-two Metrazol patients, twenty of whom had experienced some memory problems, and an additional four having "pronounced memory defects." One of these four was a sixty-six-year-old woman who had recovered from a severe agitated depression. Three days after her first convulsion, Mrs. X said: "The night before last was the first night that I seemed a little like my old self. I could let go a little from my vile thoughts. Oh, they were so terrible!" Yet Mrs. X complained: "You know there may be something wrong with my memory. There may not be. I'm having trouble thinking of what did happen this morning. I must have had breakfast but I can't tell what—I'm just trying to think." Three days after that, her depression was gone. Yet her husband said: "She appears well except for poor memory. She forgets from one minute to the next. She also sits around dazed at times." She had forgotten her homecoming dinner on the next day and did not remember her children coming to visit. The family said that over the next three months her memory returned to normal. Ziskind's overall view of the memory issue is unequivocal: "Usually the defect is minor and transient and may even escape detection if not sought for. . . . Recovery is the rule."[38]

The authorities agreed that memory loss with Metrazol was more severe than with ECT. Yet in electroconvulsive therapy as well, impaired memory was certainly an issue. In 1941, Cerletti's assistant, Giovanni Flescher, called attention in the *Swiss Archive for Neurology and Psychiatry* to what he called "permanent" memory loss as a serious side effect in some patients treated in the Rome university psychiatric clinic: "The abolition of retrograde amnesia occurs gradually and in a space of four to seven hours. Whatever [memories] are not spontaneously recalled in this lapse of time . . . we have not succeeded in evoking subsequently. Thus in these cases we should speak of a partial permanent amnesia."[39]

By 1944, Bernard Pacella documented a series of more than five hundred patients treated with ECT at the New York State Psychiatric Institute: "As a rule, the memory defect disappears or markedly diminishes after a few weeks, but occasionally the patient still complains of slight memory loss for several months subsequent to treatment." Two of the patients "complained of memory impairment for as long as a year after therapy."[40] Real but transitory was the verdict pronounced in 1946 by Paul Delmas-Marsalet, the French ECT pioneer who was a professor of psychiatry in Bordeaux: "They clear up in a few weeks and are certainly not a counterindication to continuing the treatment."[41]

In these early notations of memory loss, two themes stand out. One is that ECT produces physiological brain changes, but not permanent damage. These changes in brain activity may cause memory impairment, but they also relieve an acute state of mental illness. Second, ECT is not suited for every type of psychiatric patient, particularly those who are considered highly neurotic. These patients, by nature of their disorder, are prone to seeing a temporary memory impairment as a permanent and devastating loss.

ECT could briefly precipitate transient confusion, or in rare cases, delirium, that was called at the time "psychosis." This presumed psychosis was thought to have nothing to do with the original illness. Sakel called it a "productive psychosis," meaning therapeutic in nature, and Max Müller termed it an "exogenous psychosis," produced by external factors. Yet when Adolf Bingel at the university psychiatric clinic in Erlangen, Germany, looked at it in 1940, he found memory loss and disorientation to be a significant part of this transitory ECT-delirium. After the ninth treatment, one of Bingel's melancholic patients ceased the moaning and crying that had characterized his original illness and instead suddenly demonstrated a "conspicuous change in the symptom picture. The patient makes a perplexed impression. To the question of the clinic director whether the patient knows him, the patient responds, 'Oh yeah, you're our chairman, what do I know.' To the question where he is, the patient responds, 'Oh, it's probably in the general direction of Rothenburg. I have no idea where I am. Everything is so different. The doors have all been changed around.' How long have you been here? 'It's a few days at least, maybe one to two months, I just don't know [patient rubs his head]. I must just have forgotten everything.'" Bingel said that common to all these patients is "that after an original clear-cut improvement of the psychosis, once the ECT is continued, manifestations appear of retarded thinking [*Schwerbesinnlichkeit*], memory loss, inability to concentrate, and in extreme cases temporal and spatial disorientation that stand in no causal relationship to the original illness." He noted that the syndrome was fully reversible.[42]

In 1945, Kalinowsky pulled all this together for an American audience as a kind of transitory organic brain syndrome. He viewed memory loss as "the most constant but never the only organic mental symptom during electric convulsive therapy." He called these symptoms "organic psychotic reactions implanted on the psychosis for which the patient is being treated; they disappear within one or two weeks after the last treatment." Early on, in a kind of "organic neurasthenia," memory and intellect are impaired; later a kind of Korsakoff-picture (extreme short-term memory loss) may develop, in which the patient is disoriented, incoherent, and makes connections poorly. Kalinowsky emphasized the brevity of this "organic psychotic syndrome" and said that treatment should not be discontinued if it appeared.[43] Still, one can appreciate the concerns of patients and their families: ECT had whipped up real issues involving memory.

ECT specialists were concerned about treating the wrong kind of patient, namely psychoneurotics who would cling to claims of abolished memories. This included many patients with a diagnosis of "depressive neurosis," which, despite its label, was not the kind of depression that responds to ECT but rather a mixture of character disorder and anxiety treated then by psychoanalysis (and now by the Prozac-style "SSRI" drug class).[44] In 1950, Erwin Stengel, a psychiatrist from Vienna who at the time was at the Maudsley Hospital in London, told the Paris World Psychiatry Congress of a "hysterical" patient who developed "total amnesia" after receiving ECT.[45] Kalinowsky was quite adamant about not treating psychoneurotics with ECT: "It cannot be emphasized enough," he said in 1949, "that contrary to psychotics, some neurotics may be harmed by ECT. Anxiety, as the most frequent symptom in neurotics, is often aggravated. Many neurotics react badly to the memory impairment and complain of it long after psychological tests have shown that actually no impairment persists."[46] Years later, he returned again to the subject, saying that "after ECT for typical endogenous depressions, patients, when recovered, do not have memory complaints, whereas patients with neurotic depressions (who usually respond poorly) add memory complaints to their other anxieties."[47] Kalinowsky emphasized over the years that anxious patients should not be treated with electric shock.

In an interview in 2004, one of Kalinowsky's students, New York psychiatrist and ECT specialist Robert Levine, repeated this sentiment: "You don't give ECT to the character-disordered," he said. "If you give ECT to patients with borderline personalities or general anxiety disorder unnecessarily, they'll end up with lifelong loss of memory and headaches that won't go away."[48] The message here is that patients with anxiety may be suggestible, and that the treatment creates an impression of more memory disarray than has actually occurred.

In the 1940s and after, ECT specialists tried hard to reduce memory impairment by decreasing the amount of electricity flowing into the brain while at the same time producing an effective seizure.[49] It was once believed that there was a trade-off between memory loss and therapeutic efficacy: the less effect on memory, the less efficacious the treatment of the illness itself. This was the logic behind intensive ECT, discussed later in this chapter. The current view is that efficacy and amnesia are unrelated. In 1979, Max Fink wrote in his guide to ECT: "The elimination of amnesia should not interfere with therapeutic efficacy."[50]

Sorting out the relationship between efficacy and memory was like entering a scientific maze, with blind alleys at every turn. A first blind alley was giving the patient so little electricity that only a petit mal seizure was produced, not a grand mal. (In a petit mal the patient loses consciousness and experiences some muscle twitching but does not have a cerebral seizure that is measurable by EEG [electroencephalograph] or is clinically visible.) In 1941, Lothar Kalinowsky, Eugene Barrera, and William Horwitz at the New York State Psychiatric Institute found that of twenty-seven patients treated only with petit mals, none recovered from their original illness, and only three showed significant improvement; when the same twenty-seven were given grand mals, seven recovered fully and four were much improved. "The definite therapeutic superiority of convulsions over petit mal seizures has to be emphasized," they concluded. It was clear that the convulsion was the basic mechanism of ECT.[51]

The original Cerletti method relied on alternating current from a wall socket that pulsed from positive to negative at forty-five cycles per second (45 hertz). (Wall current in the United States pulsed at sixty cycles per second, or 60 Hz.) This form of current is called a "sine wave." Cerletti would ask Bini to turn the rheostat to around 125 volts for 0.16

seconds, which produced an electrical current of 250–600 milliam-peres, depending on conditions.[52] On an everyday basis, this amounted to the electical energy in the instant flip of a light switch off/on/off—"just enough but no more" as ECT specialists tend to put it.

In 1942, Emerick Friedman and Paul H. Wilcox, who then were a res-ident and junior staffer at the Metropolitan State Hospital in Waltham, Massachusetts, introduced the concept of unidirectional wave forms for a gentler shock. (Friedman had already made a name for himself as an early Metrazol therapist.) The investigators supposed that if they used only "half-sine waves," that is, sine waves with the bottom, or negative, half eliminated, they could reduce considerably the amount of electricity flowing into the patient. This was a "unidirectional" form of pulsating current (also called a "rectified sine wave"). Unidirectional is a form of "direct" current (DC), as opposed to alternating current (AC), which reverses its flow from positive to negative sixty times every second. In electrotherapy, *regular* direct current has a steady flow in one direction only; *unidirectional* direct current pulsates, going from positive to neutral. In the Friedman-Wilcox wave form, the duration of flow would be a bit longer. But at one second and 30–50 volts, the uni-directional technique required an electric current of only 40 milliam-peres. By flicking the switch back and forth, they could give a number of these in a row.[53] Engineer Reuben Reiter constructed the apparatus they used for unidirectional ECT and began marketing it in 1946.

Friedman and Wilcox made an innovation in the area of electrode placement in order to spare nonmotor parts of the brain (such as sen-sory and memory areas) the direct passage of electricity. Cerletti and the other early ECT specialists placed electrodes bilaterally, on either side of the patient's head, in the area of the temples. The electrodes were held on with a rubber band or a forceps-like pincer. The new method involved attaching the positive electrode to the top ("vertex") of the skull, the other just above one of the temples. The current was thought to pass in a straight line through the motor cortex, creating "motor seizures" that affected other parts of the brain only indirectly. (Of course, the electrical current diffuses in space, and these concepts were simplistic.) "From previous trials it was found that if the negative electrode was placed on the temple just above the ear and the positive electrode on the vertex of the skull at mid-obelion, convulsive electrical doses seemed to be minimal when compared to doses necessary to in-duce convulsions when the electrodes were placed at other areas."[54] The downside of this "right unilateral" technique was that it was less effective than "bitemporal" or "bifrontal" ECT, which stimulated directly these other brain areas.

Soon after this work, Friedman got a post at the Norwich State Hospital in Norwich, Connecticut, and did further research on various forms of unidirectional current on 176 patients at Norwich, including the "half-sine" form mentioned above. Two-thirds of these latter patients convulsed at doses of electricity less than 50 milliamperes per second, much lower than the Cerletti dose. Friedman concluded: "Unidirectional electrostimulation seemed to offer convulsive doses markedly less than required by techniques utilizing the alternating current."[55]

At the same time in France, Paul Delmas-Marsalet, professor of psychiatry in Bordeaux, completely independently of Friedman and Wilcox, was also working on direct current. Beginning with animal experiments in March 1941, he progressed to applying fifty-cycle direct current at doses of 50 to 100 milliamperes to an undisclosed number of patients; he spoke of "hundreds" of applications administered without incident. Published in a French psychiatry journal in 1942, the article was little noticed.[56]

Was unidirectional ("direct") current as effective as Cerletti's alternating current? Here opinions were mixed. Kalinowsky was dubious about any departure from the Cerletti-style of alternating current, to which he remained faithful all his life. In 1949, he said the patients were uneasy about the low-current techniques because not enough patients received grand mal seizures: they did not become immediately unconscious and experienced in a quite unpleasant way the passage of electricity, discouraging them from seeking repeat applications. He concluded: "ECT has the great advantage of being a surprisingly harmless procedure and any recommendations complicating its simplicity should be carefully tested as to their safety."[57]

This consciousness of flowing electrical current was often addressed using anesthesia. With Cerletti-style alternating current, anesthesia was unnecessary because the patient was instantly unconscious. Trading amperage for stimulus duration resulted in a prolonged application during which the patient did not lose consciousness immediately. With some modified ECT protocols, the seizure would take its time marching across the body, the patient still aware of the stimulus. "In order to administer [such] techniques," David Impastato explained in 1954, "it is essential that the patients be adequately anesthetized. It is impossible to administer these treatments without adequate anesthetization, because the treatment is extremely painful. If attempts are made to give these treatments without anesthesia, the patient will develop a horror of treatment and stay away."[58]

Yet there were enthusiastic voices for unidirectional current too. In 1943, Louis Wender left Hillside Hospital to become codirector with Joseph Epstein of Pinewood Psychiatric Hospital in Katonah, New York. In 1956, well satisfied with the success of unidirectional current for ECT, they compared 436 patients who had received Cerletti's alternating current with 370 who had pulsating unidirectional current (UDC). In terms of efficacy, the outcomes were about even: 78 percent of the manic-depressives recovered with AC, 81 percent with DC. Yet unidirectional current cut the complications in half: "The two most unwanted complications—namely, severe fractures and severe confusion and memory defect are almost eliminated by the UDC method." The authors concluded: "In the hospital setting, [unidirectional] has practically eliminated the anxieties and fears of relatives and patients alike, who constantly complained of forgetfulness and memory changes and worries as to the permanence of the symptoms."[59]

A second innovation in the application of unidirectional pulsating current occurred in 1944, when Wladimir ("Ted") Liberson at the Institute of Living in Hartford, Connecticut, and the pharmacology department of Yale University proposed "brief stimulus therapy" (BST). Liberson was a psychiatrist and physiologist born in Kiev and trained in Paris and Montreal. He too had noticed patients' anxieties during treatment with unidirectional direct current: "Because of the prolonged time of stimulation and only slight memory disorders, the patient develops an extreme anxiety and becomes very resistive to the treatment." A grand mal seizure could be more easily elicited if the individual impulses were greatly shortened from one-sixtieth of a second to impulses as short as one-twentieth of a millisecond. These very brief impulses, one-thirtieth the duration of Cerletti's AC impulses, were separated by relatively long, energy-free gaps, a wave form referred to as "square waves." Liberson developed a machine that could put out up to 250 of them per second. The shortening of the stimuli to fractions of a millisecond produced a great decrease in the amount of electricity necessary for a series of stimuli to produce a convulsion. When Liberson announced his first findings on BST in 1944 and 1945, he had done work only on rabbits and guinea pigs.[60]

By 1947, Liberson had been able to apply BST to eighty patients at the Institute of Living, forty-six of whom had received no previous shock treatment. He was by then using a machine designed by engineer Franklin Offner, owner of Offner Electronics of Chicago, in which the size of the pulses (stimulus amplitude) increased progressively with every cycle.[61] Using the same vertex-temporal placement of the electrodes as Friedman and Wilcox, Liberson achieved a technique that delivered only 14–40 milliamperes of current every one to one and a half seconds (as opposed to Friedman's 40–90 milliamperes). Of the depressed patients in the group of forty-six, 80 percent responded well, and almost all the patients were said to have fewer memory disturbances and to show less dramatic EEG changes than patients who received Cerletti-style ECT.[62]

By 1949, Douglas Goldman at the Longview State Hospital in Cincinnati, Ohio—one of the earliest ECT therapists in the United States (see chapter 4)—had used BST on 112 patients in the asylum and in his private practice, compared with 435 treated with conventional ECT in both settings. He popularized the right unilateral technique when he described his use of BST, one electrode on the vertex, the other on the right temporal area "to avoid excessive application of current to the important areas of speech." He noted that other researchers had preferred the left side "with the idea that some of the symptoms of mental derangement may originate in such areas."[63] Goldman's protocol involved delivering pulses at a rate of 120 per second, with the current rising over the course of the shock, which lasted from one-half to one and a half seconds, and sparing the muscles from all contracting instantaneously. He said that BST was at least as effective as the Cerletti technique and that it resulted in a "marked diminution and, at times, complete absence of confusion associated with the electric shock therapy." Continuing patient anxieties were a disadvantage, yet Goldman said they could be alleviated by giving the patients a barbiturate, Pentothal, before treatment.[64]

Brief stimulus therapy touched off a great vogue of memory-sparing procedures, in which the actual shocks might last up to two seconds (as opposed to 0.2 seconds in the Cerletti procedure) yet require only 40 milliamperes of current.[65] Swedish psychiatrist Jan-Otto Ottosson discovered in 1960 that the convulsion was the therapeutic component, and that the surplus electricity beyond that needed to produce a convulsion just added to the patient's confusion. Cross-appointed in the departments of psychiatry and physiology at the Karolinska Institute in Stockholm, Ottosson said that therapeutic outcome and memory impairment in ECT arose from different mechanisms, "the memory impairment as a side-effect from the current, the therapeutic effect from the seizure."[66]

Efforts to reduce disorientation and memory loss resulted in several innovative uses of direct current, as opposed to the considerable hit of electricity in Cerletti's alternating current. This research discredited alternating current, perhaps unfairly, as primeval and dangerous. Even today it is not clear whether brief stimulus therapy is the superior form of electroconvulsive treatment.[67] Doubts remain concerning BST's effectiveness (see chapter 11).

Returning to the debates over electrode placement in ECT as a factor in reducing side effects, a series of trials began in the late 1950s that established a unilateral arrangement (both electrodes on the same side of the brain) as the position of choice. In 1954, Bernard Pacella at the New York Neurological Institute and David J. Impastato at Bellevue Hospital would ramp up the direct-current stimulus slowly until they got a convulsion on one side, then increase the current-dose more until the fit spread to the opposite side. They noted that this technique was less effective than bilateral grand mal seizures. (The patient was anesthetized, an important modification to original ECT, given that a slow increase in the application of direct current is painful.)[68]

In 1958, a comparative trial provided striking evidence. Neville P. Lancaster, a consultant psychiatrist in Bristol, and Reuben R. Steinert and Isaac Frost, a resident and consultant psychiatrist, respectively, at Deva Hospital in Chester, England, attracted wide attention with their work on what they were then calling "unilateral" ECT. By *unilateral* they meant both electrodes were positioned closely together on the same side, in this case the right side, supposedly to spare the "dominant" left hemisphere. Of the forty-three depressed patients in the trial, twenty-one were given unilaterally induced generalized or focal seizures (the technique produces a good many "Jacksonian" focal seizures, named after British neurologist John Hughlings Jackson, starting on one side of the body and marching over to the other; these are not grand mal seizures); fifteen received bilaterally induced generalized seizures (these are grand mal); and seven got unilaterally induced "subshocks." In therapeutic terms, bilateral and unilateral virtually tied (subshocks did poorly).

Of great interest was a "memory recall test" the investigators administrated shortly after each of the four shocks that the patients received. Those who got standard bilateral ECT did poorest (score of 1 at the bottom of the scale); the unilateral general-convulsion patients scored 19, the unilateral-focal patients, 27; and the unilateral subshock patients, 24 (this latter score a bit of an anomaly, but the sample was very small). Unilateral ECT, with both electrodes on the same side, appeared to be therapeutically effective and at the same time to spare memory. The authors recommended unilateral ECT for "elderly patients . . . who are depressed and difficult with food" and for "patients of very superior intelligence and especially those who have to earn their livelihood with retained knowledge." With a certain arrogance, these elite consultants cast off concerns about memory loss among the average or learning-disabled classes. Only the memories of "superior" minds should be protected, according to their recommendations. They deemed bilateral ECT acceptable for "involutional depressives of average intellect," as well as for patients who were "actively suicidal"; catatonic schizophrenics, known to be "dangerously impulsive"; and nonresponders to unilateral therapy.[69]

In 1962, Stanley M. Cannicott conducted a randomized controlled trial of unilateral ECT versus standard ECT at the Holloway Sana-torium in London. The results suggested that unilateral ECT signifi-cantly reduced memory loss and disorientation while retaining the same therapeutic effectiveness as the standard bilateral form. Cann-icott concluded that "unilateral ECT is as effective as bilateral ECT in the treatment of depressions but produces a significant reduction in confusion and amnesia." He said it should be "the treatment of choice for all outpatients and for those intellectual workers who must earn their living by retained knowledge." The numbers of patients involved in the trial were quite small: twenty in the bilateral group and thirty in the unilateral group.[70]

In 1966, veteran ECT specialists David Impastato and William Kar-liner proposed a technique for inducing full grand mal convulsions by putting both electrodes close together on one side of the head (near the "motor strip," an area of the cerebral cortex that controls muscle move-ment). Impastato and Pacella had been experimenting with unilateral techniques since 1954, mainly producing non–grand mal focal seizures that either generalized to both sides of the body or did not. These had not been as effective as bilateral ECT with its grand mals. Now, to-gether with Karliner, Impastato was suggesting a new technique for administrating right-sided unilateral so that grand mals would be rou-tinely forthcoming. They started the rheostat at 190 volts, descending in a hundredth of a second to 97 volts. They believed the results as ef-fective as bilateral ECT, "over which it has one great advantage; namely, marked diminution of cumulative memory changes as well as practical abolition of post-treatment confusion and agitation." This made outpatient treatment "a safer and easier procedure and does not engender the fear that many patients developed following bilateral treatment." The nurses and accompanying relatives, too, were relieved to "see the patient clear and normal and not confused and babbling as after the bilateral treatment." The technique also made it possible to step up the pace of treatments, even to a daily frequency, because disorientation had ceased to be a problem.[71]

After this contribution, enthusiasm for unilateral ECT became widespread, and state legislators even contemplated enacting the procedure into law as a precondition for convulsive therapy. But bilateral placement proved more effective in treating the core illness. With unilateral electrodes, patients awakened from anesthesia with a certain clarity of mind. That same clarity occurred for patients receiving bilateral applications within a half-hour, and their memory impairment recovered in a day or two. As Kalinowsky noted in 1984: "We all tried unilateral treatment, and many have returned to bilateral ECT despite the highly undesirable effect of having patients confused during and shortly after the treatment." He pointed out that most depressions would clear with six or fewer treatments. Unilateral positioning required six to twelve. "It may be added that the double number of anesthesias is in itself a potential risk for the patient."[72]

Despite the fashionableness of unilateral ECT, bilateral placement remained the technique of choice for many hospitals. William Karliner later regretted his endorsement of unilateral ECT. As early as 1972, he began backpedaling from the enthusiasm he had expressed alongside Impastato. He said that since then he had gained further experience: "I have found that in acute depressive or schizophrenic reactions, bilateral electroshock or Indoklon remains the choice treatment." A much greater number of unilateral treatments would be required to gain comparable results.[73] Much later, in an interview, he said simply: "I tried unilateral with no effect. . . . Unilateral caused much less memory loss but it also was less effective."[74]

Indoklon: The "No-Electrocution" Therapy

Of the three physical therapies to emerge in the 1930s and early 1940s, only ECT was practiced with any regularity by the 1950s. But concerns over ECT prompted the development of a different, nonelectrical, convulsive therapy. In 1957, John C. Krantz Jr. and coworkers in the department of pharmacology of the University of Maryland discovered that an odorless anesthetic gas, flurothyl, known popularly by its brand name Indoklon, elicited convulsions in lab animals when inhaled. Encouraged by the absence of side effects in the animals (as measured by EEG), they administered flurothyl to four patients, three of whom had standard ECT-style seizures. The patients recovered uneventfully with no clouding of memory. "It is possible," the authors concluded, "that this comparatively simple procedure of the inhalation of hexafluorodiethyl ether might be found useful in the treatment of certain types of mentally ill patients."[75]

The following year, in collaboration with psychiatrist Albert A. Kurland and another colleague at Spring Grove State Hospital in Catonsville, Maryland, the Krantz group described in the *Journal of the American Medical Association* a randomized trial of Indoklon versus standard ECT involving seventy-five patients. The principal finding was that patients seemed to find Indoklon less threatening and experienced less postictal (postseizure) confusion.[76] Pennwalt Chemicals obtained a preparation patent for the substance in Britain in 1959, and the Air Reduction Company procured a separate patent in 1962 (Air Reduction officials had been involved in the research from the beginning). It was Air Reduction that would market Indoklon in the United States through its subsidiary Ohio Chemical, although Smith Kline & French also sought to develop the drug.

The true motor behind Indoklon's progress was that it did not have to be presented to patients as "electroconvulsive therapy." Gas sounded more benign than electricity. And the term "convulsions" was either omitted or downplayed in small-type advertising copy for the drug. Indoklon's most prominent early trial in the United States was rather inauspicious, conducted between 1957 and 1958 at the New York State Psychiatric Institute. After going to Spring Grove for an orientation, on December 7, 1957, William A. Horwitz, the principal clinical psychiatrist at PI, together with Alvin Mesnikoff, a senior psychiatrist there, and resident David R. Lyons, initiated Indoklon treatment at PI. "Since electricity was not used to induce the seizure, it was possible that patients would be less concerned with 'electrocution fears,'" wrote Horwitz later in the PI *Annual Report*. Yet the result of the trial in eight patients was discouraging: one of the patients fractured several vertebrae and several others became fearful after the first treatment. The following year the group abandoned Indoklon research as offering no real advantage over ECT, and Smith Kline & French withdrew its support.[77]

In 1958, Indoklon research passed to ECT specialists William Karliner and Louis J. Padula at the West Hill Sanitarium in the Riverdale district of the Bronx, who basically revived Meduna's 1934 ideas about chemical convulsive therapy. Asked by Smith Kline & French to administer it to a series of thirty-three patients who had a mixture of diagnoses, they obtained more convincing results than the investigators at PI. They used a barbiturate to quell the patients' anxieties in addition to succinylcholine, a relaxant, to abolish the muscle thrashing. In 1960, they called it "equally as effective as electroshock in depressive disorders." In "schizo-affective disorders" it was indeed superior to electroshock, they said.[78] This research launched Indoklon in American psychiatry, with Karliner as its chief advocate. Pushed by his anesthetist Salvatore Dell'Aria, Karliner began giving Indoklon by intravenous injection as well. He did so partly in the belief that it was quicker, as he said later in an interview.[79] Karliner also noted in a 1963 article that "patients are more prone to accept the intravenous route than that of inhalation. Less apprehension and fear were noted when intravenous rather than inhalation Indoklon was mentioned as the method of treatment."[80]

For a while, it seemed Indoklon would replace ECT as an effective somatic therapy. It required less apparatus and was ideal for the outpatient setting. "Most of my patients fall into the lower middle-class income bracket," said Karliner, "and the cost of private hospitalization is prohibitive. It is necessary, therefore, to treat these patients, even the severely disturbed ones, on an ambulatory basis."[81] If Indoklon equaled ECT in efficacy and safety, there was no reason for not replacing it. In 1964, the FDA approved inhalational Indoklon, and its brief career in the world of mainstream psychiatry commenced.[82]

Yet in the end Indoklon was put aside. Smith Kline & French was said to have lost interest in it. And although the gas required less apparatus, the procedure itself involved more steps and preparation. As early as 1961, Max Fink and colleagues in the research department at Hillside Hospital found electrically induced convulsions on par with Indoklon from the viewpoint of efficacy and memory, but superior to Indoklon in terms of ease and cost.[83] In 1972, Joyce G. Small and Iver F. Small, then in the department of psychiatry of Washington University in St. Louis, said the "cumbersome method of induction with Indoklon makes it a less useful procedure for routine application" than ECT, although it should be reserved as a second-line treatment.[84] *Cumbersome* and *ease* may be code words for something less innocuous. It was Max Fink who much later pointed out another reason, one that would rarely be mentioned in the scientific press yet was crucial: "Flurothyl has the distinct odor of diethyl ether. When two or more patients were treated, the air in the room carried the odor and the staff was no longer willing to treat patients. Having seen the efficacy of a few breaths of flurothyl in patients, they themselves feared the induction of a seizure."[85]

Fractures

Fractures were the bane of unmodified ECT. Fractured femurs and "broken backs" represented powerfully undesirable side effects, and unless they could be eliminated as a risk factor, ECT would never be accepted as a tool of mainstream psychiatry. A high fracture rate had been the kiss of death for Metrazol. As mentioned in chapter 4, in 1939, Phillip Polatin and his coworkers at New York's PI discovered that, in an X-ray study of fifty-one patients who had received Metrazol, 43 percent had compression injuries of the spine. Many of the fractures were slight cracks in the anterior part of the upper surface of the vertebral body, an apparent consequence of the patient's suddenly arching forward in a clonic contraction.[86] It did not matter that most of the vertebral fractures were asymptomatic and healed quickly. Many clinics discontinued Metrazol therapy after these statistics appeared.

It was hoped that ECT would produce a lower injury rate than Metrazol because the convulsions were thought less violent. Late in 1940, Cerletti reported with pride that his university psychiatric clinic had experienced no fractures, and only two dislocations of the temporomandibular (jaw) joint.[87] Almansi and Impastato in the first report of their experiences claimed they had "not had a single complication" in about one hundred ECT cases.[88] Such reports were overshadowed by mounting data that ECT did, indeed, lead to fractures. At a meeting of the Royal Society of Medicine on convulsive therapy in London in January 1940, Donald Blair said that "it was disappointing to learn that fractures occurred in electrically induced convulsions. In the cases first treated by Cardiazol it was supposed that no fracture of the vertebrae occurred, but afterwards it was discovered that there were quite a number of such fractures."[89] When Bingel in Erlangen reported on ECT in 1940, he warned of a variety of fractures. "Electroconvulsive therapy is not so lacking in complications as it appeared from the first reports of the Italian authors Cerletti and Bini, and Sogliani."[90]

In a statistical study, Lauren H. Smith and coworkers in the Department for Mental and Nervous Diseases of the Pennsylvania Hospital in Philadelphia found that 5 percent of their 156 ECT patients had experienced fractures (eight fractures, of which five affected the vertebrae). Their Metrazol fracture rate was about 22 percent.[91] At Shanley Mental Hospital in England, the ECT fracture rate stood at 2.8 percent in the 420 patients treated at the time that radiologist Eric Samuel studied them in 1943. He allowed that the figure might be low, as all patients did not receive a postictal X-ray.[92] So the fracture rate was, in fact, considerable, and merited concern.

The ECT specialists themselves found the statistics exaggerated and the risks to the patients minimal. As Kalinowsky protested to Bini in 1940, the Metrazol fracture study that came from his own institution had been badly damaging. "With the same radiological technique we also found some cases after electroshock, yet a much lesser percentage. The patients don't complain about any pain and this business had created a huge resistance to any convulsive therapy. Certainly, it's not of any practical matter."[93] Kalinowsky remained exasperated about the preoccupation with vertebral fractures and viewed other kinds as rare. As he said in 1941: "It must be stated that [these X-ray findings] have a limited or no clinical significance at all. . . . The psychologic factor of the 'broken back,' however, considerably discredited a method that is of definite help in psychiatric treatment."[94] When in 1948, Phillip Polatin and Louis Linn at the New York State Psychiatric Institute did a follow-up study of patients who had experienced vertebral fractures ten years previously, they found virtually no long-lasting consequences.[95] Yet something had to be done. Even if such events occurred to only one patient in a hundred, shattered teeth, broken backs, and humeral fractures had an intimidating effect on doctors and patients alike. And in a treatment extended to hundreds of thousands of patients, one-in-a-hundred was still a formidable statistic.

The most practical solution to the problem of the patient's pitching forward and fracturing a vertebra was hyperextending (bending backward) the spine by putting something under the small of the back. Victor Gonda was first to describe this, placing his patients atop a barrel stave, thus curving the spine backward and making it much more difficult for them to arch forward. "To prevent injury to the vertebrae," Gonda wrote in 1941, "[the patient] is placed in bed with a blanket-covered wooden base placed under his back. This wooden base is merely a stave from a large barrel, and is so placed that the maximum convexity is under the middorsal spine. This hyperextension separates the anterior vertebral edges, which are most vulnerable to compression injuries."[96] The following year, in 1942, Kalinowsky described a similar hyperextension of the spine that they had introduced at Pilgrim State Hospital in Brentwood, Long Island: "Three large sand bags are placed beneath the patient's middorsal spine. The shoulders and hips are then manually applied to the table with some force, producing hyperextension to the greatest degree that this relatively rigid section of the spine will permit." They x-rayed their first sixty ECT cases after introducing this procedure and found no vertebral fractures.[97]

The sandbag method seems to have been highly effective, although it looked terrible.[98] As Baltimore psychiatrist Frank Ayd recalls: "The first ECT treatment I ever saw was on one of my own relatives [in fact, Ayd's father]. I was at St. Joseph's Hospital in Baltimore then, and the ECT was done in the radiology department with sandbags under his back. There was no ECT machine as we have now, no succinylcholine, no Brevital sodium, nothing. You saw what a real grand mal seizure was and the scream, not really a scream of pain, but as the air was inspired. Quite an experience. It was a horrible one for me." But with eight treatments his father recovered.[99] (There were other ways to prevent the patient from pitching forward aside from sandbags. Around 1945, Nathan Savitsky and Karliner started tying a sheet about the patient's chest and attaching it to the table, leaving the limbs free to twitch or thrash. They called it a "modified straitjacket.")[100]

The advent of psychopharmacology gave the problem of fractures a definitive solution with the introduction of curare into ECT practice. Curare is a botanical drug derived from the *Strychnos* genus of Amazonian climbing vines that blocks the nerve-muscle junction, effectively preventing the voluntary muscles from moving. In the 1930s, curare had just started to be used in medicine for spastic disorders, and in 1939 Harold Palmer, a psychiatrist at St. Thomas's Hospital in London, suggested that it might be used in blocking fractures caused by Metrazol convulsions.[101]

Meanwhile, in Omaha, Nebraska, psychiatrist Abram Bennett was working with the Squibb company to develop a stable curare preparation for use in convulsive therapy. (As early as 1939, he had experimented with a spinal anesthetic for preventing spinal fractures in Metrazol therapy.)[102] Squibb had the dimethyl ether extract of purified curare in development and would market it as Intocostrin. The particular form of curare Squibb used was called *d*-tubocurarine, one of the main alkaloids of the plant. Curare was a dangerous substance without doubt. As the standard pharmacological guide of the day advised: "In view of the extremely potent nature of curare and the ever-present danger of respiratory muscle paralysis . . . the safe employment of the drug is restricted, as a rule, to experienced anesthesiologists who are thoroughly acquainted with resuscitative procedures such as tracheal intubation."[103] Many psychiatrists would have reservations about using it. In 1940, Bennett described the use of curare for "preventing traumatic complications in convulsive shock therapy" with Metrazol. "Care must be used not to allow the patient's head to fall backward, as his neck muscles are powerless." A much softened version of the standard convulsion takes place, and the only precaution needed was a tongue guard.[104] In effect, the drug achieved a flaccid paralysis of all the muscles. Patients under its influence would experience no further traumatic fractures.

Extending the application of curare from Metrazol to ECT was an obvious step, and by June 1942, convulsive therapist Byron Stewart at the Compton Sanitarium in California was curarizing all of his ECT patients.[105] By 1950, the benefits of curare in abolishing surgical complications had become evident. After curare was introduced at the South Hospital in Stockholm, the vertebral fracture rate dropped from 37 percent among men and 7 percent among women (men being more muscular were more susceptible to musculoskeletal damage), to none among men and 4 percent among women.[106] Yet an undercurrent of uneasiness accompanied curare use. It could easily be deadly. Calculating a precise therapeutic dose was tricky: doses of natural substances varied in potency, and individuals responded differently to equivalent doses. ECT was a remarkably safe procedure, in the sense that there were almost no deaths associated with the treatment. Yet of the eight deaths in eleven thousand cases that had occurred by 1943, four were associated with curare.[107] Kalinowsky thought curare "more dangerous than the complications it is supposed to prevent."[108] The New York State Psychiatric Institute prided itself on never having adopted curare.[109] Much later, Arthur Gabriel said that curare "came into disfavor when it was realized that it sometimes converted potential morbid complications into fatal complications."[110] Was there no better solution?

In 1951, the problem of fractures was solved with the introduction of succinylcholine. Succinylcholine chloride, otherwise known as "sux," was a muscle relaxant that Nobel Prize–winner Daniel Bovet, head of the laboratory of chemotherapeutics at the Superior Institute of Health in Rome, first described in 1949 in an Italian journal.[111] It was patented in 1952 by an Austrian company and marketed in the United States by Burroughs Wellcome and Company under the brand name Anectine. In February 1951, Carl Gunnar Holmberg of the department of psychiatry of the Karolinska Institute in Stockholm, and Stephen Thesleff, of the departments of anesthesia and pharmacology, introduced into ECT a Swedish version of sux (succinylcholine iodide) as a short-acting blocker at the neuromuscular junction. (It "depolarizes" the motor end plate that attaches to muscle.)

Holmberg and Thesleff first gave an intravenous injection of a barbiturate. "When the patient had fallen asleep, succinylcholine was injected rapidly intravenously. . . . When the maximum effect was apparent after about 80 seconds, the shock was given. With this procedure we obtained complete muscular relaxation with none of the unpleasant sensations that always accompany a 'curarization.'" They then changed to injecting sux and the barbiturate simultaneously, mixed together in the syringe, giving the shock about 20 seconds after the end of the injection. They simultaneously administered oxygen. "When it is evident that the patient's breathing is regular and that there is a free airway, he may return to the ward. Further supervision . . . is then superfluous."[112] This corresponds roughly to the procedure used in ECT today.

Holmberg and Thesleff's article, published in the *American Journal of Psychiatry* in May 1952, transformed the practice of ECT, taking it from what was later judged a "brutal" spectacle of uncontrollable thrashing to a calm scene in which scarcely a muscle moved, the clinicians' only clue to a cerebral seizure taking place being the twitching of the patient's big toe, a blood pressure–style cuff having been wrapped about the calf to ensure that the sux would not reach the muscles that control the toe, so that evidence of a fit would be visible. (Max Hamilton at Leeds introduced the cuff method, a simple maneuver to verify adequate seizures before the EEG method of demonstrating the seizure replaced it.)[113]

Succinylcholine drew along with it the use of anesthesia in ECT. Previously, in Cerletti-style ECT, small amounts of barbiturate had been given to sedate the worried patient or to manage postconvulsive episodes of excitement. (Some direct current techniques did entail anesthesia by design.) With sux, large amounts of barbiturate were given as full-scale anesthetics in all forms of ECT.[114] Why did giving anesthesia become almost obligatory with sux? Many patients disliked the transitory sensation of not being able to catch their breath as they felt the sux take hold. Though they were never in danger of asphyxiation, a barbiturate (such as methohexital sodium, "Brevital," or thiopental sodium, "Pentothal") was used to block this momentary feeling from their consciousness and ensure that they would return for subsequent treatments. Max Fink later said that when they introduced sux at Hillside Hospital in 1953, they did so initially without giving the patients any anesthetic. The patients started screaming: "I can't breathe, I can't breathe." Then somebody said to Fink: "You should give her a barbiturate first. You put them to sleep first and then give them succinylcholine." "So the anesthesia came in," Fink said, "not because we wanted anesthesia for the ECT; it came in because we wanted amnesia for the succinylcholine."[115]

Among the earliest to use sux in the United States were Benjamin F. Moss, Corbett H. Thigpen (of *The Three Faces of Eve* fame), and William P. Robison of the department of neuropsychiatry of the Medical College of Georgia, practicing at University Hospital in Augusta. They administered Pentothal and sux in quick succession through a single syringe (obviating a second needle puncture) and gave pure oxygen during the seizure itself. "No untoward effects have yet been observed in over 300 electric treatments," they said.[116] The problem of surgical fractures in ECT had now been solved. English psychiatrist Max Hamilton said in 1976 that he had not seen a single spinal fracture since they started giving muscle relaxants in 1952.[117] The modification of ECT was complete.

Yet in retrospect it is possible to wonder if much of the modification was really necessary or rather if it reflected mainly cosmetic changes rather than therapeutic progress. The blessings of sux, of course, were apparent, and as time went on virtually all muscle movement was suppressed. Veteran ECT specialist Zigmond Lebensohn of Washington, D.C., scoffed in 1999 that in reality "the primary reason for the excessive use of muscle relaxants . . . was to placate the nurses, who might recoil from viewing an unmodified grand mal seizure."[118] Kalinowsky had figured out during the war that simply hyperextending the patient on a pile of sandbags would reduce vertebral fractures to almost zero.

With anesthesia and barbiturates as part of the procedure, ECT now has to be done in a hospital. Barbiturate anesthesia depresses a patient's respiratory centers (respiration is already interrupted for forty seconds or so by the shock itself) and entails the presence of an anesthetist, in case resuscitation is necessary. This is in addition to the psychiatrist who delivers the current and the nurses who administer the air bag and monitor the electrocardiograph and electroencephalograph machines that ensure a convulsion had actually occurred and that the patient's vital signs are fine. The unilateral treatments are not as effective as the bilateral and must be administered twice as often for the sake of minimizing an otherwise brief period of memory loss and disorientation.

So what has this cascade of interventions actually accomplished? It has had the effect of converting ECT from a relatively accessible outpatient treatment to a cloistered hospital procedure available only to a few. Whether this is a plus for the public health remains debatable.

"Brain Damage"

In the scientific uncertainty that accompanies any new therapy there was speculation that the new somatic treatments damaged the brain. After all, investigators reasoned, patients experienced convulsions, which were usually a consequence of epilepsy or a cerebral lesion, such as caused by a tumor, stroke, or advanced syphilitic infection. Postictally, patients often displayed the kinds of abnormal reflexes associated with brain lesions, such as a "positive" Babinski sign (big toe goes up when lateral margin of plantar surface of foot is stroked with a pointed instrument; normally the big toe curls down). Were the therapeutic gains of insulin coma and of convulsive therapy being purchased with permanent and irreversible harm to the brain?

Cerletti and Bini in 1940 provided strong evidence of an absence of brain damage with ECT. They examined the brains of thirty-four dogs divided into three groups: those that received the same dose of electricity as humans; those that received a series of shocks; and those that received very large amounts of electricity. Five other dogs served as controls and received no electrical stimulus. In animals of the first group that were sacrificed immediately after the experiment, there were some minor anatomical changes, mainly slight edema; in the animals of the first group sacrificed a month later, these changes had reversed themselves. Similar negative results were found for the other groups. Thus, these early Italian investigators concluded that full-strength (sine wave) ECT, as practiced in humans, produced no lasting brain changes.[119] Published in Italian, during a war, this report failed to enter the international literature.

The first American investigators therefore began from scratch. In 1940, Phillip Polatin, Hans Strauss, and Leon L. Altman reported on five patients at PI who had experienced "severe fog and forgetfulness" following prolonged insulin coma or Metrazol treatment. It seemed as though they must have been harmed. Yet in the three on whom EEG studies had been performed, the patients' brain function was soon restored to normal. Nonetheless, the authors speculated: "It may consequently be inferred that some residual cerebral damage existed which could be elicited only by . . . finer laboratory techniques."[120] For Eugene Ziskind in Los Angeles, the memory defects he observed following Metrazol treatment could be associated with organic brain damage. In 1941, he argued: "There is probably actual injury to nerve cells, the damage being reversible in early, or milder, stages and irreversible in the later, or more pronounced, states." There might even be, he speculated, "decortication and decerebration," or a massive occurrence of brain cell death, clearly something the patients and their doctors would find unacceptable.[121]

As insulin and Metrazol faded from clinical use, most discussions of brain damage concerned only ECT. It was Manfred Sakel, keen to sabotage competition to his beloved insulin therapy, who first suggested to the nonmedical public the notion that convulsive therapy caused brain damage. In 1942, he told the *New York Times* that the "indiscriminate use" of ECT could "lead in some cases to an impairment of the personality and possible damage to the brain itself." Convulsions alone, he said, were a terrible idea. Insulin should first be used to "prepare the ground" and "in most cases convulsions are not needed at all." When memory losses occurred in ECT, he told the reporter, they resembled "a symptom that we see only in two brain diseases, both malignant, namely, in paresis [syphilis of the central nervous system] and progressive arteriosclerosis of the brain, in which serious brain damage takes place."[122]

At the Paris World Psychiatry Congress in 1950, when Sakel raged so dramatically against Metrazol and ECT, he repeated that convulsions were useless—and damaging in schizophrenia: "The damage done, particularly to the Schizophrenic patients . . . is still going on, a fact which forces me again to bring up this matter." "The convulsion is not only useless in Schizophrenia but possibly even damaging if applied in great number." He said that he had called this to the attention of "the main advocates of this misconception" in personal letters as early as 1937 (there is no evidence that he actually did so). "But now I feel it necessary to speak publicly since I have seen that damage is being done to schizophrenic patients and no other way is left to me."[123] This was the first time the "brain damage" charge reached an international scientific audience, and it reverberated widely: ECT harmed the brain!

When later in the Paris session Kalinowsky arose to refute Sakel, it was with an awareness that in the intervening years there had been a number of studies demonstrating that ECT did not cause brain damage. In 1942, he himself had been part of a team of investigators at PI who studied the electroencephalograms of ECT patients and the postmortem pathology of rhesus monkeys given ECT. As for the ECT patients, the group concluded that transitory changes in brain function did indeed occur following ECT, but that they were temporary, brain function returning to normal: "In general, the electroencephalographic abnormalities associated with electric shock treatments are for the most part 'reversible' in the sense that they gradually disappear."[124] The authors were ambivalent on the subject of underlying cortical changes. The twelve laboratory monkeys who received shock therapy did display some brain changes, but the control monkey who had not received any ECT also showed the same changes, a probable consequence of captivity rather than electrotherapy.[125]

There were in these years a handful of similar animal studies: some showed small histopathological changes following ECT; others did not. In 1944, at the end of this series of contributions, N. William Winkelman and Matthew T. Moore, psychiatrists affiliated with the neuropathology lab of the University of Pennsylvania, reported their own painstaking research on cats receiving ECT at standard human doses (the cats showed no tissue changes). The authors said that some of the previous research had not been properly performed, the animals' heads banging about during the procedure or their nutrition not properly controlled (postictally, animals may stop eating). In any event, they dismissed the whole notion of ECT causing brain damage.[126] And Ziskind in California had changed his mind. In 1945, he said there was no evidence of brain damage among their sixty-nine convulsive therapy patients who were in remission: "Reports on the working ability of our recovered patients reveal . . . that it is as good as, or even better than it was in the prepsychotic period. One gains the impression, therefore, that there cannot be any serious impairment to the brain, the reports of their performance being as good as they are."[127]

Despite these scientific findings, brain damage became an allegation that refused to go away. As will become clear in chapter 9, members of the antipsychiatry movement and the Church of Scientology continued to promote this idea throughout the 1960s and 1970s. Most of the scientific establishment lost interest in ECT during those years, and it was only in 1984, at a scientific symposium devoted to the question

"Does Electroconvulsive Therapy Cause Brain Damage?" published in *Behavioral and Brain Sciences,* that neuroscientists and clinicians again refuted the entire assertion. Richard Weiner, a psychiatrist at Duke University, delivered the main paper, the gist of which was a rather timid "not really."[128]

The various authorities called on to comment were much more emphatic. Joyce G. Small and Iver F. Small, then at the Indiana University School of Medicine in Indianapolis, noted that the use of ECT had been increasing in the late 1970s and early 1980s precisely because it was "safer and more effective than drug or other methods of treatment." They pointed to the "long-lasting and sometimes irreversible impairments in brain function induced by neuroleptic [antipsychotic] drugs. In this instance the evidence of brain damage is not subtle, but is grossly obvious even to the casual observer!"[129] Steven F. Zornetzer at the Office of Naval Research in Arlington, Virginia, invited "concerned and interested clinicians and scientists [to] stop obsessing over the problem of possible ECT-produced brain pathology (based on such scanty evidence)." A more interesting subject, he said, was "the *changes* in the brain, rather than the *damage* to the brain." He noted that psychiatrists who prescribed ECT "need no longer beat their breasts over the possibility of doing great harm to their patients."[130]

Max Fink, scarcely able to contain his exasperation with Weiner, seized on Weiner's use of the slippery word *substantial:* "If there is no *substantial* evidence for brain impairment, then there is *no* evidence for brain impairment. . . . If considerable investigation finds *no* evidence, then the possibility of rarely occurring cases is not a reasonable conclusion. While there is always a possibility of anything, such kowtowing is inappropriate in a review that endeavors to be definitive." Fink noted that the main study on which Weiner hung his reservations was that of Larry R. Squire and Pamela C. Slater in 1983.[131] "These conclusions hinge on a study in ten patients and seven controls, and the maximum impairment was related to two items—events on the day of hospital admission and questions about the Watergate political fiasco. What trivia on which to base a conclusion of persistent brain damage!"[132]

Stunned, perhaps, by these combative declarations of the safety of ECT, Weiner was considerably more affirmative about the procedure in his rebuttal than he had been in his original report. He said that over the years, such ECT critics as Washington, D.C., psychiatrist Peter Breggin had slid from the assertion that ECT produced brain changes to the conclusion that ECT "*always* produces serious brain damage as manifested in the acute organic brain syndrome." This kind of bait-and-switch, said Weiner, "suggests that a couple of martinis or a few beers, in producing a delirious state, always leads to serious brain damage."[133]

In 1991, Edward Coffey and his colleagues at Duke University reported a definitive study pertaining to the question of brain damage and ECT. (The initial findings were presented at the meeting of the American Psychiatric Association in 1989.) They did before-and-after magnetic resonance imaging (MRI) studies of thirty-five depressed patients, using the brief-pulse (Liberson) bilateral technique. In a sophisticated analysis of the images, they found no changes in brain structure immediately after ECT or even six months later. "Our results confirm and extend previous imaging studies that also found no relationship between ECT and brain damage," they concluded.[134]

As though the phantom of brain damage were Dracula and required a stake through the heart, a team of researchers from the departments of biological psychiatry and neuroscience at the New York State Psychiatric Institute led by Andrew J. Dwork, and including such internationally known ECT investigators as Harold A. Sackeim and Sarah H. Lisanby, randomly assigned twelve *Macaca mullata* monkeys to either ECT, magnetic seizure therapy, or sham treatment (in which no stimulus is administered but the other physical or preparatory conditions of treatment are conducted). As they said in their article in the *American Journal of Psychiatry* in March 2004: "We avoided the confounds of earlier studies by using general anesthesia, muscle relaxation, oxygenation, seizure and physiological monitoring, and formalin perfusion before removal of the brain." The group found no anatomical lesions in the monkeys in any group, concluding that "the absence of pathological findings provides empirical evidence that routine use of convulsive therapy does not produce structural brain damage."[135]

The half-century-old myth about ECT and brain damage had been pushed decisively back into its tomb. Yet the discredited theory continued to be perpetuated in the nation's public discourse. In a 1976 decision striking down key aspects of California's notorious anti-ECT legislation, the Court of Appeal of California justified upholding part of the contested law on the grounds that "possible risks include permanent brain damage."[136] (See chapter 9 for further details on the California laws.) It was an interesting, if unpleasant, demonstration of the notion that ideas have consequences.

Making a Virtue of Necessity? Several Treatments a Day

Shortly after the end of World War II, the mother of a Hindu princess brought her daughter to Oscar Forel's private clinic in Prangins, Switzerland:

> "I have consulted the best neurologists and psychiatrists in England," said the mother. "Nobody has been able to cure her, and her state is now so grave that her husband is thinking of renouncing her. Doctor, you are my last hope."
>
> Forel considered: "Madame, I would like to save your daughter, but I am going to ask you to share with me some grave risks. I am proposing that you leave your daughter with us and then that you travel elsewhere for three weeks. With your permission we are going to give her some sessions of electroshock. In a sense, we are going to decerebrate her. It is a brutal treatment, but in a case as desperate as this it holds out some chance of success."
>
> "If it were your daughter," said the mother after a long silence, "would you do it?"
>
> "I wouldn't hesitate," Forel responded.
>
> "Very well then," said the mother. "You have carte blanche."

Forel began the treatment immediately, administering a series of successive shocks in close intervals. This produced an arrest of all higher mental functions. "For a number of days, the patient's life was thus reduced to so-called vegetative functions. Then, little by little, her mental activity resumed, and equally her memory. At first she regained her memories of the long distant past, then progressively the more recent recollections and some insight into herself." The upshot was that the princess recovered, "despite the traumatism of her marital life . . . that had completely upset her."[137]

What Forel described was known as "intensive" or "regressive" ECT. The impression it created was poor, yet it had a record of some success and may be considered one of the last technical innovations in ECT. But its purpose was to maximize memory loss rather than to minimize it. The logic was first articulated in 1942 by Hans Löwenbach, an émigré psychiatrist who had trained in Germany at a prominent brain research institute and had come to Duke University: "If the patient becomes almost immediately his pre-shock self," he said, "then the therapeutic procedure has been in vain." He argued that confusion and disorientation were essential to ECT results.[138] In a later article, Löwenbach and Edward A. Tyler explained that in January 1942 they had started giving up to four shocks a day, "sometimes for several days in succession." It was their impression that "patients who had an extended period of post-convulsive confusion tended to improve more readily than patients in whom this effect was absent."[139] This, then, was the rationale for intensive ECT: making a virtue of, indeed maximizing, the confusion that would inevitably follow standard ECT.

Giorgio Sogliani at the provincial mental hospital in Sondrio, Italy, first proposed intensive ECT in 1939, saying that he practiced ECT in "a rhythm more intense than is customary for Cardiazol therapy, thus daily."[140] Elsewhere he said that he might give several shocks in a row without the patient regaining consciousness in between.[141] In 1944, Lucio Bini at the university psychiatric clinic in Rome started administering what he called, in one of the most unfortunate coinages of postwar medicine, "annihilation therapy" (*metodo dell'annichilimento*). In reality it consisted of daily ECT treatments. Bini gave it for such "psychoneuroses" as neurasthenia, obsessive-compulsive disorder, and "hysteria."[142]

Lauretta Bender at New York's Bellevue Hospital, the founder of the study of childhood schizophrenia in the United States, reported in 1947 that over the previous five years her Children's Ward of the Bellevue Psychiatric Division had administered daily treatments to some ninety-eight children ages four to eleven for a typical course of about twenty treatments. Although the basic illness had not been relieved, the children had become much more sociable, composed, and able to integrate in group therapy as a result of the daily ECT.[143]

These early attempts at intensive ECT appear timid, however, in comparison with what came later. W. Liddell Milligan, a staff psychiatrist at St. James Hospital in Portsmouth, England, began using "the intensive method" in 1941, giving patients up to four treatments a day. "In some cases it is necessary to reduce the patient to the infantile level, in which he is completely helpless and doubly incontinent." They employed intensive ECT for "psychoneuroses," at least those serious enough to warrant hospitalization, and claimed excellent results without sustained memory loss.[144] Milligan is considered the initiator of regressive ECT, even though he did not use the term.

Intensive ECT acquired a certain following in the ensuing years.[145] The New York State Psychiatric Institute, the premier American center, experimented with it in 1947, although it did not have enough nurses to conduct the treatment properly (it involved large amounts of nursing care, as the patients had to be spoon-fed and toileted).[146] Two years later, Kalinowsky directed the intensive treatment of several female patients who had the diagnosis "tension," the outcome being unsuccessful.[147] In the mid-1950s, Reginald Taylor of the Psychiatric Institute's department of experimental psychiatry studied the EEGs "of Sing Sing prisoners [in Ossining, New York] receiving massive and prolonged electrical convulsive therapy," but the EEGs apparently were little different from regular electroencephalograms in ECT.[148]

In 1948, Cyril Kennedy and David Anchel at Kings Park State Hospital in Kings Park, New York, formally labeled the Milligan approach "regressive" ECT, and elaborated some details. For them, the preferred patient population was schizophrenic nonresponders and not "psychoneurotics." The investigators induced two to four convulsions daily "until the desired degree of regression was reached." "We considered a patient had regressed sufficiently when he wet and soiled, or acted and talked like a child of four." The patients became confused, could not take care of their physical needs, and had to be spoon-fed. As soon as the treatment was stopped the patients "returned toward their chronological age levels," their behavior "essentially normal and symptom-free."[149] In other words, the circumstances of the entire thing were ghastly, yet the treatment seemed to work on patients who otherwise would have been candidates for lobotomy.

In these years, the controlled trial in clinical research was just beginning to serve as the gold standard of evidence, and in 1952 Ephraim S. Garrett and Charles W. Mockbee at the Veterans Administration Hospital in Chillicothe, Ohio, conducted regressive ECT on a group of thirty chronic schizophrenic patients, with an equal number serving as matched controls. The schizophrenics in the experimental group had all failed previous insulin and ECT treatment, and some were very ill indeed: "All of these, except one, were almost completely withdrawn from reality. Sixteen soiled themselves; six ate their own excreta; twelve were actively combative; while three were on suicidal status. All were actively reacting to hallucinations." The patients received three grand mals daily, five days a week, "until the patient reacted like a child of 3 to 4 years of age," with the soiling and spoon-feeding. "Several were fed from a bottle and many apparently received pleasure in playing with dolls or other childish games." The gains one year later were apparent mainly in the realm of ward behavior, rather than discharges, yet of the sixteen who before treatment had soiled themselves, only two did so daily post-treatment ("and one only on rare occasions"). "Only one of the six now rarely eats his excreta."[150] The control group had not shown any changes. The regressive ECT had not touched the underlying psychosis, yet it did have some impact on the illness, moderating the more bizarre features of its force.

Regressive ECT retreated after the introduction of antipsychotic drugs in 1954 on the American market. Yet many chronic schizophrenics did not respond to medication, and in 1977 psychologist John E. Exner at Long Island University and Luis G. Murillo at Stony Lodge Hospital in Ossining conducted a follow-up study of twenty-eight Stony Lodge patients on regressive ECT versus sixteen on antipsychotic medication. The numbers were very small, and the results meant little statistically, yet it is of interest that the two treatments tied in terms of outcome, regressive ECT actually beating chemotherapy soundly in terms of the ultimate result of getting off therapy entirely: at the twenty-four- to thirty-month follow-up, only one-quarter of the drug group but two-thirds of the ECT group had "terminated all forms of treatment."[151]

By the 1970s, regressive ECT became ultimately impossible to perform for political reasons, stoked by allegations of widespread abuse. D. Ewen Cameron, head of psychiatry at McGill, was driven from office for his use of regressive ECT combined with continuous sleep, an approach that he called "depatterning."[152] In retrospect, regressive ECT was probably a technique that held some kind of a key to improvement in chronic psychotic illness—an area notoriously resistant to treatment even today, where keys are in short supply. Was it brutal and inhumane? Many colleagues thought so, and the opinion of two English psychiatrists responding in the *Lancet* to early reports of regressive ECT offers a sample of the vast flow of condemnation that was later to sweep over ECT altogether: "We find that the statement . . . that such traumatic clouding is therapeutically valuable to be one which fills us with something akin to horror."[153]

A third approach to intensive ECT was outlined by psychiatrist Paul Blachly of Portland, Oregon, in 1966. Blachly was not interested in regression but in ameliorating side effects. He proposed giving a whole course of ECT basically in one sitting rather than at separate intervals spread out over the day, as in regressive ECT. Because his technique involved simultaneously monitoring the patient's heart with an electrocardiogram and brain activity with an electroencephalogram, Blachly called it "multiple monitored electroconvulsive treatment," commonly

abbreviated as MECT, followed by a numeral for the number of treatments to be administered in a session. He typically would give another
stimulus three minutes after the conclusion of the previous seizure, before the patient awakened from the anesthesia, and administer three to
eight stimuli per session.[154] Advocates of this method claimed that the
memory side effects were comparable to those of regular ECT (unlike
regressive, where they were huge); the duration of treatment was, of
course, much shorter. Blachly drowned tragically in a canoeing accident in 1977 while trying to save his son and never had the opportunity
to serve as a resolute partisan for his approach. Richard Abrams and
Max Fink dismissed the single-session version of it in 1972 as having
lots of side effects and offering no real therapeutic advantages.[155]

Some of these accounts sound awful. Did these clinicians not know
at the time that it was a bad idea? One never knows something like this
amid the roar of events. As Fink later said: "The problem at the beginning was what is necessary for an effect. It was very easy to get seizures.
But they didn't know what was important, so they tried subconvulsive,
they tried convulsive, they tried multiple seizures, they tried different electrode pairs, with drugs, without drugs, daily treatments, twice
daily." [156] There were no institutional review boards to assess ethics in
those days, no protocols minutely determined in advance. These early
researchers did not realize that history would later judge their efforts
as "abuses"—and damn the entire therapy.

When the ECT enterprise later came to be condemned by the media
intellectuals, it was these efforts at delivering multiple treatments close
together—treatments that seemed worth trying at the time—that were
cited as horrible outrages. It was a philosophical, not a scientific, judgment. When Max Fink applied for an NIMH grant to study multiple
monitored therapy, the institute sent a colleague, an epileptologist, for
a site inspection. Fink told her about his plans. She replied: "Max, you
cannot do this because you are doing a lobotomy!" The site visit that
was supposed to last a day lasted ten minutes.[157]

Progress in ECT research stopped. It is notable that most of the technological development of ECT basically came to an end in the early 1950s
with Holmberg's introduction of succinylcholine and the anesthesia and
oxygenation that were necessary with it. Subsequent changes have been
minor, mainly adoption of monitoring the convulsion with an electroencephalograph—introduced in 1940 into American ECT practice by
Renato Almansi and David J. Impastato at Columbus Hospital in New
York City.[158] (They asked émigré neurologist Hans Strauss to conduct

the EEG studies for them, who had already published an EEG study of Metrazol.)[159] In Europe, EEG monitoring was introduced by two German investigators in 1941, then by Jean Delay in France in 1944.[160] Cerletti and Bini began tailoring the dose of electrical current to fit the patient so that the seizure threshold would not be grossly exceeded, and this too became generalized. All other subsequent innovations have either failed to pan out, such as intensive ECT, or have remained controversial and unproven, such as the assertion that unilateral is superior to the bilateral placement of the electrodes. (The only other widely adopted innovation was changing the wave form from sine wave to brief pulse stimulus.) What this lack of progress really demonstrates is the failure of research to lead to new approaches to treatment and to suggest new mechanisms of action. This is the result of psychiatry's massive disengagement from ECT after the 1960s as a result of stigma.

CHAPTER SEVEN

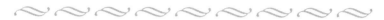

"They're Going to Fry Your Brains!"

In October 1983, an internationally renowned scientist at a prominent East Coast campus was in Copenhagen on sabbatical. There, he started to feel ill. He was depressed, fearful that he could not keep up with his students. New symptoms began to develop, as researcher Michele Greenwald, who had access to the family's notes of the illness, tells the story.[1] The scientist experienced what seemed like permanent insomnia, feelings of guilt, decreased energy, and thoughts of death. Then at an international scholarly meeting in Copenhagen he flipped into mania, jumping up and "animatedly explaining exactly what the speaker had really intended to say." His thoughts raced as he worked on a paper.

Then he crashed again, and by the end of December he was despondent at the thought that death was approaching. He had somatic delusions, convinced that a fungus had grown on his skin and was spreading to his buttocks. "By February 1984," explains Greenwald, "his weight had dropped from 180 to 150 pounds. He felt sure that he was starving to death, but could not seem to eat enough. In addition to a fungal rash, he believed that he had a strong body odor, though he bathed nightly." His wife became alarmed, telephoned the psychoanalyst the scientist had been seeing in Copenhagen, and the analyst made an appointment for him to consult Professor Tom Bolwig, who was in charge of the ECT service at the university hospital.

Bolwig tells the story at this point:

> I was in the hospital when the scientist—let's call him X—was admitted, and I had a room in an open ward arranged for him. To have him accept admission was not easy, and his wife, who had worked as

a psychiatric nurse, very explicitly, and before treatment options had been mentioned, expressed a protest against ECT being given to her husband. The staff nurse called me to the ward to talk with the couple. The situation was very difficult. X was in a dreadful condition, and I had him transferred to a closed ward. I and a senior resident discussed giving ECT the next day, and later that same evening the resident informed the family of these considerations.

During the preceding hours X's son and his ex-wife had discussed the situation, and all family members vehemently protested against ECT. The son called me at home and told me that he was very agitated. X was at that time calmer, had eaten a large meal, and was under close supervision. On that background, we decided to cancel ECT and await the situation the following day.

My considerations were: To give ECT in a not immediately life-threatening situation with hostile relatives may be hazardous for the therapy of any patient, and in the case of X the resistance from the family was indeed pronounced, and would not have given him the necessary support and might have induced mistrust of the staff. Further, nobody was against continued stay in the department. Therefore I cancelled ECT that night.[2]

The following morning X heard he might receive ECT. Researcher Greenwald explains: "Knowing little about ECT, [the scientist] took this as a pronouncement of execution. He had seen an empty bed with a strap over it outside his room and assumed this was where they strapped patients down as they sent large currents of electricity coursing through their bodies. He wondered how they got rid of the smell of burnt flesh." The scientist's condition worsened. He warned fellow patients that their food was infested with fungus and that his ex-wife had hired a TV crew to film him in hospital. He was briefly discharged, then readmitted.

This time he shared a room with a man who had previously experienced a depressive illness with paranoid thoughts and was now returning from his job in Greece for a refresher treatment. The man explained there was no smell of burning flesh. Bolwig raised the ECT issue again in a conference with the scientist, the scientist's wife, and another colleague who had come to Copenhagen to do research with X. The other colleague said that ECT seemed the only resort, so the scientist, who was in no condition to make the decision on his own, consented. The scientist's ECT treatment was commenced June 4, 1984. He had a three-week course of electrotherapy, three times a week, and did surprisingly well. "After eight treatments, he was released from the hospital feeling like a new man." He gained back his (excellent) memory, much of which he had temporarily lost during his depression.

In this very ordinary story of a good therapeutic response to ECT in psychotic depression, there is only one real question: Why did the family say no?

The Strange Decline of ECT

In 1959, only twenty-five years before the scientist's story, ECT was considered such a straightforward procedure that Group Health Insurance in New York City made a public announcement that it would allow coverage for "ten electroshock therapy treatments, in or out of the hospital," for each subscriber annually.[3] Even in the late 1950s, ECT was merely one psychiatric treatment among others. It was no big deal.

Then the wind began to change, and ECT would face a thirty-year decline. With a remarkable clinical result in treating devastating mental illness, it is difficult to fathom the underlying rationale for society's sudden and increasing aversion to it. It is as though penicillin had suddenly gone into a decline in the absence of any objective circumstance that might discourage physicians from prescribing it or patients from accepting it. There are various explanations for the growing disfavor of electric therapy that began in the 1960s, such as the success of psychopharmacology. In addition, an emerging antipsychiatry movement deplored the use of ECT for such repressive missions as making gay people straight (which notably failed punk-rocker Lou Reed).[4] And hostility to ECT was rising among psychologists. But coupled to these individual factors there was the overall climate that boded poorly for ECT. With the upheavals of culture and lifestyle that began to churn American society in the 1960s, institutions of the older generation were everywhere assailed. Some of these changes led to important reforms in education and rights for African Americans and women, for example. Others led to strange innovations and institutional decline. For the "flower children" of the 1960s, there would be no place for sending jolts of electricity through someone's brain. ECT, representing all that was brutal and inhumane in clinical medicine, began to acquire a massive stigma.

In the absence of a national ECT registry, it is difficult to measure how great the decline was. Yet scattered shards of data point to a sharp drop in use. In Monroe County, New York (which includes the city of

Rochester), the rate of electroconvulsive therapy declined from 50.4 per 100,000 population in 1963, to 32.8 in 1968, to 24.6 in 1973. (The decline for women was particularly notable, from 67.7 per 100,000 in 1963 to 29.5 in 1973.)[5] In Missouri in 1971, seventy patients received ECT at one of the state hospitals; in 1975, only eighteen did so. Two other Missouri state hospitals performed virtually none in those years.[6] Max Fink, who directed the Missouri Institute of Psychiatry in St. Louis in the early 1960s, noted that even then: "ECT was dead, outside of a few academic centers like Barnes Hospital." He did not even think of opening a program in convulsive therapy in Missouri and instead focused on developing one in psychopharmacology.[7] According to National Institute of Mental Health (NIMH) data obtained between 1975 and 1980, recourse to ECT in the United States as a whole decreased by 54 percent, remaining most popular in general hospitals and private psychiatric clinics. In public mental hospitals, where the vast majority of inpatients lay, ECT had virtually disappeared by 1980. The authors of the analysis wrote: "We find ECT is largely used as a treatment for patients who are white, voluntary, and paying their way in private institutions."[8] Between 1979 and 1984, according to a survey of the International Psychiatric Association for the Advancement of Electrotherapy, the number of ECT practitioners declined in a third of all academic centers; in 41 percent of them there was no training at all in ECT.[9] By 1986, no state hospital in the Pacific Northwest offered ECT any longer.[10]

ECT became a treatment that only the privileged could buy, not one that the poor might deserve. Look at the contrast between two hospitals on Long Island: Hillside and nearby Long Island Jewish. Sam Bailine, a prominent ECT specialist, conducted convulsive therapy at both. He noted that in the mid-1970s, 12 percent of the (largely middle-class) private patients at Long Island Jewish got ECT on its twenty-bed unit. At Hillside, only 1 percent of the (mostly poorer) patients received ECT; rather, Hillside offered mainly psychotherapy or medication.[11] (At the state hospitals patients would not have received psychotherapy, but Hillside had a long tradition of psychoanalysis as the treatment of choice.)[12] In 1979, after looking at several surveys of ECT use, a group of researchers in the Department of Mental Hygiene of New York State concluded that, far from being "a mechanism of social control for the poor, powerless, or racial minorities committed to State mental hospitals[,] . . . ECT is administered largely in non-public facilities to a relatively advantaged population of white, middle-class females whose treatment is covered by private insurance."[13]

ECT declined similarly in Britain. At the Maudsley Hospital in London, its use went from 34 percent of all admissions in 1956 to 21 percent in 1968 to 5 percent in 1987.[14] At Bethlem Hospital (the former "Bedlam," merged administratively with the Maudsley), so many difficulties and restrictions were encountered that the frequency of ECT dropped off severely. As one historian of Bethlem said: "The junior staff did not see the importance of the treatment and often failed to attend sessions. It was admitted that ECT, even if it went well, which was rare, proved nerve-racking."[15] In 1988, when Max Fink asked London neurologist Oliver Sachs, author of *Awakenings,* his opinion of ECT, Sachs said that the treatment was "horrible." "We sat at the same table and when I asked him why ECT had not been considered, he shuddered."[16]

There is no question that in these years people shied away from ECT. Once when psychiatrist and ECT specialist Michael Taylor was on vacation in Montana, two guests began talking to him about their mother, "who was clearly melancholic and had not been responding to medication treatments." He told them: "Well, what you are describing to me is someone who probably needs ECT. I give ECT and she might benefit from it, but she should be seen by somebody who knows." One of the guests looked at him in horror from across the table and said: "You don't do that, do you?"[17]

In a conversation between Boston psychiatrist Elissa Ely and a lawyer representing a patient who had asked the court for permission to have a course of ECT, Ely described the patient, who had stopped speaking, eating, or drinking: "If he were eighty years old, you might have called the lack of light in his face a demented vacancy. But he was forty." The lawyer finished the patient's affidavit and asked Ely: "You want to give him ECT?" "That's right," she replied. "Between you and me," said the lawyer in a tone that implied she was risking a confidence, "wouldn't you rather have a tube in your stomach for the rest of your life than shock therapy?"[18]

For patients, the stigma was awful. Psychologist Martha Manning, who became depressed and received ECT, wrote the following account in her diary in 1991, which was later published as an illness narrative: "Telling people I've had ECT is a real conversation killer. People seem to be more forthright these days about discussing depression. Things have loosened up, even talking about medication. . . . But ECT is in a different class. For months, in my conversations with most people, I have glossed over ECT's contribution to the end of my depression." But recently, she said, she had started telling them about her ECT. "My admission is typically met with uncomfortable silences and abrupt shifts in topics." An acquaintance she met at a party became outraged. "How could you let them do that to you?" Manning bristled: "I didn't let them do it to me. I asked them to do it."[19]

Worse, patients who themselves were in the depths of depression began to shun ECT. At the age of sixty, novelist William Styron became depressed, for the first time in his life. It was full-fledged melancholic depression, beginning as a kind of hypochondriacal foretaste of what was to come, a premonition in which "nothing felt quite right with my corporeal self." Then in a Connecticut farmhouse he finally understood Baudelaire's phrase—"I have felt the wind of the wing of madness." He became riveted with fear at the sight of a flock of Canada geese above the trees. "I stood stranded there, helpless, shivering, aware for the first time that I had been stricken by . . . a serious illness whose name and actuality I was able finally to acknowledge." In the depths of illness he became suicidal: "What I had begun to discover is that, mysteriously and in ways that are totally remote from normal experience, the gray drizzle of horror induced by depression takes on the quality of physical pain." This was true psychotic depression, which responds beautifully to ECT. But did he accept ECT as deliverance from his misery? No. He congratulated himself on *avoiding* ECT. Once he was hospitalized, the staff thought him a suitable candidate for the procedure. Yet Styron mused: "It is plainly a drastic procedure one would want to avoid."[20] He had come within a hair's breadth of destroying himself, yet he shunned the treatment of choice for his depression.

Carmela X, thirty-nine, a resident of Massachusetts, did in fact commit suicide, pushed over the edge at the thought that she was about to undergo ECT. In 1975, she received a diagnosis of cancer and had a mastectomy. She was admitted to the New England Deaconess Hospital, actively suicidal. A staff psychiatrist recommended that she have ECT, which she was to discuss with her husband when he visited later that evening. Yet when the husband came by, she told him the place was a "nuthouse"; he stomped away "disgusted" with her. Later that night, apparently preoccupied with concerns about the ECT treatments that would begin in two days' time, she drowned herself in the bathtub in her room.[21] These were tragedies that arose only because the notion of ECT had bloated into such a terrifying concept. "They're going to fry your brains!"

Hospitals that might, under other circumstances, readily have offered ECT declined to do so because of public sentiment against it. The

New York Times asked Dr. Hong Cho, director of psychiatry at South Nassau Communities Hospital in Oceanside, Long Island, what the results were in ECT. "Excellent," said Dr. Cho, "when we apply this to deeply depressed patients whose onset is middle age or later, who are having a first breakdown." A colleague then added that they could push their response rate in depression to 90 percent, "but we don't because of the public outcry against it." [22]

So fierce was the public turn against ECT in these years that entire sections of the community rejected it; this was true of African Americans in particular. According to a 1980 survey: "Nonwhite [psychiatric] admissions were much less likely to receive ECT than were white admissions, even when the number of admissions of whites and nonwhites was controlled for." In some hospitals in the survey, almost no blacks received ECT. In the sample of 1,221 patients in state hospitals who received ECT in 1980, there was not a single nonwhite. [23] A study of almost eighteen thousand admissions to the adult inpatient psychiatric service of the Johns Hopkins Hospital in Baltimore between 1993 and 2002—a hospital that serves a predominantly African American population—found that 21.9 percent of the white patients with affective disorders received ECT, but only 5.6 percent of the African American patients. For the authors of the study, the reasons for the disparity were a mystery. [24] It is possible that there is a stigma among African Americans about the "depression" diagnosis. [25] Yet these black patients at Hopkins must already have accepted the depression label, or they would not have been in the psychiatric service. In this demographic group, it was ECT and not just the depression label that bore the greatest stigma.

In 1979, the Chicago Medical School, heavily identified with the Jewish community, was seeking affiliation with a university hospital; the department of psychiatry there as well needed a clinical affiliation. Michael ("Mickey") Taylor, then head of psychiatry, said: "Among the affiliations that I arranged was with Jackson Park Hospital, which was in the southeast part of Chicago serving an African American community." A prominent black psychiatrist there was very interested in the affiliation.

> "Everything was going just great," said Taylor. "He and I would periodically meet and talk about the things we wanted to do. I make rounds and I see a lot of depressed people. I see that you don't have an ECT unit—how about setting one up?"

The Jackson Park psychiatrist said: "That's a good idea. When I was trained, we gave ECT treatment. Let me talk to the people on the board of the hospital and see what we can come up with. I will get back to you."

A couple of weeks passed and the Jackson Park psychiatrist came to Taylor's office highly embarrassed. "Mickey, I can't do it. I can't get the ECT unit for you. I just can't do it."

"How come?" Taylor asked.

"The community won't stand for it. They went up in arms, they would just not stand for it."

Taylor said, "Don't they know it's a good treatment?"

"They don't care about that."

"Don't they have all these depressed people?"

"They don't care about that."

Taylor asked: "What was the problem?"

The Jackson Park psychiatrist said: "They don't want Jewish doctors shooting electricity into the brains of black people. It's racism. That's not what I think, but that is what I have to deal with. I can't do it for you."[26]

Interestingly, the black community in Greenville, North Carolina, had the same attitudes when psychiatrist Conrad Swartz, whose specialty was electrotherapy, arrived there in 1992. He made many allies. "We had a couple of black nurses. And they did really help, and we got those black patients on ECT. There was one patient in particular. She was a law student from a major city several hundred miles away, and she had believed she was dead, and she was going to prove to everybody that she was dead. That she would be able to cut off her head with a chainsaw and still be able to continue talking. So she came to see me with a scar on her neck. But after the ECT I gave her, she was just raving about how wonderful it was, and she came hundreds of miles for follow-up. And she was so happy."[27]

Yet the law student was the exception that proved the rule. In a survey conducted in Texas in 1995–1996, the ECT population was overwhelmingly white—accounting for 87 percent of all ECT cases, compared with 3 percent for blacks and 9 percent for Latinos.[28] (According to the 2000 U.S. Census, whites constitute 52 percent of the Texas population; Latinos, 32 percent; and blacks, 11 percent.)[29] In the United States by the 1990s, the massive rejection of ECT among the poor and the marginalized meant that ECT had acquired the same social profile that

psychoanalysis once enjoyed: the typical ECT patient was highly educated, middle-class, and urban.[30] What accounts for this peculiar decline of a safe procedure that was more effective than any other used in
psychiatry? Why did it become reserved for the affluent and the dominant, denied to the poor and those outcast in state asylums? Received
in the 1940s and 1950s in a relatively neutral manner as one therapy
among many, ECT became massively stigmatized in the 1960s. This
discouraged many from seeking treatment and made the therapy itself
widely unavailable whether physicians wished to prescribe it or not.

ECT at the Movies

The problem is that ECT lends itself beautifully to cinematic drama-
tization. There is the gurney, the weird music as the electrotherapist
reaches for the button, the searing electrical storm as the patient's body
writhes from the electric shock, the hollowed features and lifeless eyes
afterward. No movie has ever depicted ECT administered with a muscle relaxant or an anesthetic. Said New York psychiatrist Louis Linn:
"Hollywood has frightened the shit out of everybody about ECT."[31]
From the get-go, Hollywood depicted ECT as a scene of horror. The
first movie to feature electrotherapy was *The Snake Pit*, released early
in 1949, in which Olivia de Havilland gave a luminous performance as
the protagonist of Mary Jane Ward's 1946 novel of that title. Ward had
been a patient at Rockland State Hospital in Orangeburg, New York.
She resented the shock therapy she had received there and made the
staff psychiatrist Gerard Chrzanowski, who had attempted psychotherapy with her, into "Dr. Kik," the novel's caring hero. The movie's depiction of ECT was anything but sympathetic, and a shot of de Havilland,
the face of madness just behind her, on the cover of the December 20
issue of *Time* magazine in 1948, represents the initial media stigmatization of convulsive therapy.[32]

After 1948, ECT appeared sporadically in the movies and always in
the same fashion—with the gurney, the music, and so forth, as though
The Snake Pit had provided the only conceivable template for representing the treatment.[33] In *Shock Treatment*, for example, in 1964, actor Stuart Whitman, faking insanity, endures horrible ECT treatments while
trying to learn where an asylum inmate has hidden a sum of money.
But the film that blew the horrors of ECT right into the face of the great
moviegoing public was *One Flew over the Cuckoo's Nest*, a dramatiza-
tion of Ken Kesey's 1962 novel that director Milos Forman launched in

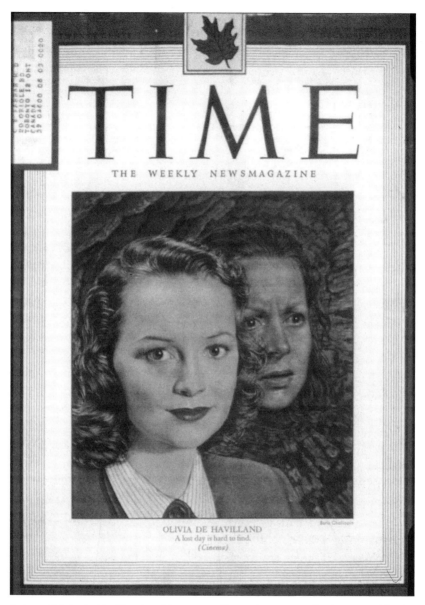

TIME

THE WEEKLY NEWSMAGAZINE

OLIVIA DE HAVILLAND
A lost day is hard to find.
(Cinema)

Actress Olivia de Havilland on *Time* cover, December 20, 1948. She starred in the movie *Snake Pit* (released in 1949), which gave an unsympathetic portrayal of ECT. TIME Magazine © 1948 Time Inc. Reprinted by permission.

1975. It was United Artists's biggest hit up to that time and swept the Academy Awards of that year by winning all five main Oscars. "Randle P. McMurphy," played by Jack Nicholson, had somehow wandered into a mental hospital in an effort to avoid prison and is given ECT as a way of keeping him in line. McMurphy emerges from shock treatment and a lobotomy a virtual zombie. The movie seared public opinion, becoming the popular guide to what happened in convulsive therapy.

Patients and their families began to refuse electrotherapy on the grounds of having seen the film. Jason Pegler, a straight-A student at Manchester University in England, experienced a psychotic break one night when he started thinking he could save the world from impending nuclear war. "At 4 A.M.," he said, "I thought I'd call Snoop Dogg to ask for his help. There was an emergency number on the back of the Doggystyle CD cover." He was hospitalized, then later hospitalized again for mania and offered ECT. As the London *Sunday Times* reported: "Pegler had seen *One Flew over the Cuckoo's Nest* where Jack Nicholson is given the electric-shock treatment; he flatly refused."[34]

Elissa Ely recommended ECT for an elderly male patient who had not been helped by a series of antidepressant medications. She spoke to his daughter, the patient's legal guardian. Ely said the words "electroconvulsive therapy," but the daughter heard "shock treatment." Ely commented that "I think she thought I was condemning him to a gulag." The daughter declared: "Absolutely not. He's an old man. His bones could break. He might have brain damage. He'll lose his memory. It's like that movie."[35] What could one say? A movie, a Hollywood fantasy, had become the public's guide to medical treatment.

Fantasy's dominance of the public discussion reached a pinnacle when medical reporters themselves started taking *One Flew over the Cuckoo's Nest* as an authoritative account of electroconvulsive therapy. In 1999, Josephine Marcotty, a staff writer for the *Star Tribune* in Minneapolis, gave readers an overview of the ghastly history of ECT: "The treatment, a terrifying and painful procedure at the time, was overused and misused. Powerful voltages coursed through the body, sometimes breaking bones or causing burns or even death. As 'One Flew over the Cuckoo's Nest' pointed out so graphically, it was sometimes used to punish and control inmates in mental institutions."[36] Thus, for some journalists, scientific evidence was a waste of time; movie evidence was the most reliable source.

Later, Mickey Taylor reflected about the sources of ECT's stigmatization. An interviewer asked him: "Why did society not see what you saw?" (namely, the benefits of the procedure). Taylor answered: "Because they didn't see ECT as a treatment. They didn't see patients. They saw Hollywood. . . . They saw Jack Nicholson overacting, being dragged into a room, screaming and getting ECT over his objection."[37] There is no doubt that in its fantastical depictions of ECT, the movie industry played a capital role in stigmatizing the procedure, and a terribly irresponsible one from the viewpoint of public health.

The Intellectual Class Turns against ECT

Veteran ECT specialist Richard Weiner at Duke University in North Carolina recalls a visit from the producers of the television show 20/20. "They wanted to talk to a patient about ECT," said Weiner, "someone to talk about memory, so we referred them to some patient who said: 'Yeah, I'll talk to them.' It was a professor. They said: 'Did ECT affect your memory?' And he says: 'Oh yeah, it did. . . . It made my memory better.' [Laughter.] It wasn't really what they wanted to hear."[38]

At some point in the 1960s, the intellectual class decided that ECT was really a very bad idea. Previously silent on the subject of most psychiatric therapies except psychoanalysis, academics, journalists, and literary figures now took up arms against a medical therapy that they suddenly had begun to notice. Why convulsive therapy appeared on the radar of the intelligentsia thirty years after its introduction is a bit of a mystery. But almost certainly this astonished discovery is linked to the general intellectual tumult of the 1960s. The first postwar generation was coming of age and decided to break with much of what they considered the conservative, repressive past. In sexual morality, in attitudes toward pleasure and authority, and in styles of dress the break was quite clear: the hippies were opening a new chapter. ECT, involving as it did the apparent imposition of medical authority and the use of physical energy over reasoning-style therapies, became a particular object of hatred. Then Kesey's 1962 novel, *One Flew over the Cuckoo's Nest*, foregrounded ECT as an issue for public intellectuals, who conflated it with lobotomy. It was a most fateful convergence of zeitgeist and belles lettres.

Of course the equipment and the physical reaction associated with the procedure, especially in the film version, made ECT vulnerable to caricature. A new cultural sensitivity found these elements—electrodes, mouth guards, thrashing limbs, straps, and strongholding assistants—unpleasant at best, and horrific, brutal, and sadistic in the worst characterization. These same critics clearly had never witnessed a forceps delivery or a hip amputation, for these procedures as well would have been outlawed, as ECT virtually was, in the state of California. But they had read the book and seen the film: Kesey's portrayal became the primary source of information on ECT for most of the liberal intelligentsia. In their view, ECT must be evil because the image of flailing bodies and thrashing limbs was so awful. It mattered little that the era of flailing bodies had ended in the mid-1950s with the universal acceptance of anesthesia and muscle relaxation in standard ECT. A great campaign thus began against ECT in antipsychiatry circles, on university campuses, and in the newsrooms of the quality press. It succeeded in driving a valuable medical procedure almost out of existence. What transpires in elite intellectual circles is often a matter of no great public import. Yet a transmission line runs from the senior common rooms or "salons" through the newsrooms of the quality press directly into the nation's most literate and influential living rooms. This pathway was crucial in stigmatizing ECT as the work of the devil.

The intellectual class received a warning signal about ECT in 1961, with the death of novelist Ernest Hemingway. In the summer of 1960, Hemingway was in the grips of a psychotic depression and was reluctant to leave his New York apartment because, as he told his wife, Mary: "They're tailing me out here already. . . . Somebody waiting out there." He also had made several suicide threats. On November 30, 1960, he entered the Mayo Clinic in Rochester, Minnesota, and was treated at the psychiatric unit of St. Mary's Hospital, which is part of the clinic. In December 1960, he received a course of convulsive therapy. What other treatment he might have had is unknown. But the ECT did not work for Hemingway; his delusions persisted. Yet on January 22, 1961, he was discharged from the clinic, possibly on a course of antipsychotic medication (his biographer A. E. Hotchner reports that his "writing became severely cramped, the letters so small and tight it was difficult to read the words"—an evident sign of the Parkinsonian side effects of the phenothiazine-class of antipsychotic drugs, such as chlorpromazine).[39]

On April 25, he reentered the clinic and again had a course of electrotherapy. It is inconceivable that he was not also prescribed medication, to which he evidently was not responding or simply refusing. He was discharged June 26, drove back to his home in Ketchum, Idaho, and shot himself two days later. In addition to being a great personal tragedy and loss of an international literary figure, Hemingway's death became almost immediately associated with the ECT treatment he had received, a treatment that the intellectual class began to think of as "murderous." *Time* magazine exposed the story of his depression and his shock treatment at the Mayo Clinic in its obituary on July 14, 1961; the piece debunked his wife's claim that the death was accidental.[40] Hotchner's memoir, published in 1966, further revealed the story of Hemingway's debilitating depression and suicidal death, searing these details into the public's consciousness.

One must bear in mind, however, that Hemingway was a chronic alcoholic; alcoholics have a high seizure threshold and often are unresponsive to ECT. He would have had a barbiturate anesthetic, increasing the likelihood of an inadequate seizure. It is unclear that ECT played a role in his death, except perhaps, by exacerbating his despondency as a result of the memory loss he might have suffered (which would in all likelihood have shortly cleared). One of Hemingway's biographers, in an account hostile to ECT, theorizes: "He realized his memory had been virtually destroyed."[41] This is improbable, and it is more likely that his depression made him think his memory was shaky. The argument that Hemingway was killed by ECT is simply untenable.

Another famous suicide, that of novelist and poet Sylvia Plath in 1963 at age thirty-one, also crystallized an image of ECT for the many who had read her work. Plath received ECT in the early 1950s at McLean Hospital outside of Boston, but her suicide occurred the week after starting a course of an antidepressant, phenelzine.[42] The fact of her suicide became known only later, following the publication in 1971 of the American edition of her semifictionalized autobiography, *The Bell Jar;* an English edition under a pen name had appeared in 1963. The novel contains what are evidently autobiographical ECT scenes in which she remains semiconscious as the machine shrills: "Whee-ee-ee-ee—ee, through an air crackling with blue light, and with each flash a great jolt drubbed me till I thought my bones would break and the sap fly out of me like a split plant [in the early 1950s, the treatment would have been unmodified, that is, without the benefit of anesthesia and muscle relaxants]. . . . I wondered what terrible thing it was I had done," she wrote.[43] The depiction of ECT in *The Bell Jar* had the effect of scaring the wits out of anyone who read it. What was underappreciated was the poetic license of this loosely biographical work, nor was it generally understood that the technique of ECT had changed.

Plath, Hemingway, Kesey—the intellectual class began to openly criticize electrotherapy. In an admiring review in the *New York Times* in 1964 of Thomas Szasz's book *Law, Liberty, and Psychiatry,* Edward de

Grazia, a Washington, D.C., lawyer and literary figure, scorned "treatments" (the ironical quotation marks were his) such as "electric shock, lobotomy and indeterminate [prison] sentences" as "barbaric old vindictive criminal punishment."[44] This was a new tone. Intellectuals were not hurling these kinds of thunderbolts in the 1950s.

In 1968, the novelist and songwriter Millen Brand, who had cowritten the screenplay of *The Snake Pit* in 1948, brought out *Savage Sleep*, a novel about psychiatric misadventures that prominently highlighted ECT: "The nurse smeared salve on her temples. . . . She looked aside as Dr. Wellman grasped the electrodes. The electrodes closed their goring clamp on her temples, a switch was snapped, and she moaned or the outrush of her breath sounded of itself. Her eyeballs turned back. As her convulsions began, her body rose in the middle and jerked."[45] *Savage Sleep* was a bestseller. Book reviewer Thomas Lask said: "Those who know of others, especially close ones, who have undergone shock treatment will certainly want to read this book—if only for a starter."[46] Indeed. Who would want such a therapy? Who could even contemplate it for a loved one?

The assault on ECT accelerated in the 1970s. Doris Lessing savaged the treatment in her 1971 novel *Briefing for a Descent into Hell*, and Joan Didion, in a *New York Times* review of the novel, obligingly noted that ECT had "obliterated" the protagonist's memory.[47] These were two of the biggest names in literature, and ECT was suddenly in their target. The following year, the psychologist and feminist Phyllis Chesler, in *Women and Madness*, made ECT sound like some kind of male plot against women. The book was well received among the burgeoning feminist movement. Reviewer and poet Adrienne Rich said that a woman who accepts the "help" of ECT becomes "more than ever bound to the patriarchal script which has compounded her difficulties."[48] Other personal revelations began to pour forth. Actress Gene Tierney, who had been nominated for an Academy Award in 1945 for *Leave Her to Heaven*, had been in and out of mental hospitals over the years. She told the story in her 1979 *Self-Portrait*, detailing the "barbaric" nature of her electroconvulsive therapy. Those who missed the book caught up on the atrocity in a major review by Seymour Peck, the cultural editor of the *New York Times*.[49]

Journalists themselves began to cover ECT in a negative way. The media spin on electrotherapy before 1970 had been largely approving, the few critical stories mainly reporting Manfred Sakel's attacks on ECT because it rivaled his own insulin therapy.[50] But in the 1970s, the same hostile wind began to blow through the newsrooms that had touched other venues of discourse. In 1970, a piece in the *New York Times* dwelt on "the many side effects of electroshock treatment," singling out memory loss.[51] Journalist Elizabeth Wertz, who herself had had ECT in the 1950s, chose 1972 to come out against it in a harrowing account of victimization in the *Washington Post*.[52] She had interviewed Washington psychiatrist Zigmond Lebensohn, who in an astonished, subsequent letter to the *Post* said that in no psychiatric hospital in the country was ECT administered as she described it.[53] The litany of horror intensified. In the *New Yorker* in 1974, veteran medical journalist Berton Roueché featured ECT victim "Natalie Parker," later identified as antipsychiatry activist Marilyn Rice, who claimed to have had all her memories blotted out by the procedure.[54] She later became a staunch supporter of the anti-ECT movement (see chapter 9).

Then came the Eagleton story. In 1972, the Democratic ticket lost its vice presidential nominee amid circumstances that would focus media attention on ECT as bizarre and radical. George McGovern's running mate was a senator from Missouri named Thomas Eagleton. Eagleton had been reticent with McGovern about having had several previous occurrences of depression between 1960 and 1966. He was treated during two of these episodes with ECT, once at Barnes Hospital in St. Louis; a second time at the Mayo Clinic.[55] He would fly home from Washington on a Thursday evening for treatment at Barnes on Friday and Sunday, then return to D.C. by Monday for congressional sessions. When the story broke, the public outcry was such that Eagleton had to step down from the ticket. The press clucked about ECT as something really beyond the pale: if you had been treated with ECT, you were manifestly unfit for national office. When Eagleton was asked why he had not disclosed the episodes earlier, he replied: "Electroshock is simply something you don't go around talking about at cocktail parties."[56]

In 1977, the *New York Times*'s editorial page called for federal controls over ECT. It asked why millions of "vulnerable" Americans could "not be systematically protected against electrodes or cockroaches or rape?" The nation's newspaper of record asserted that ECT was a menace comparable to cockroaches and rape; there one had it.[57] Then on May 26, 1977, ABC aired its special, *Madness and Medicine,* narrated by Howard K. Smith. Strongly slanted against the somatic therapies, the program included interviews with such antipsychiatry activists as Peter Breggin and David Richman, author of *Dr. Caligari's Psychiatric Drugs.* Richman, for example, offered a view of ECT as "absolutely barbaric and a gross misuse of electricity to say nothing of the poor people whose brains get fried. . . . Yes, you can electrically shock someone out of their so-called crazy mind but you don't shock them back into their right mind, you shock them into a shock mind." For balance, the program did offer Oregon psychiatrist Paul Blachly, an important ECT innovator, who insisted that the procedure was quite safe and effective. Yet Smith's narrative and the bulk of the footage was stridently antipsychiatric. Of the patients interviewed, none had been helped by ECT, and all claimed to have lost their memories.

The American Psychiatric Association was so upset at the program's lack of balance that it threatened ABC with a lawsuit.[58] In gathering material for the legal battle, the APA discovered that the program's producer, Phil Lewis, had envisioned a slanted account from the beginning. In an affidavit, Dwayne DeLong, a peace officer of the Napa State Hospital in Imola, California, where Lewis had filmed, said that he had heard Lewis "indicate that he was interested in presenting an exposé on psychiatry. Other comments made by Mr. Lewis in my presence clearly conveyed the impression that he intended to portray psychiatry in a negative light."[59] Indeed, at Napa the ABC crew had demonstrated an interest only in the sickest of the patients, and their footage showed nothing positive about the hospital.

When the ABC crew visited the clinical psychopharmacology unit of the Massachusetts General Hospital, Lewis let it be known that "he'd like to put psychiatry out of business." The hospital refused permission for the shoot.[60] At the office of New York psychiatrist Leonard Cammer, the ABC crew had the opportunity to show that ECT could in fact make patients better. As Cammer subsequently wrote to Lewis: "You witnessed several dramatic, unrehearsed events in my office—a severely agitated attorney whose wife was much concerned that he might kill himself in order to obtain relief. You witnessed the improvement in his state of mind after treatment; you saw how mild the treatment is and that there was neither confusion nor horror." Yet Lewis refused to put any of this material on the air, because, as Cammer believed, doing so would be "'inconsistent' with the purpose of your film." Cammer concluded his letter with a statement that serves as a collective sigh from the discipline of psychiatry about the highly politicized media of the 1970s: "For a change I would like to see a documentary made that does not start off with an antipsychiatry, antibiologic, anti-ECT posture. My experience to date is that such a statement is unlikely in the present climate."[61]

Looking back a number of years later on the stigmatization of ECT in the 1970s, Richard Weiner remarked tongue-in-cheek: "With all the bad press ECT has received, as well as . . . the unholy trinity of electricity, convulsion, and memory loss, it may be to some a wonder why ECT continues to be tolerated at all." His conclusion was that the public was probably somewhat wiser than the media: "That experiences of the 'silent majority' of ECT patients, who feel helped rather than hurt by ECT, are acting to quietly encourage a more liberal attitude toward ECT." [62] In fact, as we see later on, he was right.

Psychiatry Abandons ECT

It was the mid-1960s. Anthony D'Agostino had just graduated in medicine at the University of Illinois in Chicago; he went away for a year to intern, and when he came back he found that "a radical change" had occurred in his father's mind. [63] "His appearance had changed dramatically. He was 52 but looked over 70; he had lost over 20 pounds and was anxious and agitated." Even though D'Agostino was just a first-year resident in psychiatry, he diagnosed a depressive illness in his father and sought help. At the first hospital they turned to, the father was diagnosed with "chronic brain syndrome" (it is unclear what the doctors had in mind) and discharged when he refused psychotherapy. The father had now "stabilized somewhere around absolute zero," so the son contacted a second hospital, the one where he himself worked. Overcoming his personal feelings of shame—in those days many psychiatrists considered illness the result of faulty family dynamics— Anthony D'Agostino had his father admitted. The father did not do badly on medication, but the mother had him removed because she did not like the attending physician's unresponsiveness to her own questions. At yet a third hospital, this one an institution guided by theories of the community health movement, the clinicians recommended "day hospital" rather than admission. Anthony groaned to himself and continued the search.

"Finally, my mother took matters into her own hands. Living in a small, lower-middle-class suburb, she took Father to see a psychiatrist practicing in the town. He saw Father for a few minutes and recommended hospitalization and electroconvulsive therapy," which Anthony's father received at a fourth hospital—one considered to be "of marginal repute." Six weeks later Anthony's father was working again. At Anthony D'Agostino's own hospital, the second one that his father visited seeking help from acute depression, he was the only resident who had treated a patient with ECT. "And the treatments had to be stopped after three sessions because the patient was a black man and the staff wondered whether I wasn't simply torturing an already sufficiently oppressed citizen."

By the late 1960s, ECT was replaced by psychoanalysis, community psychiatry, and a nascent practice of psychopharmacology. Many psychiatrists had never really trained in ECT. As one older clinician put it in 1959: "It is almost impossible for younger psychiatrists to imagine the impact which the advent of shock treatments made on the morale and on the outlook of the working psychiatrist." He said that the psychiatrist had once been "a contemplative individual who liked to sit in an armchair discussing philosophy or listening to a patient talking. When the advent of electric shock forced him, if he was conscientious, to become a physiologist, an anaesthetist, a physicist and an internist, his reaction was something similar to what would have happened if cardiologists had been told that as their patients' troubles were 90 per cent psychological in origin they must all become psychoanalysts."[64] So it is not as though the entire profession waved ruefully goodbye to ECT as societal stigma swept it away. Many were glad to see it go.

And evaporate from training programs it did. ECT virtually disappeared from university psychiatric residencies in the years from 1960 to 1980, and few psychiatrists trained in that period are familiar with it.[65] As Max Fink pointed out in an interview in 1993, in the changes sweeping psychiatric training: "ECT was largely left out of psychiatry and was hardly taught in this country. We can't find any good endorsements in textbooks from about 1955 to the late 1970s. Most medical schools and psychiatric residency training centers ignored ECT completely."[66]

In the 1960s, the psychoanalysts, having yet no idea of the pharmacological express train bearing down at them, believed that they had won. Zigmond Lebensohn, an ECT-friendly psychiatrist in Washington, D.C., said that analysts' attitudes toward ECT went "from overt antagonism to smug condescension." "The psychiatrist who still administered ECT was often viewed with the same gaze that gynecologists used to reserve for their colleagues who performed abortions in the days before legalization."[67]

But it was not merely the traditional analysts who were skeptical. The newly fashioned biological psychiatrists were equally dubious about the advantages of ECT (see chapter 8). At a meeting of the American College of Neuropsychopharmacology (ACNP) in 1985, Robert Friedel, a veteran ECT specialist from the University of Alabama, stood up to give a paper. Friedel reported that, of his nine schizophrenic patients who had failed to respond to antipsychotic medication, eight had responded to ECT.[68] Friedel then sat down. Seymour Kety, the dean of American neurophysiology, sitting next to Max Fink, leaned toward him and said: "Impossible to be true." Somebody else raised his hand and said: "What did you actually do?"[69] Younger psychiatrists had no knowledge or experience with ECT; it was as if penicillin had somehow vanished from the medical armamentarium and a generation's memory of its very existence had been somehow erased.

In the entire decade of the 1970s at the National Institute of Mental Health (NIMH)—the nation's premier research center in psychiatry—only nine patients were treated with ECT, all by an outside consultant, psychiatrist John Nardini, who would arrive with a portable apparatus. Each of the nine had serious depression. Steve Paul, at the Clinical Psychobiology Branch of NIMH, reported with wonderment that eight of them recovered and stayed well for at least a year following the treatments. None complained of memory loss. Paul concluded: "It is likely that the high morbidity and mortality associated with affective illness could be reduced by early treatment with ECT in selected patients rather than by turning to it as a last resort."[70]

In 1981, Matt Rudorfer came to NIMH and began doing ECT on a regular basis, simply because he had learned it as a resident at Washington University of St. Louis. When he arrived, he discovered they had a machine just "gathering dust" that had never been used. Rudorfer was selected to resume electrotherapy there, after the practice had lapsed when Nardini was forced to retire because of illness. Rudorfer's first patients were those who had failed to respond to multiple medications, because, as he said in an interview: "I was the only one in the neighborhood who knew anything about ECT." NIMH undertook a multitreatment study with ECT as one of the arms, comparing it with various drugs. A paper detailing the findings was submitted to the *Archives of General Psychiatry.* But after editor Danny Friedman's death in 1993, it was never published. Rudorfer conducted ECT for NIMH until about 1990, when he went to the "extramural" side (administering outside grants). After Rudorfer, no one took up ECT at NIMH.[71]

In this manner, ECT faded away at many institutions. It was lost at Bellevue Hospital in New York in 1962 when the head of the anesthesiology department decreed that henceforth the sodium amytal anesthesia must be administered in an operating room near the anesthesiology service, which was three blocks away from the psychiatry department. So the patient would have to be strapped to a gurney and wheeled to an operating room, accompanied by the psychiatrist and a nurse who would perform the treatment, wait in the recovery room until the patient had regained consciousness, and then trundle back to the psychiatry department. Sometimes they would arrive to find the operating room occupied with an emergency case and have to return to the ward needing to reschedule. The entire business became so burdensome that the ECT program was cancelled.[72] Another example: when Alfred Stanton, a big believer in psychotherapy and in the hospital as a therapeutic milieu, arrived at McLean Hospital in Belmont, Massachusetts, in 1955, he permitted the ECT service to dwindle to virtually nothing: two or three patients a year. ECT had arrived at McLean during World War II and had achieved some stunning successes; then it was gone.[73]

Starting in the 1970s, mental hospitals all across the United States began to close as deinstitutionalization, the great discharge of psychiatric patients from inpatient care to "the community," gained traction. These were often the only source of ECT for an area, unless patients could afford one of the private clinics. Most of the community mental health clinics that Congress had mandated in the Community Mental Health Centers Act of 1963 did not offer ECT. So the closing of a mental hospital meant the end of access to convulsive therapy for the people of that area. Harvard psychiatrist Mandel Cohen recalled of the Boston area: "There was a time when, if I had a patient with depression and she needed to be in a hospital, I would send her to a State hospital where she could get electrotherapy. But now, since these hospitals have closed, there is no place to send them." Cohen blamed "an intense crusade among the psychoanalysts and in the State [mental health] department not to use ECT. . . . Then they formed these clinics and Mental Health Centers run by psychoanalysts, where there were also social workers and others who were all opposed to hospitalization and electrotherapy. The problem was that the patient couldn't get treatment; there were too many people who were opposed to this."[74]

It was mainly from the commanding heights of psychiatry in the 1970s that ECT was dying out; it was vanishing in the academic departments caught up with psychopharmacology and psychoanalysis. Down in the trenches, among the community psychiatrists, ECT retained even in these years a considerable following. In a nationwide poll of psychiatrists that the American Psychiatric Association commissioned in 1977, fully 61 percent of the 2,973 respondents replied that they were "generally" or "decidedly" favorable to its use. Seventy-two percent agreed with the statement that it was the "most effective form of treatment" for many patients. And the great majority felt that psychiatric hospitals should offer it (even though it was rapidly disappearing from many hospitals). One in six had personally treated a patient with ECT in the previous six months, and 11 percent had referred patients for convulsive treatment.[75] The statistics show that a good many doctors retained a considerable fondness for convulsive therapy—regardless of what the discipline's leaders thought—because these practitioners needed urgently to make their patients better again. And they knew how useful ECT could be.

CHAPTER EIGHT

The End of "Bedlam" and the Age of Psychopharmacology

Stigma alone would not have sufficed to marginalize electroconvulsive therapy. Physicians have a kind of gut-wrenching responsibility for patients with serious illnesses and, generally speaking, do not lightly discard a useful therapy. For years, shock had been virtually the only effective treatment of depression and psychosis. Clinicians would not have let the cinematic image of Jack Nicholson as "McMurphy" deter them from prescribing a remedy of benefit to their patients. But they could easily discard a treatment if an apparently superior one came along. This is essentially what happened within medicine to ECT: it was put aside in favor of pharmacological treatment. Only later would psychiatrists realize they had abandoned shock therapy for drugs that were not, in fact, better for treating many forms of mental illness.

In 1954, two drugs were introduced that changed fundamentally the treatment of psychiatric illness, transforming the field from one based on psychoanalysis and shock to one based on pills and injections. Chlorpromazine, the first of the phenothiazine antipsychotics, was licensed in the United States by the Food and Drug Administration (FDA) in March 1954.[1] And a month later, in April, psychiatrist Nathan Kline, research director at Mary Jane Ward's "snake pit" asylum, Rockland State in Orangeburg, New York, proposed a botanical compound called reserpine—derived from the plant *Rauwolfia serpentina*—for the treatment of psychotic illness.[2]

In a conference that Kline organized in December 1954, Winfred Overholser, the superintendent of St. Elizabeths Hospital in Washington, D.C., called the two drugs "harbingers of a new era." Previous psychiatric drugs were unsatisfactory, he said, because "they quieted the patient at the expense of clouding his consciousness or even rendering him unconscious." But chlorpromazine and reserpine "have the unusual quality of sedating the patient, reducing his overactivity, and allaying his anxiety," while at the same time he remains conscious and accessible to psychotherapy.[3] (This was an era when everyone believed that the ultimate restorative in psychiatry was psychotherapy.) These were, and remain today, remarkable achievements: a treatment that diminished anxiety, restored sleep, and calmed psychotic excitement, while making it possible for a patient to work, have amicable social relations, and lead a normal life.

The Antipsychotics and ECT

Reserpine was discarded relatively early from psychiatric practice because of its side effects. Yet chlorpromazine went on to become the cornerstone of the new biological psychiatry that in the mid-1950s was just starting to profile itself. Conventionally, the antipsychotics are seen as distinct from the antidepressants, even though they greatly overlap. In our discussion as well, we separate the antipsychotics and the antidepressants in tracing their impact on shock therapy. But at the same time we ask the reader's pardon, because many observers think that the distinction between the two drug classes is a false one—more a commercial marketing device, actually—just as the distinction between serious depression and psychosis is also discussable. Yet together, the two new drug classes pulled the rug from under ECT.

The effectiveness of chlorpromazine was recognized in Paris in 1952. The Rhône-Poulenc drug company, building on its success with the new antihistamines, came up with a compound that had a "central" effect, that is, on the brain and the mind. In 1952, three psychiatrists at the Val-de-Grâce military hospital in Paris discovered the effectiveness of the new drug in a patient with mania. Then a professor of psychiatry, ECT specialist Jean Delay, together with his assistant Pierre Deniker, tried chlorpromazine in a series of psychiatric patients and in June 1952, reported their findings.[4] In the space of three months, chlorpromazine had transformed life at the Ste. Anne mental hospital, where Delay held a chair. As Delay and Deniker commented afterward: "The most remarkable effect is, without doubt, the change which has taken place in the entire atmosphere of these hospital wards. In a few hours, in a few days at the most, the patients are calmed without being somnolent."[5]

At Ste. Anne's, the windows facing the street were opened in the spring and summer, and the clamor of patients would normally be audible along the rue d'Alésia in the fourteenth arrondissement. After June 1952, the local merchants began pulling aside Jean Thuillier, one of Delay's assistants, and asking him with wonder: "Doctor, what are you doing with the patients up there? We don't hear them anymore." "I'm not killing them," Thuillier would reply. He recalled a patient who had a hallucinatory psychosis. "She was tormented by voices saying to her she was a bad woman. She was one of the first people I gave chlorpromazine to and there was quite a change. She said that now she was well and she needed to go home and go to work."[6]

In 1953, Paul Brouillot worked as a pharmacist in Lyon for Spécia, a branch of Rhône-Poulenc that developed pharmaceuticals. He went to the Vinatier Hospital in search of evidence of side effects related to chlorpromazine. "Side effects?" said a staff psychiatrist. "We haven't had any of those." (This was decidedly premature.) Instead, the psychiatrist took Brouillot around the wards. Brouillot remembered a psychotic patient who had been hospitalized for five or six years. "He was a farmer, who now following treatment was quite well and wanted to go home to see his wife and to the farm. This was almost a resurrection. Someone who all of a sudden wakes up and says, 'What am I doing here?'"[7]

In 1955, Delay and his assistants presented data at a conference on chlorpromazine on the drug's superiority to ECT in treating mania. The average duration of hospitalization for mania before the introduction of ECT was 122 days; with ECT, 95 days; with chlorpromazine, 59 days.[8] Hearing these results, two psychiatrists from Bordeaux, students of ECT specialist Paul Delmas-Marsalet, asked themselves: "Is insulin dead?" They answered the question, essentially, "Yes, thank God!"[9]

Delay's explanation of how chlorpromazine therapy—which he called "neurolepsis"—differed from shock therapy is interesting. Shock, he thought, mobilized the central nervous system; it provoked "an alarm reaction." "By contrast, in neurolepsis a general mobilization of defenses is not sought, but rather a sort of demobilization, not an alarm reaction of the nervous system but a reaction of détente" is desired, producing a central-nervous "truce."[10] The mechanism of neither chlorpromazine nor ECT is understood even today—putting aside all the musing about "monoamine theories"—and Delay's ideas stand as an effort to achieve a great somatic synthesis about the central nervous system in the days before ECT receded from clinical use.

The first use of chlorpromazine in Switzerland was in 1953. Raymond Battegay, then on staff at the Basel University Psychiatric Clinic, recalled a schizophrenic woman who thought she was a military colonel. After four weeks of treatment with chlorpromazine, she said: "You do not have to call me colonel any longer. I know that I was sick."[11] Samples of chlorpromazine were distributed to psychiatric clinics in England during the winter of 1952–53 by W. R. Thrower, the medical director of May and Baker, a company affiliated with Rhône-Poulenc. When he came to Joel Elkes's newly created Department of Experimental Psychiatry at the University of Birmingham, he got Joel and his psychiatrist wife Charmian to agree to run a double-blind, randomly controlled clinical trial of chlorpromazine against a placebo, one of the first such trials in psychiatry; it was actually Charmian Elkes who led it.[12] The German émigré psychiatrist Willi Mayer-Gross, who had organized the ECT service at the Scottish asylum in Dumfries, joined them for the study. At the international conference that took place in Paris in 1955, Mayer-Gross reported in general on the logic of a controlled trial, the beginning of systematic evaluation in psychiatry of treatment effects.[13] In disentangling the question of which was better, chlorpromazine or ECT, this kind of trial should have been the gold standard. Yet few were ever done.

The first samples of chlorpromazine came to the United States directly from Germany in 1953. Paul Hoch and Sidney Malitz at the New York State Psychiatric Institute apparently gave the drug to the wrong patients, and without significant results they lost interest in it. But others soon began administering the drug, distributed in the States by Smith Kline & French under the trade name Thorazine. Sometime in 1953, Henry Brill, the commissioner of the New York State mental hospital system, called a meeting of state psychiatrists at Creedmoor Hospital. Max Fink, representing Hillside, attended: "In presentation after presentation during a long and exciting day, doctors from the state services described the remarkable effects of chlorpromazine in relieving excitement, aggressivity and psychosis. . . . The descriptions were so congruent that each of us in the audience avidly sought samples from the representative of Smith, Kline & French."[14]

N. William Winkelman, who had a private and a hospital practice in Philadelphia, published the first U.S. trial in 1954, a mixture of inpatients and outpatients. He found that chlorpromazine could reduce anxiety, diminish phobias and obsessions, abolish psychosis, quiet mania, and "change the hostile, agitated, senile patient into a quiet, easily managed patient."[15] That same year, Heinz Lehmann in Montreal published the first North American trial involving large numbers of hospital patients. Lehmann compared chlorpromazine favorably to ECT (which he detested): "Many of us have in recent years lost sight of our essential task of understanding our patients, as we subject them to a sequence of comas, shocks, convulsions, confusion, and amnesia, all of which render them incapable of relating to the psychiatrist in a consistent and meaningful manner." By contrast, he called chlorpromazine "the most reliable psychiatric agent in the control of symptoms of psychomotor excitement. . . . Unpleasant side-effects with chlorpromazine are of minor significance. . . . Perhaps the greatest advantage of this drug lies in its power to quiet severely excited patients without rendering them confused or otherwise inaccessible."[16]

Thus chlorpromazine, and with it psychopharmacology, began its ascent to dominance in American psychiatry. While academic centers were still firmly wed to Freudianism, state hospitals and private nervous clinics quickly embraced the new medicines. In U.S. asylums in those years, there were about three hundred thousand patients with severe psychiatric illness (all of whom were labeled "schizophrenics"), filling half of the nation's mental hospital beds. A drug that had the ability to release them, in part at least, from the grip of illness and let them return to the community would have a stunning impact on public health. The medical testimonials to chlorpromazine have the quality of a religious revival. In the mid-1950s, Donald Klein was at a Public Health Service hospital in Lexington, Kentucky, in charge of a ward for veterans of World War I. "These people had been psychotic for 30 years. They were out of it completely. We gave some of them chlorpromazine and I remember a guy who hadn't said anything for 30 years comes over to me after a few weeks and said, 'Doc, when am I getting out of here?' It was Rip van Winkle. He had remembered nothing. The last thing he remembered was in 1916 going over the trenches. That was an honest to God miracle."[17]

At the Yankton State Hospital in South Dakota, the "back wards" now had television sets, "as well as potted plants, glassware, and many other items we would never have dared put within reach of these patients before. And practically nothing has ever been slightly damaged. We have gotten all of our patients out of seclusion cells and wearing clothing and our attendants are no longer complaining of torn shirts and bruises inflicted by combative patients. We just don't have combative patients anymore."[18]

For Leo Hollister at the Veterans Administration hospital in Palo Alto, California (where Ken Kesey had been an orderly), controlled studies to prove effectiveness were unnecessary. "All you had to do was look at your patients and improvement was obvious. People who were mute began talking. People who were attacking ward personnel were no longer hitting people." Hollister asked one of his colleagues: "Would you like to have some more of your patients treated with chlorpromazine?" The colleague replied: "Leo, I have so many patients talking to me now who never talked to me before that it's all I can handle to keep up with them." [19]

Scores of patients with schizophrenic illness were brought back to life with a pill, pushing electrotherapy to the margins. In 1957 at Hillside Hospital, Max Fink and his colleagues did a randomly controlled trial of chlorpromazine versus insulin. [20] In terms of effectiveness the two treatments were equivalent, but chlopromazine was so much safer and easier to administer that within six months the Hillside insulin unit was closed. ECT services also closed down. Fritz Freyhan, a German émigré psychiatrist who in the 1950s was clinical director at the Delaware State Hospital in Wilmington, cast aside ECT as soon as the new drugs came in. Freyhan spoke of the end of "bedlamism." [21] Frank Ayd in Baltimore, once an ECT specialist of some repute, turned his back on the procedure completely when he testified to Congress in 1968, saying in a hymn of praise for psychopharmaceuticals, that ECT "offered little or no improvement" for sick patients. [22]

Even in institutions where ECT was not abandoned for treating schizophrenia, it was almost never used exclusively, as a method of choice. Rather, it was applied either simultaneously or consecutively with drugs, to augment their effect. In a rather audacious review that Philip May of the Neuropsychiatric Institute at UCLA wrote in 1967 for the annual meeting of the American College of Neuropsychopharmacology, he suggested that all positive reports in which ECT showed better results than drugs must "be viewed with suspicion." Yet he allowed that if electrotherapy must be administered, "it is generally more prudent to give ECT and drugs consecutively rather than concurrently." [23]

The 1950s and 1960s were a golden age of drug discovery. By 1969, there were at least nineteen important drugs for schizophrenia on the American market, including haloperidol, perphenazine, and thioridazine. [24] Congresses, conferences, symposia, and trade fairs occurred with dizzying frequency, their proceedings rushing into the medical mailboxes of the nation. Within psychiatry, a subculture of psychopharmacology formed in which all treatments except pharmacotherapy were excluded from the clinicians' visual field. It is not that the psychopharmacologists weighed ECT against drug treatment in every patient they saw, wondering which would be better. They simply forgot about ECT. It ceased to exist as a therapeutic option in this subculture.

For Seymour Kety, one of the most active and influential scientists in American biological psychiatry in the 1960s and 1970s, with posts at NIMH, Johns Hopkins, and Harvard, ECT was completely off the radar. Max Fink recalled: "He considered ECT too messy an intervention and none of his students ever had anything to do with it. When he dominated U.S. psychiatric research—and he did for two or more decades and he is considered the father of the neurohumoral [neurotransmitter] basis for mental illness—ECT was easily rejected."[25]

Psychopharmacology also ushered in a period of new thinking about the basic mechanisms of psychiatric illness. Knowing the chemistry of a particular drug, coupled to a clinical picture of a drug's effect, led to speculation about the brain's own chemical systems in causing disease. It quickly became a matter of faith that the key to mental illness lay in the neurotransmitters and their receptor molecules. A malfunction in dopamine metabolism led to schizophrenia, and when dopamine-receptor blockers like Thorazine and Haldol were given, a patient would be on the path to recovery. For depression and anxiety, a defect in the brain's serotonin levels could be cured by Prozac-style drugs, the SSRIs (selective serotonin reuptake inhibitors). (Psychopharmacology has since become more sophisticated about mechanisms, identifying cellular "second messengers," receptor subclasses, and other neurochemical signaling activities both within and between neurons.)

Many ECT specialists were skeptical about these neurohumoral explanations, and a scientific wedge regarding the underlying mechanisms of illness separated members of the ECT community from the psychopharmacologists. ECT obviously was a very powerful treatment, but some felt that neurotransmitter explanations alone were not enough to account for its action. Max Fink deplored the lack of interest of the psychopharmacologists in ECT and said: "Unfortunately, our leaders are prisoners of the belief that the brain neurohumors are the site of mental illnesses and their relief."[26] Fink and Jan-Otto Ottosson felt that some kind of hormonal ("peptide") discharge from the hypothalamus and the pituitary gland might be the key to the action of ECT.[27] In other words, conventional psychopharmacology might be pointing away from the mechanism of ECT's effect.

In their conception of how things worked inside the brain, it was as though ECT specialists and psychopharmacologists were speaking different dialects. But in contrast to the psychoanalysts—who spoke a different language entirely—researchers in ECT and psychopharm both spoke the language of basic science and agreed that the route to relieving illness passed through the valley of research. "The purpose of chemistry," said Paracelsus, the pseudonym of a sixteenth-century Swiss physician who stood at the boundary between alchemy and pharmacology, "is not to produce gold, but to study the basic sciences and use them against disease." Within this subculture of psychopharmacology, as Spanish psychiatrist Félix Martí-Ibáñez and his colleagues put it in 1956, chlorpromazine was seen as "a crystallization of Paracelsus' dream." [28] In truth, "[You felt like] the medieval priest who could drive out delusions," said Hartford psychiatrist Benjamin Wiesel about the 1950s. "When you could influence delusional thinking in schizophrenics with this new drug, you could treat them in a general hospital. . . . It was a whole new game." [29]

The Antidepressants and ECT

The antipsychotics pushed out ECT for the treatment of schizophrenic illness, but the story with antidepressants was different. ECT was demonstrably so effective for depression that it was never completely bested by pharmacotherapy. In a review of the literature, Per Bech at Frederiksborg General Hospital in Hillerod, Denmark, looked at how much various treatments reduced the symptom count on the Hamilton Depression Scale (HDS), the standard instrument for measuring depression. He found that, at four weeks, placebo treatment reduced the HDS only ten points; the tricyclic antidepressants, sixteen points; and ECT, twenty points. [30] The question for clinicians therefore was, do the side effects of ECT outweigh its benefits, given the availability of pharmacotherapy for depression? And increasingly the answer was yes.

The concept "antidepressant" dates from the amphetamines of the 1940s, when doctors wrote thousands of prescriptions for stimulants to treat depressive illness. Amphetamine is highly addictive and is rarely prescribed today, yet it is effective for treating mild depression and obesity. It is much less suitable for deep depression—the kind of depression that ECT can reach. In 1957, two new drug classes were introduced: the "tricyclic antidepressants" by the Geigy company in Basel, and the monoamine oxidase inhibitors as "psychic energizers" by a team from

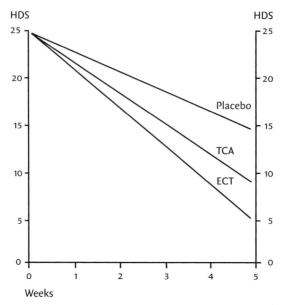

ECT outcomes in depression are considerably superior to those of antidepressant medication (TCA = tricyclic antidepressants), and certainly to placebo, as this figure illustrates. The lower the HDS (Hamilton Depression Scale) score, the better the outcome. Per Bech, "A Review of the Antidepressant Properties of Serotonin Reuptake Inhibitors," *Advances in Biological Psychiatry* 17 (1988): 58–69, fig. 1. Per Bech is a professor of psychiatry at Frederiksborg General Hospital, Hillerød, Denmark. Courtesy of S. Karger AG, Basel.

Rockland State Hospital headed by Nathan Kline in research that won him his second Lasker Medical Research Award.

Like schizophrenia, *depression* is a term for a number of different clinical entities. In the mid-1950s, Geigy designated psychiatrist Roland Kuhn at the Münsterlingen asylum in Switzerland to test an antihistamine that it hoped would have the same success as chlorpromazine. Kuhn and his colleagues gave the compound to patients with a variety of illnesses, to no particular effect. Then, just to be complete, toward the end of the trial Kuhn gave the drug to several patients who had what German psychiatrist Kurt Schneider described in 1920 as "vital" depression. Vital depression, in Schneider's view, was not just a lowness of mood, but a condition that seized the entire body, sapping the patient at a somatic level.[31] It is also known as "endogenous" depression, affecting not only mood but all autonomic body functions. Kuhn was steeped enough in the German psychopathological tradition to recognize vital depression when a patient with it responded to the new drug. According to Paula X's chart on January 21, 1956: "For three days now, it is as if the patient had undergone a transformation. All of her restlessness and agitation have vanished. Yesterday, she herself observed that she had been in a complete muddle, that she had never acted so dumb in all her life. She did not know what had caused her behavior, but she was just glad to be better again."[32] Geigy marketed the drug in Switzerland in November 1957, as imipramine, under the trade name Tofranil. It was launched in the United States in 1959, the first of the tricyclic antidepressants. Geigy called it a "thymoleptic," and when nobody understood what that was, the company changed its marketing strategy and advertised it the following year under the slogan "lighting the road to recovery in 80 percent of cases" of depression.[33]

Meanwhile, at a regional meeting in April 1957 of the American Psychiatric Association in Syracuse, New York, Kline and two colleagues from Rockland State announced their finding that a derivative of hydrazine, synthesized in 1952 called iproniazid (marketed by Roche as Marsilid), was psychoactive. It was the first of the antidepressants that acted by inhibiting the breakdown of brain monoamines (such as serotonin); the drug class became known as the monoamine oxidase inhibitors, or MAOIs. Their efficacy in depression was discovered when the mood of patients being treated for tuberculosis with iproniazid was seen to lighten. Kline published these results the following year, in 1958.[34] Until the tricyclics and the MAOIs appeared on the scene, ECT had no serious competitors for endogenous depression. "To date there has been no satisfactory replacement for electroshock therapy in the typical depressive state," wrote Benjamin Pollock in 1959 at Rochester State Hospital in New York, who had led one of the early trials of imipramine.[35]

As with chlorpromazine, the initial reaction to the new antidepressants was stunned disbelief. Bernard "Steve" Brodie, a pharmacologist at the National Institutes of Health who was involved in antimalarial work and the development of Tylenol, was initially a total skeptic. "For several years my good friend, Dr. [Willi] Haefliger from Geigy, Basel, kept pressing me to carry out studies on the nature of the antidepressant action of imipramine. Frankly, I was not particularly interested. . . . I did not believe the clinical reports. When the symptoms of endogenous depression were translated to me (from the German), my only thought was—no drug can possibly cure that!"[36]

Early reports bolstered imipramine as more useful than ECT, and more compatible with psychotherapy. As one English psychiatrist put it at a symposium in 1959 in Cambridge: "If, for example, you treat the depressive patient with imipramine you can be, as it were, with the patient all the way through the illness until recovery, for he remembers all that takes place and does not undergo a rapid series of changes [as with ECT]."[37] In June 1959, Anthony Sainz, director of research at Marcy State Hospital in New York, told the *New York Times* that a related MAOI called phenelzine (Warner-Chilcott's Nardil), "could possibly supplant electroshock." The *Times* headline singled out this theme: "Energizer Is Said to Relieve Depressions and to Curb Need for Electroshock."[38]

Fritz Freyhan, on the verge of abandoning ECT at Delaware State, traveled to Germany in 1959 to lecture to the Berlin Psychiatric Society. He told them that he had tested imipramine at Delaware State in the autumn of 1957. It "may be described as an antidepressant." "If you compare Tofranil with a key, it fits best into the cyclothymic [manic-depressive] keyhole."[39] A small trial of imipramine at a New Jersey mental hospital led by J. Richard Wittenborn found that imipramine was generally preferred to ECT, having a "much shorter latency."[40]

Still, ECT was found to be overwhelmingly superior to any drug for the treatment of serious depression. In 1960, Linford Rees at the Bethlem Royal and Maudsley Hospitals in London did a trial of iproniazid. The results were shattering for the drug when compared with ECT: "Eighteen patients who did not benefit from Iproniazid were given electroplexy [the English term for ECT]. Of these, sixteen responded immediately making a complete recovery and one showing improvement but not full recovery. Thus only one patient failed to improve with electroplexy. The response to electroplexy was so striking regarding speed and in the degree and quality of recovery, that it left no room for doubt regarding the supremacy of electroplexy over Iproniazid in these patients."[41]

After a trial of four MAOIs in 1963, two English psychiatrists at the Harrow Hospital near Bristol, concluded: "The recovery rate with [severely depressed] patients is not sufficiently satisfactory with the present group of drugs to warrant their substitution for electrical treatment."[42] In 1965, after a survey of the literature on six new antidepressant drugs conducted at the Massachusetts Mental Health Center in Boston—part of a larger NIMH drug study then under way—Milton Greenblatt and his coworkers concluded: "EST [electroshock] appears to produce more improvement than all of the medications; placebo less."[43] None of the new drugs was inferior to placebo, but none could top the treatment Cerletti had introduced in 1938. In 1974, McGill

University psychopharmacologist Thomas Ban addressed the question of which antidepressant group was better. The tricyclic antidepressants on balance performed better than the MAOIs, he said. "On the other hand, ECT seems to exert a more rapid and radical effect than tricyclic antidepressant drugs."[44]

The public-relations people at Lakeside Laboratories must have been clenching their jaws as Boston psychiatrist and veteran psychopharmacologist Jonathan Cole took the floor at a meeting they sponsored at Columbia University in 1970 on current trends in depression research. "In my judgment, both the antianxiety agents and the antidepressant agents suffer from overpromotion," he said. He acknowledged that the tricyclics probably had some effect. "On the other hand, a lot of depressions, particularly neurotic depressions, get better anyway, and severe retarded endogenous depressions did well with electric shock before the antidepressant drugs ever came along. A cynic might say that these drugs provide the psychiatrist with something to give the patient, while waiting for the depression to go away." Cole mused about what would happen if the FDA suddenly found all existing drugs too toxic for further use. "Would they really be missed?" Maybe the chlorpromazine-style drugs would be, "while the antidepressants and the antianxiety drugs could be adequately replaced by electroconvulsive therapy and selected barbiturates."[45] The situation has not really changed since Cole spoke these words in 1970. The SSRI-class, which includes Prozac, Paxil, and Zoloft, also has not had a track record better than ECT since these drugs became available in the 1980s.

Clouds on the Psychopharmacology Horizon

Despite a general atmosphere of jubilation in 1953 at the Basel symposium on chlorpromazine, there were several isolated notes of alarm: some of the patients had developed the symptoms of Parkinson's disease with its muscular rigidity and slowing. Felix Labhardt at the Basel University Clinic of Basel Canton, who had brought chlorpromazine back to Switzerland from Delay's clinic in Paris, noted at the symposium: "Among many of the patients there occurred in the first weeks of treatment a singular stiffness and slowing of movement and facial expression, that to be sure could be related to the underlying illness, especially catatonia. Nonetheless, in a condition such as this there is always the thought of a mild Parkinsonian syndrome."[46] Several other Swiss psychiatrists commented on similar Parkinson-like symptoms among their chlorpromazine patients. Richard Avenarius, for example, at the private sanatorium in Oberwil, Zug Canton, reported on a thirty-three-year-old patient who, from the third week of treatment on, demonstrated "rigid facial features, muscular rigidity with cogwheeling [tremor at passive movement of a rigid joint], and lessening size of the handscript."[47] The following year, there were two formal reports on Parkinsonism associated with chlorpromazine by two Swiss physicians: Hans Steck, a professor of psychiatry at the Prilly Psychiatric Hospital in Céry near Lausanne, and Hans-Joachim Haase, a young psychiatrist who, like Avenarius, worked at the Oberwil sanatorium.[48] These are generally considered the first articles on the subject in what would become a vast literature.

It was soon realized that Parkinson-like symptoms were a serious problem with chlorpromazine and the phenothiazine-class of antipsychotics (and in some other classes too). Many clinicians, unfamiliar with the French and German literature, discovered the side effect independently. In 1955, at the symposium in Philadelphia that Smith Kline sponsored, George Brooks at the Vermont State Hospital in Waterbury, volunteered: "Our feeling has been that all patients who are on large doses of Thorazine for any length of time show some signs of basal ganglion dysfunction; not perhaps full-blown Parkinsonism, but some loss of associated movements, loss of facial mobility, etc. We have begun to feel that quite frequently the greatest improvement coincided with the development of these symptoms."[49] In other words, when patients developed Parkinsonism, clinicians could be assured that the medicine was actually working.

The philosophy that one must drive up the dose of antipsychotics until Parkinsonism appeared characterized the American approach to drug therapy. According to Vernon Kinross-Wright at Baylor University in 1954: "The average maximum dosage, the point at which we level off, is about 2000 to 2400 mg daily."[50] In Europe, 200 mg daily was seen as a lot. "You Americans!" said Hy Denber, who had practiced on both sides of the ocean. "In America, everything is big; you have big skyscrapers and big automobiles, and it is the same thing with chlorpromazine!"[51] There was a direct relationship between the size of the dose and the appearance of Parkinsonism. Patients on small doses were not immune from rigidity and slowing, but they were much less likely to experience it. Jean Sigwald in Paris, who initiated outpatient treatment with chlorpromazine in 1952, usually gave less than 150 mg per day and said he had never seen extrapyramidal (Parkinsonian) symptoms in his patients.[52]

Schizophrenic patients early acquired a distaste for a medication that gave them such unpleasant symptoms—including the tongue protrusion and muscle twitching of tardive dyskinesia—and often refused to stay on their medication. It must be emphasized that most patients must remain on medication for long periods if they wish to control their symptoms. Going off one's meds usually means a relapse will occur. It is a measure of their distress with drug therapy that, despite the risk of relapse, schizophrenic patients tended to be highly noncompliant with medication regimes. Frank Ayd said that even hospital patients often did not take their pills. "I was in a hospital recently," he said in 1969, "and saw some patients playing poker—using chlorpromazine tablets for stakes."[53]

Pharmacotherapy, especially chlorpromazine, would have a chance to rival ECT *only if the patients took their medicine.* Few patients were enthusiastic about ECT, fearing as they did unconsciousness. But few were keen about antipsychotic medication either, and the complaints about Parkinsonism were just the tip of a side-effects iceberg that included many other symptoms. The early appearance of Parkinsonism was a cloud on the antipsychotics' horizon that with time would loom much larger. Today, around a fifth of schizophrenia patients are noncompliant with medication,[54] and even those who remain on pills often dislike them so much that, according to one study, only 12 percent stay on the same drug for an entire year.[55] ECT would be a reasonable option for the symptoms of some of these individuals, but it is no longer available in many places.

ECT and the Pharmaceutical Industry

It is a gauge of how grinding commercial competition has changed the pharmaceutical industry that, when both the industry and ECT were young, the sector did not turn its back on electrotherapy in the same sovereign manner as it does today. Now, one can search in vain for sessions on ECT at industry-sponsored meetings. There is no vast conspiracy. It is merely that the drug companies have no interest in publicizing the existence of a potentially aggressive competitor. At the beginning it was quite otherwise. For one thing, none of the firms had any idea what a mammoth industry psychopharmacology would become. The field went from a number of family-owned businesses marketing "long line" chemicals to a concentration of wealth and power rivaling the oil industry. Nobody could believe that drugs could improve mental illness; the only restorative factor was thought to be psychotherapy. As Paul Janssen, research director of a family firm by that name in Belgium, said: "When I was young one of the definitions of psychosis included incurability. If the psychosis disappeared, this was indicative of a misdiagnosis. The idea that it could be cured with a pill was ridiculed as simply too childish an idea."[56]

With depression as well, the idea of a successful physical treatment seemed inconceivable. Depression was too context-dependent, a response to loss. What could a pill do for grief or emotional pain? Pharmacotherapy for anxiety made some sense, given a fifty-year history of success with barbiturates. But drug treatments for depression were not something the industry pursued until Kuhn approached Geigy, and even then Geigy responded with anything but alacrity. It was only after Kuhn gave one of the directors of Geigy some imipramine for his depressed wife that the company took notice.

Nor was there a lot of excitement in the United States when Rhône-Poulenc proposed chlorpromazine. Several U.S. drug companies turned the French company down before Smith Kline finally bit. As Janssen explained, it was "because they didn't believe it and because they couldn't see a market. Schizophrenia was completely unknown to them."[57] So early on, the commercial potential of drugs was not apparent, and the industry could be more relaxed about competitors such as convulsive therapy.

Smith Kline's first advertisements for chlorpromazine in 1955 mentioned ECT as the main competition. In the journal *Diseases of the Nervous System* the company claimed: "Thorazine reduces need for electroshock therapy," and cited the virtual abandonment of the procedure at Rochester State Hospital with the advent of the company's drug. There was a big picture of bilateral ECT in the ad, together with an ECT apparatus.[58] This was certainly different from ignoring ECT. At the chlorpromazine symposium that Smith Kline sponsored that year, a company executive cheerily offered: "We need to know more about the use of the drug in conjunction with electro-shock and insulin shock."[59]

Merck with its rival tricyclic antidepressant amitriptyline (Elavil) conceded in an ad in 1965: "Some depressed patients still need EST [showing an older woman with electrodes]. With ELAVIL some patients need less EST [showing a younger woman] . . . and many don't need EST at all [showing a quite young woman]."[60] Another company, Roche, marketed its MAOI isocarboxazid (Marplan) as "compatible with EST."[61] Geigy even admitted that ECT was "the most effective treatment" in hospitalized depressed patients.[62]

After the mid-1960s, public references by the industry to competing electrotherapy came to an end. It may be that physicians were simultaneously losing confidence in ECT, so the companies felt no further need to mention a procedure that was going onto the back burner. Or it may be that the dollar amounts involved in the sale of psychopharmaceuticals were by then so overwhelming that caution was the watchword: don't throw away millions of dollars in sales by reminding doctors that there is an alternative to pharmacotherapy. After all, by 1961, Thorazine and a related drug called Compazine (prochlorperazine) accounted for 39 percent of Smith Kline's total sales;[63] the sales volume of chlorpromazine in 1960 was almost $21 million, making it one of the first blockbuster drugs.[64]

In this era of wildly successful drugs, the financial stakes for a company are enormous. When a company depends so heavily on retaining the market share that the drug generates, its role as a guarantor of scientific integrity is questionable. Events early in the twenty-first century have made this apparent: evidence has been mounting for forty years that antidepressant drugs may induce suicide in certain vulnerable populations. Right from the start, some of the senior figures in the field saw the risk, but it was not until 2004 that the issue exploded into public consciousness and the FDA acknowledged the danger. That the disclosure took forty years is based in part on the companies who have vigorously defended their huge profits.[65]

As physicians wrote prescriptions and profits rolled in, ECT became the object of a great industry-produced silence. It was left out of controlled trials and comparison studies. Nobody at meetings of the FDA's Psychopharmacological Drugs Advisory Committee ever asked: "How does this drug compare to ECT?"[66] ECT specialists, although they know a great deal about depression, are almost never invited to academic (industry-sponsored) meetings on depression. As Oregon psychiatrist and ECT pioneer Paul Blachly noted somewhat dolefully in 1976: "Because of the great hopes for psychopharmacology, ECT has been neglected for many conditions where it can be helpful and where the patient now views a spectre of apparently interminable chemotherapy."[67]

Between roughly 1960 and 1980, ECT disappeared from the awareness of most doctors, except insofar as they read negative and stereotyped references to it in the popular press. Drugs became the main treatment of psychiatric illness, sometimes in connection with psychotherapy, but more often as a single method. As New York psychiatrist Arthur Zitrin mused later: "Compared to writing a prescription, ECT is a big deal! But there are times when you need a big deal."[68]

CHAPTER NINE

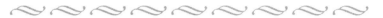

The Swinging Pendulum

The Effects of Politics, Law, and Changes in Medical Culture on ECT

Reform movements have punctuated the history of psychiatry. From the celebrated loosening of the chains of the inmates of the Bicêtre Asylum in Paris by Philippe Pinel in the 1790s, to the policies of nonrestraint in the mid nineteenth century, and to the revisions of the committal laws during the twentieth century, practices and theories of mental illness have responded to broader contexts of social change. These reforms are often lumped together with the upheaval in psychiatry during the 1960s that has been termed *antipsychiatry*, but 1960s antipsychiatry was fundamentally different from anything that had gone before.[1]

Antipsychiatry

Previous reforms focused on conditions within the asylum and did not threaten medical claims that the conditions being treated were mental illnesses; indeed reform essentially involved a medicalization of what previously had been seen as social problems. Antipsychiatry in the 1960s, however, hinged on the notion that mental illness did not exist, or at least not in the form that psychiatrists claimed. The antipsychiatrists argued that, in fact, society itself had gone mad and that those suffering from mental illness were only its most apparent victims.

From our vantage point in the twenty-first century, this is an argument that the antipsychiatrists seem to have lost. Today increasing numbers of people take psychotropic medication of one sort or another: Ritalin, Valium, Zoloft, just to name a few. Increasing numbers of illnesses are identified and listed in handbooks such as the *Diagnostic and Statistical Manual of Mental Disorders,* fourth edition (*DSM-IV*).

Media coverage of all topics related to mental illness and consumer advertisements of psychotropic medications have exploded in recent years—clearly, the public attributes some notion of reality to the idea of mental illness. But arguably the claims of antipsychiatry have been proven rather than disproven by these developments: although the headline claims of 1960s antipsychiatry focused on the acutely mentally ill who were committed to asylums, in fact, the real concern was for the rest of society who for the first time were exposed on a mass scale to the attentions and ministrations of psychiatry.

Despite the deinstitutionalization of patients from hospitals that began in the 1950s with the development of chlorpromazine and the psychopharmacological revolution, there are in fact no fewer patients in service beds now than there were fifty years ago. Before World War II, few people were at risk of being committed to an asylum, and most knew no one in professional treatment for mental illness. Now we all know plenty of folks being treated with Prozac, Paxil, and Zoloft, and these medications are prescribed for people of all ages, including young children. Since the 1950s, there has been a tripling of the rates of detention to psychiatric facilities, and since the early twentieth century, a fifteenfold increase in the number of patients who are admitted to a mental health service bed even in remote parts of Britain—which, compared with the United States, have scanty service provision for mental illness.[2] Arguably, those who were really deinstitutionalized were psychiatrists and other mental health therapists rather than their patients.

It was a recognition of this extension of the psychiatric reach that motivated the antipsychiatrists of the 1960s, although in focusing on ECT and the seriously mentally ill they missed their target. The medical doctors who had previously run the asylums (the "alienists") and had worked secluded within the asylum walls, from the 1960s onward were increasingly likely to serve as office psychiatrists running community clinics. Access to the new pharmacology was by prescription only; in order to get help, people had to engage with psychiatrists in a way that they had not had to do before. Personal, private lives became the purview of psychiatrists. And who are they to make ethical judgments about aspects of an individual's life? How can we know whether their views are correct that certain behaviors are manifestations of psychological disorder rather than stemming from political concerns or social injustice?

We return again to the case of Randle McMurphy, the hero of *One Flew over the Cuckoo's Nest* in Ken Kesey's 1962 book and in a 1975 film starring Jack Nicholson (see chapter 7). Kesey compares life on an asylum ward to the political state in which we all live, an increasingly all-controlling, oppressive, big government that you have to protest against in order to survive. McMurphy is then punished for bucking the system; the ECT and, later, the lobotomy he receives are a means of quashing rebellion and ensuring conformity. But the ultimate message is that if this can happen to someone like Randle McMurphy, it can happen to you. As Kesey makes very clear from the start, McMurphy does not have mental illness in any traditional sense. Rather, he feigns mental illness to escape a jail rap. This anticipated a famous experiment undertaken by sociologist David Rosenhan in the late 1960s, in which volunteers posed as mentally ill and had themselves committed in order to experience life through the lens of psychopathology. It turned out to be frighteningly easy to fool medical staff and get detained in a hospital, and indeed, in some cases it was difficult to get out afterward.[3] The message was that psychiatrists did not know what they were doing and there was little that could stop them from doing it to almost anyone they chose.

The antipsychiatry movement of the 1960s and early 1970s fed the currents of cultural revolution in the West. Civil rights for African Americans, equal rights for women—a deeper meaning of democratic process took hold with new intensity. Whereas democracy before referred to the ability of people to cast a vote, now women organized to resist the colonization of their minds by men and demanded equal representation in the processes of government, in the ministry of churches, and in opportunities at work and within the law. It was a time when ethnic groups challenged the hegemony of the white elites of Western countries and argued that the acceptance of established views risked an internalization of white imperialism. Teenage rebellion was seen as resistance by the young to having their minds manipulated by their elders. Against the backdrop of World War II, the Cold War, and the Vietnam War, this resistance to the "wisdom" of a previous generation not only made sense but felt like a necessary struggle for survival.

Many of the most heated moments of protest and outrage took place at universities. In Paris and Tokyo, students marched on the universities, particularly medical departments of psychiatry. In Paris, the offices of Jean Delay, the discoverer of chlorpromazine, who also had worked prominently on shock therapies in the early phase of his career, were ransacked and occupied for three months. More than anyone else in Europe, Delay was the symbol of psychiatry's new physical therapies. He was forced into retirement. The department of psychiatry at Tokyo University was occupied for ten years, and all research there came to an end. Hiroshi Utena, the head of the department, who was closely linked with research on the use of physical treatments, was also forced to retire.[4]

In the United States, as in Kesey's novel, antipsychiatry involved a much greater element of protest against the state than it did in Europe and Japan, and student demonstrations there were linked to activism against the Vietnam War. The state was the ultimate source of malfeasance, corruption, and conflict of interest. Indeed, the notion of a conflict of interest was born in the 1960s. Today we use the term to refer to a supposed corruption of research by private interests; in the 1960s and 1970s the most obvious and threatening conflicts of interest were perceived to be the funding of research and education by the state.[5] Eisenhower's vision of a tightly integrated military-industrial complex was the original source of concern about conflicts of interest and threats to our liberty.

Psychiatrists and philosophers using psychiatry as a metaphor for the rest of society provided the public face of the upheavals. Ronald D. ("Ronnie") Laing and David Cooper in Britain; Thomas Szasz, Erving Goffman, and Herbert Marcuse in the United States; and Michel Foucault and Frantz Fanon in France represented a cadre of influential thinkers who, in differing ways, offered visions of the confinement of deviance within the mental health system, of the need for individuals to resist therapy in order to stay in tune with their true selves, and of the revolutionary potential of the oppressed. The disturbances in Tokyo erupted after Szasz and Laing visited the university in 1968.

In 1969, Szasz cofounded the Citizens Commission on Human Rights (CCHR) along with the Church of Scientology. A key event in this founding centered on Viktor Gyory, a recent Hungarian immigrant detained at Haverford State Hospital in Philadelphia, where he was held in seclusion, forcibly medicated, and then given ECT. Szasz interviewed the man in Hungarian and was prepared to testify in court that Gyory was not ill, only unable to communicate in English. Rather then face a challenge to the laws on detention in Pennsylvania, the hospital released Gyory. CCHR and the Church of Scientology have since been the most sustained critics of psychiatry, and especially of ECT, within the United States.

Szasz's vision that mental illness did not exist, and in particular that people designated as mental patients needed to assert their basic rights

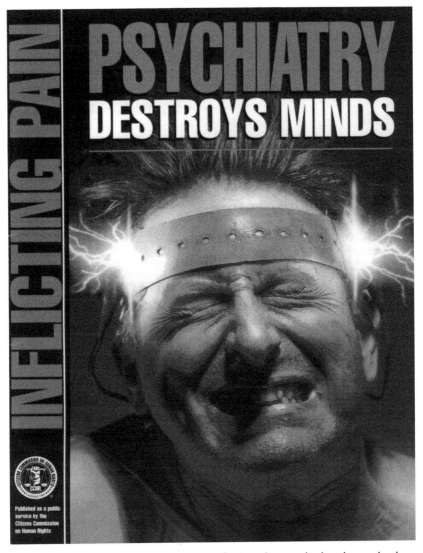

"Psychiatry Destroys Minds": the Church of Scientology and related organizations such as the Citizens Commission on Human Rights, which it co-founded in 1969 with antipsychiatrist Thomas Szasz, campaigned systematically against ECT using ads such as this one. Courtesy of the Citizens Commission on Human Rights International.

as citizens, was a key driver in American but not European antipsychiatry.[6] Taking inspiration from some of these themes, in 1970 the Insane Liberation Front was established in Portland, Oregon, followed in 1971 by a Mental Patients' Liberation Front in Boston and a Mental Patients' Liberation Project in New York. For a number of reasons,

ECT became a focus for all these groups. One reason was the simple salience of the treatment. Another was its symbolic value. A third reason was that some of the most coherent patients critical of psychiatry were individuals who had undergone ECT. But taking on ECT meant taking issue with a treatment that many thought clearly worked for severely ill patients, which was strategically a very different matter from taking on a treatment that did not have such a track record, such as psychoanalysis, or the widespread and indiscriminate usage of SSRIs today. ECT, however, was more readily portrayed as a treatment that had been "survived" than psychoanalysis or Zoloft.

Survivors

One of the first psychiatric "survivors" was Leonard Roy Frank. Frank had moved to San Francisco in 1962, where typical of the 1960s he dropped out, became a vegetarian, and developed an interest in religion. His Manhattan parents were horrified and had him compulsorily detained in Twin Pines Hospital in Belmont, California, for eight months from 1962 to 1963, just as Kesey's book was published. There, he was labeled a paranoid schizophrenic and was first treated, fifty times, with insulin coma. He then had thirty-five electroshock treatments under the care of Doctors Norman Reider and Robert James. Frank claimed sparse recollections from this period of time, and he spent five years trying to regain the knowledge that he believed the shock treatment had destroyed. He also began to learn more about psychiatry, and in doing so, came across an early article by Szasz.[7] From there he gravitated toward the new survivor network that was emerging.

In 1972, Frank joined Madness Network News, which had been started by Sherri Hersh and David Richman in 1971. This was an early, pre-cyber version of the Internet forums that psychiatric patients at the turn of the century would gravitate toward. In 1974, Frank and Wade Hudson founded the Network against Psychiatric Assault (NAPA) in San Francisco. They became heavily involved in a campaign against ECT at Langley Porter Neuropsychiatric Institute aimed at prohibiting forced shock treatment, psychosurgery, and drug treatment in California. This eventually led to the passage of a statute in California that severely limited the use of ECT (see chapter 10).

In the course of this legal action, Frank accessed his medical records and wrote up the story, which appeared in a book on shock treatment.[8] Nothing about these records provided good evidence for a diagnosis of paranoid schizophrenia, and both the records and Frank's subsequent life suggested that he had had little more than a spell of injudicious usage of marijuana. Fired up, he began assembling the first edition of *The History of Shock Treatment,* a compilation of both academic and lay articles on various aspects of shock treatment and biological psychiatry.[9] In a review of the book, Szasz wrote: "What the rack and the stake were to the inquisition, what the concentration camp and the gas chamber were to National Socialism, the mental hospital and electroshock are to institutional psychiatry. *The History of Shock Treatment* is a carefully researched documentation of psychiatry's final solution."[10]

Leonard Frank's case was emblematic of wider trends. The period from the late 1960s through the 1980s gave rise to a large number of patients' groups. Some were self-help groups taking their inspiration from Alcoholics Anonymous, which had been founded in 1935. A second type were the consumer groups who, as elsewhere in medicine, were concerned to ensure equitable access to decent facilities and the latest treatments.[11] These latter organizations were part of a tradition of improving mental health care that included figures such as Dorothea Dix and Clifford Beers.[12] But a third category was more political, with its groups taking their inspiration from Szasz and the antipsychiatry movement, and they saw it as their mission to protest against the abuse of individual rights that seemed endemic in psychiatric practice.

Another influential survivor was Judi Chamberlin, who in her early twenties had been hospitalized for depression in the mid-1960s. As a psychiatric patient she discovered she had no legal rights. This led her, in 1971, to cofound the Mental Patients' Liberation Front in Boston. She later became affiliated with the Boston University Center for Psychiatric Rehabilitation, which helped underpin a series of Ruby Rogers Advocacy and Drop-in Centers.[13] These centers had a booklet outlining patients' rights, which even as late as 1994 stated: "Where is it possible to be imprisoned although you have not committed a crime? Where can you be held without bail and denied a trial? Where can you be deprived of your rights and stripped of your human worth? Where can you be put in solitary confinement, physically abused and given drugs whether you want them or not? In the American South in 1850s? In Germany in the 1930s? In a mental hospital in the United States in the 1990s?"[14]

Somewhat later, in 1980, the National Association for Rights Protection and Advocacy (NARPA) was founded by a group of patients' rights advocates, some of whom were lawyers, with a mission to promote the rights of psychiatric patients. Today this association is a mix of lawyers, nonlegal advocates, and former patients. NARPA takes the view that mental health advocates were deliberately split into consumers on the one hand and survivors on the other by federal funding programs for the consumer side alone, and that this had led to a virtual elimination of the survivor movement.[15]

Similar movements developed in other countries. In Britain, a National Association for Mental Health (NAMH) was set up in 1946 from a number of preexisting groups.[16] Initially building on thinking like that of Beers and Dix, this group was keen to see a provision of more psychiatrists and helped sponsor the first social workers interested in supporting discharged patients in the community. Its approach to mental illness was almost identical to the position it took on mental retardation. In 1969, NAMH found itself under attack from the Church of Scientology, who accused it of being a tool of organized psychiatry. NAMH rejected what it perceived to be attempts at infiltration by Scientologists, but it also began to change character: in 1972, it was reborn as Mind, whose brief was one of explicit patient advocacy. For Mind, just as for NARPA and other groups in the field, ECT has been a major battleground (see chapter 10).

From its birth, antipsychiatry had opposed ECT. The possibility that this antagonism might be having an effect came into focus in an editorial in the *British Medical Journal* in 1975, which explicitly linked antipsychiatry and ECT: "Among the effects of the wide publicity given to criticisms of current psychiatric methods by the 'antipsychiatrists' has been an increasing reluctance to acknowledge the value of physical treatments such as electroconvulsive therapy—ECT. . . . Other professions besides medicine are taking an increasing part in therapy. . . . Rightly or wrongly these professions see their work as being to help people with problems rather than treat patients with diseases, and their weapons are psychotherapy, group therapy and alteration of social conditions."[17]

Informed Consent

Another factor that distinguished 1960s-style antipsychiatry from organized opposition to psychiatry in the past—and the reason it has lessons for the rest of medicine—lies in the parallel evolution of informed consent.

Physicians have informed patients for centuries about treatment options and have sought their written consent to procedures for more than a hundred years. So, on the face of it, the 1957 case of Martin Salgo against Stanford University would not be expected to offer anything fundamentally new or of far-reaching consequence to medicine. Salgo suffered permanent paralysis following a routine spinal X-ray at the Stanford University hospital, and he sued in a case of argued negligence.[18] In finding for Salgo, the court created a requirement for informed consent, which obliged doctors to disclose "any facts which are necessary to form the basis of an intelligent consent by the patient to the proposed treatment."[19] This judgment enshrined the notion of informed consent for the first time and fundamentally changed health care.

There were legal precedents for what happened in *Salgo*. A famous 1914 battery case resulted in a verdict that weighed in the later debate: "Every human being of adult years and sound mind has a right to determine what should be done with his own body. When a surgeon performs an operation without his patient's consent he commits an assault."[20] Battery (assault) is the tort involved when a person is touched or one's privacy is invaded without one's consent. Negligence is the result of a failure of due care, and it assumes that physicians are generally acting in good faith and that any injury is more accidental than intentional. In the case of negligence, a legally established duty must be breached resulting in an injury, measurable as damages, and this injury must be causally and proximately related to breach of duty. But until 1957 nobody had ever considered that a breach of duty might stem solely from not informing patients sufficiently.

There have been two main historians of the informed consent movement. Martin Pernick has argued that informed consent is not something novel, pointing to the prior existence of consent forms and the abundant evidence of physicians taking care to describe truthfully the hazards behind treatments.[21] Jay Katz (and others), however, contest that these forms and any truth-telling imply informed consent, in that, before 1960, patients simply did not give permission to doctors in the same way they now do.[22] The key difference lies what happened before 1960, when patients, informed of their risks, refused to accept a treatment. Before then, throughout the eighteenth and nineteenth centuries, physicians informed patients, often in great detail, but the primary reason for doing so was in order to educate patients about their recommendations and therefore motivate them to comply with treatment. Patients were not informed about procedures or options on the basis that they might then opt not to comply. Benjamin Rush, an advocate of educating patients, argued in 1811 in "The Duties of Patients to Physicians":

"the obedience of a patient to the prescriptions of his physicians should be prompt, strict and universal. He should never oppose his own inclination nor judgment to the advice of his physician."[23]

It was this position that underpinned medical willingness to deceive patients in their own interests if a doctor thought the patient might not be able to handle trickier, complex information, which could occur if he or she were not enlightened, well educated, or stable enough to deal with the emotional threat disturbing information might pose. This was a beneficence model, under which a physician's responsibilities of disclosure and consent-seeking were linked to the primary medical obligation, which was to make the patient well. This primary obligation to help the patient surpassed any obligation to respect what would now be called the patient's autonomy. If the truth were not going to be beneficial to the patient, then it would be unethical to tell the truth. Medicine was about instilling in the patient confidence, gratitude, and respect for the physician in order to enable the physician to do the best he could for acutely ill patients. It was not about treating the patient as an equal partner, in part because medicine until recently had few chronically ill patients who had the time and liberty to consider their options.

Few discussions of informed consent recognize that until recently, there was a lack of commonly accepted scientific knowledge that could be imparted to the patient. The information or evidence base that the physician used until the 1950s was primarily his or her own experience. There was not an objective body of evidence written with nonphysicians in mind to which patients or others could be directed. The idea that patients could be brought up to speed about a knowledge base that it had taken a physician a lifetime to acquire was considered bizarre. In contrast, the knowledge that we now think should be shared with patients is an entirely different and publicly available thing, stemming from published trials of treatments. More recently, the Internet has further fed patients' appetites for medical knowledge.

Faced with a directive from the court that seemed to many physicians to come out of the blue, the medical profession, and not just psychiatrists, reacted with a mixture of hostility and bafflement.[24] It was deeply offensive to them to be told that their failure to seek consent meant little distinction could be drawn between the abuse of medicine in Nazi Germany and abuses in the course of research or clinical practice in the United States. A good example of the medical response came from Carl Fellner and John Marshall, who investigated why anyone would opt to donate a kidney, for example. They concluded that donation was an "irrational" process that failed to meet the requirements of informed consent,[25] with the implication that most of medical practice in such a context was equally absurd. As of 1982, 70 percent of physicians in the United States continued to define informed consent as providing information to the patient rather than indicating a mandate to seek explicit permission based on full disclosure. The courts had instituted a radical break with tradition in 1957 that would take decades to feed through into day-to-day clinical practice.

Mitchell and Informed Consent

It is widely noted that with the rise of modern hospitals as sprawling institutions with corporate interests and the intrusion of ever more technology into the process of medicine, the relations between patients and physicians began to change. In the process, it became less acceptable for physicians to decide for patients without consulting them. But this new relationship did not come about simply because hospitals and machines were bigger; it stemmed in part from the availability of a new, public form of research evidence from randomized controlled trials (RCTs).

The issue came to a head in 1966 in a *New England Journal of Medicine* article on informed consent written by Henry Beecher, a professor of anesthesiology at Harvard University.[26] Beecher outlined a series of research practices in some of the best-known hospitals in the country and undertaken by some of the most distinguished clinicians and researchers. In twenty-two separate research studies, patients who thought they were receiving normal clinical care were, in fact, research subjects and they were receiving clinical interventions that were quite problematic. No one study was singled out as involving poor practice as such, but their combined weight indicated that in some cases, treatment-related injuries had been inflicted on patients who were unaware of the risks. Patients who had trusted their physicians had become research subjects without being aware of it. There was an outcry. Within a year the FDA, NIH, and other federal bodies had put in place requirements for experimental subjects to be informed as to the nature of any care they might be receiving and the risks that any research element of that care might pose.[27]

Beecher's article had an even greater impact than the *Salgo* case. Once let out, the genie of informed consent could not be contained within the bottle of research. Nowhere was this clearer than in the treatment of breast cancer and the administration of ECT. In the case of breast cancer, for three-quarters of a century, women had undergone mutilating surgery at the hands of physicians on a mission to eradicate cancer.[28] In the zeal of their mission, surgeons removed ever-increasing amounts of tissue, including lymph nodes, the remaining healthy breast, and often the muscles of the chest wall. In the 1960s, women became aware that some surgeons had been questioning such practices since the 1950s, and that there was a great deal of evidence to show that less severe operations were just as successful. This was the era that gave rise to modern feminism, and the battle cry went up that male surgeons were inflicting their will on women's bodies. Women who had gained knowledge about alternative procedures and best outcomes found themselves dismissed with scorn and derision as simple housewives.

Following *Salgo*, the next significant case concerning informed consent involved Irma Natanson, who sued her physician in 1960 for failing to inform her of the risks linked to a new form of radiation therapy—cobalt therapy—following breast cancer surgery.[29] In 1955, when cobalt therapy was a new and untested procedure, Irma Natanson became one of the first women in the United States to have the treatment. Whereas previous negligence cases had judged physicians in the context of their peers, in ruling against the physician, the *Natanson* case introduced a new standard—whether the physician had "explain[ed] . . . to the patient in language as simple as necessary the nature of the ailment, the probability of success or of alternatives, and perhaps the risks of unfortunate outcomes."[30] Two days after *Natanson*, a second legal judgment involving ECT and insulin coma, *William Mitchell v. Wilse Robinson*, affirmed the same principle with even more far-reaching consequences.[31] But before discussing *Mitchell*, let us consider perhaps the most famous judgment in British medicine—the *Bolam* case.[32]

In 1954, John Hector Bolam was advised by Dr. C. Allfrey, a psychiatrist at Friern Hospital in London, to have ECT. He signed a form of consent to the treatment, at a time when consent forms were not a universal feature for ECT. But he was not warned of the risk of a fracture, and during the procedure he was not treated with a muscle relaxant then widely but not universally in use. Many psychiatrists in 1954 thought that muscle relaxants, and the general anesthesia their use entailed, posed their own risks and that their use should be reserved for people where the risk of fracture was particularly great.

Should the patient—someone who was depressed—have been warned about this risk beforehand? Many eminent practitioners around London were called to testify on the case. Dr. Alex Anthony Baker, the deputy superintendent at Banstead Hospital, said: "I have to use my judgment. Giving the full details may drive a patient away. I would not say that a practitioner fell below the proper standard of medical practice when failing to point out all the risks involved." Dr. Page, the deputy medical officer at Three Counties Hospital, Bedfordshire, said: "Every patient has to be considered as an individual. I ask them if they know of the treatment. If they are unduly nervous, I don't say too much. If they ask me questions, I tell them the truth. The risk is small, but a serious thing when it happens; and it would be a great mistake if they refused benefit from the treatment because of fear. In the case of a patient who is very depressed and suicidal, it is difficult to tell them of things which you know would make it worse."

Dr. John B. Randall of Nethern Hospital, when asked: "if you feel . . . as a doctor that it is the only hope of relieving this illness, would you think it wise to discourage the patient by describing to them the possible risk of serious fractures?" answered thus: "I suppose one has to form some opinion whether the patient is likely to be influenced by it. Depressed patients are often deluded about their bodily health, and nothing will alter their attitude. Taking that distortion of judgment into account, it is probable that to tell a patient that a risk of fracture exists will not materially alter his attitude to treatment or his attitude to his illness."

The jury decided that Dr. Allfrey was not negligent in keeping silent about the fracture risk. The view was taken that the practice of not giving relaxant drugs was not unusual for the time (although by 1957 it was very unusual). But the bottom line was twofold. First, a medical practitioner who is behaving in a way that is consistent with, at least, a respectable minority of his or her peers, cannot be found guilty of negligence when outcomes are adverse. Second, it was thought reasonable that if a person was depressed, the risk that he or she might misinterpret the information given was such that not all risks needed to be conveyed.

The *Bolam* case raised what many still think are obstacles to informed consent: what to do when a patient is irrational. This, though, is only the tip of an iceberg. If it is conceded that informed consent does not apply when the patient is irrational, where do we draw the line when patients become emotional? The case that Irma Natanson brought to the U.S. courts seemed to belong to an almost different universe than Bolam's, and seemed irrelevant to cases like *Bolam*. Natanson's treatment was highly experimental; ECT was an established and widely used procedure. Few other women in the United States had received cobalt therapy, but she was not informed of this—there was no disclosure of information. The court was cleared while she exposed her radiation-burnt chest wall, where even the bones had been eroded to the point that her heart could be seen visibly beating. Despite this, the court had qualms about putting the rights of the patient ahead of those of the doctors. Lawyers, after all, have to consider that what happens in one profession can happen to others, including their own, soon after.

The vast divide between the worlds represented by *Bolam* and *Natanson* was bridged by *Mitchell v. Robinson,* a Missouri case that involved shock treatments. In the United States as of 1953, practice standards for outpatient ECT had specifically advocated getting written consent from a patient's family, after attention had been drawn to the fact "that fractures sometimes occur in this treatment . . . , and many patients undergoing electroshock develop a temporary memory impairment." This consent, however, was aimed more at informing a family about issues to be managed rather to debate the merits of treatment.[33]

Against this background, William Mitchell was treated in 1951 by an old schoolmate, Jack DeMott, a physician at the Neurological Hospital in Kansas City, Missouri, run by Wilse Robinson. Mitchell was troubled by depressive disorder, alcohol abuse, and a crumbling marriage. DeMott recommended a combination of ECT and insulin coma treatments. During his seventh coma, the patient had a convulsion in which he fractured a vertebra. Mitchell filed suit in 1952, but the case did not come to trial until 1958. He offered no testimony "to show that the insulin therapy administered to [him] failed to conform to the required standards." He did not "question the technique of administering the insulin, nor does he deny it should have been administered." The record continues:

> Furthermore, there is no question here as to the plaintiff's consent to the treatment or claim that the procedure extended beyond that contemplated by the consent. . . . The plaintiff's principal claim here is that "There was evidence of a negligent failure to disclose to plaintiff the hazards of insulin treatment" and . . . that plaintiff would not have consented to the treatment had he known of the dangers. . . .
> Thus, the serious hazards being admitted, the problem is whether

in the circumstances of this record the doctors were under a duty to inform their patient of the hazards of treatment, leaving to the patient the option of living with his illness or of taking the treatment and accepting its hazards.[34]

The *Mitchell* case returned a verdict for the plaintiff. Although this was contested in 1960 and 1962, the implication was that in the United States, at least, the cozy world in which it was almost impossible to get a judgment against a doctor was gone forever. The standard to which doctors would be held in future was not one in which their practice was deemed acceptable if some of their peers would have done things the same way, but rather one in which they had to assume that the formerly private transactions between physicians and their patients had to make sense to an increasing number of lay parties. Informed consent in this sense all but transforms patients, who endure whatever their illness or doctors inflict on them, into consumers.

What Right Does Someone "Paid for by the Public" Have to Informed Consent?

In the case of ECT, just as in the case of breast cancer, these issues played out most clearly in Massachusetts. Fred Frankel was born and educated in South Africa. In 1952, he spent a trainee year at Massachusetts General Hospital with Stanley Cobb, who had once been a pathologist and who was appointed to supervise the creation of a research department. Following that Frankel returned to South Africa to a clinical practice in psychiatry very much in the British style—an eclectic mix of patient support, practically oriented therapy, drug treatment, and ECT. His close contemporary in South Africa was Isaac Marks, the later founder of behavior therapy, psychiatry's most pragmatic treatment.[35]

When in 1962 the political difficulties between ethnic groups in South Africa exploded in Sharpeville, Frankel and his family left the country. Massachusetts General was happy to have him back. But Boston and Mass General looked somewhat different after ten years' experience in clinical psychiatry. Cobb had been replaced by Eric Lindemann, who was one of the most famous analysts in the United States and one of the founders of the community mental health movement. Nobody at Mass General under Lindemann gave ECT. Most of the other teaching hospitals affiliated with Harvard no longer administered ECT either. This was a world in which psychoanalysis had taken over completely. Even patients with schizophrenia were treated with therapy by some of the most famous analysts in the United States such as Elvin Semrad.[36]

But while Harvard kept its analytic hands clean, private hospitals such as Bournewood, Glenside, Charles River, and Baldpate gave ECT to up to 60 percent of the patients referred to them.[37] Patients referred for schizophrenia, anxiety, substance and alcohol abuse, or personality disorders were all likely to receive ECT. In Boston, therefore, the treatment you got depended on whose door you knocked on. The split was complete, with neither side talking to each other, sharing forums, publishing in the same journals, or presenting at the same meetings. The state hospitals caught in the middle frequently complied with the new Harvard norms out of fear. By the end of the 1960s in Boston, the climate was comparable to the one that existed in northern California a few years later, which lead to a ban on ECT. Frankel was struck by the ideological nature of the conflict—especially in contrast to the way it played out in Britain or South Africa. Something about the American psyche, as he saw it, pushed for closure on issues and the sense of certainty that went with closure. There was an intolerance of ambiguity.[38] The only time American psychiatry seemed to be at the midpoint was as the pendulum was swinging past it from one side to the other.

Few alarm bells rang in 1967 when Utah became the first state to pass a statute controlling the use of ECT. But they sounded in earnest in 1971 when restrictions were placed on ECT in Alabama.[39] In *Ricky Wyatt v. Dr. Stonewall B. Stickney,* commissioner of mental health for Alabama, Judge Frank M. Johnson placed a series of restrictions on treatment with ECT, which Alabama state hospitals were still giving in unmodified form. These limits were regarded by many psychiatrists as effectively outlawing ECT. Johnson's judgment is probably better understood as having been aimed at improving appalling conditions within the state hospital system. Because patients were unlikely to get the kind of clinical care they needed before and after ECT, the treatment itself could not be considered a therapeutic option. Johnson's certification and reporting restrictions on ECT forced the state to put in place many treatment provisions that had previously been lacking. As Johnson put it, anticipating the later credo of the psychiatric consumer movement, if not the survivor movement: "To deprive any citizen of his or her liberty upon the altruistic theory that confinement is for humane and therapeutic reasons and then fail to provide adequate treatment violates the very fundamentals of due process."[40]

In response to these developments, in 1971 Milton Greenblatt, the commissioner for mental health in the State of Massachusetts, approached Frankel. Both were aware that within the Massachusetts Psychiatric Society and in the Massachusetts legislature, there was a strong push to outlaw ECT, just as there was to be shortly afterward in California. Greenblatt decided to step in preemptively, whereas the commissioners in other states did not. He organized a task force to report on the use of ECT in Massachusetts, to be chaired by Frankel. While not averse to ECT, Frankel at this stage was primarily a psychotherapist. Against the advice of many colleagues who felt that this would be detrimental to his career, Frankel accepted the post.

A series of questions needed to be addressed, such as whether ECT was appropriately given to patients with schizophrenia, whether it should be combined with psychotropic drugs, whether it caused memory problems or even brain damage, whether it should be given to children, and more to the point, what techniques and apparatus should be used to deliver ECT. As a psychiatrist who had administered ECT, Frankel supplied the standard advice that memory difficulties may be present following ECT but that they, in general, improved over subsequent weeks and months. He, like others, had had the experience of giving ECT to the conductors of orchestras, to academics, to business people, and to others who came from work on an outpatient basis for ECT, returning to work soon after. Although this was received wisdom, no one knew for certain—through carefully designed and executed randomized, controlled studies—whether some patients might not be affected more profoundly than others.

A potential divide here was emblematic of the times. Psychiatrists saw the dramatic improvements in cognitive function in patients who might one day be sitting mute and stuporous in a chair and the following day were doing crossword puzzles. There seemed little doubt that ECT produced benefits—indeed, cognitive benefits. Patients at home, however, months later, conceivably might suffer subtle deficits of memory function, for example, about which only they could provide leads.

Also controversial was ECT for children. As Greenblatt later said, one of the issues had been a plea from child psychiatrists who "were having confused or disorientated youngsters dumped on them following multiple shocks."[41] ECT for children as young as three or four had been pioneered by Lauretta Bender in New York. In her view, children might experience various symptoms characteristic of the prodromes of schizophrenia, and just as children now will be put on methylphenidate or other stimulant drugs in a manner that may well appear extraordinary in decades to come, children then were treated enthusiastically with ECT by some practitioners.

A questionnaire was devised and sent out to 650 psychiatrists in Massachusetts to map ECT usage in the state. Sixty-six responded. Frankel drew up a committee to analyze the data and help him address the issues.[42] Shortly after the task force convened for the first time, Senator Thomas Eagleton, who had been picked as George McGovern's running mate in his 1972 presidential bid, was reported as having received ECT on two occasions (see chapter 7). Eagleton was forced to stand down as vice presidential nominee. Who knew what it might mean to have a man with his finger on the button who had previously had ECT?[43] With Eagleton's rise and subsequent fall, ECT was in the spotlight as never before.

In the introduction to the subsequent task force report, Frankel indicated that the study had come about because of civil rights pressures in general, the uncertainty about the appropriate use of ECT, and the possible effects of the treatment on memory.[44] The problem for the task force, as for later task forces, was to reconcile differences of opinion in the absence of evidence—because for most of the issues there simply was no evidence. Ultimately, the logic of the data in Massachusetts, where some hospitals were giving ECT more than a hundred times a year to some patients and others were simply not giving ECT at all, forced the committee back to a set of first principles. The key principle was diagnosis: it should drive treatment. They achieved consensus that a diagnosis of severe or psychotic depression might reasonably lead to ECT, even at Massachusetts General, whereas a diagnosis of substance misuse or depressive symptoms in the context of another diagnosis or trauma should not lead to ECT, as they believed was happening frequently in the private hospital system. This was a principle on which all of the task force members could unite, although they disagreed on the question of ECT for schizophrenia, for instance. Following this principle, they reasoned that ECT should be rarely, if ever, used for children.[45]

The second principle that Frankel introduced was that of informed consent. On this matter, one of the replies to his questionnaire stated frankly: "Somebody getting paid for by the public, what right do they have to informed consent?" Informed consent was certainly an issue for Frankel, as he had sat on the committee set up by Henry Beecher in 1966 that attempted to drag informed consent into research, but for many psychiatrists this was the first they had heard of the concept. Few, if any, realized what a strange world they worked in. None seemed to appreciate that psychiatry allowed the committal and detention of patients, while simultaneously depriving them of the kind of rights to which anyone who was criminally committed was entitled. Detention in a mental hospital involved a more comprehensive loss of liberty than committal in the penal system, despite the fact that patients being treated had committed no crime.

Even in the 1960s, psychiatric care involved patients' being told what to do. They took their Thorazine and tranquilizers when told to do so. And in the 1970s there was still no ethical debate about the wisdom of introducing long-acting intramuscular antipsychotics to enforce compliance. It would be another decade before patients won the "right" to refuse antipsychotics.[46] Earlier, patients had typically been sent for lobotomies without being consulted, and they had ECT, perhaps after being informed, but not with an option to refuse.

Following the publication of Frankel's report in 1973, Massachusetts became the first state to issue a set of administrative regulations (as opposed to laws) on ECT. Hospitals within the state were required to report the number of ECT allocations monthly, to strictly follow consent procedures, and to limit the number of treatments a patient could receive each year to thirty-five or fewer. The rules resulted in a 50 percent reduction in the number of patients receiving ECT and an increase in the average age of those receiving it. By 1983, twenty-six out of the fifty states had passed statutes regarding ECT, and regulations of the sort adopted in Massachusetts had been established in six others.

But the critical developments happened in California. In the late 1960s, consent requirements were tightened in the state, and were later reined in even more.[47] In April 1974, State Representative John Vasconcellos introduced a bill, coded AB 4481, imposing a further set of regulations on ECT as part of the Lanterman-Petris-Short Act.[48] This statute required that ECT could be given only after "a) the patient gives written informed consent; b) the patient has the capacity to consent; c) a relative . . . has been given a thorough oral explanation; d) . . . all other treatments have been exhausted and the treatment is critically needed; e) there has been a review by three appointed physicians who agree with the treating physician that the patient has the capacity to consent."[49] AB 4481 was signed into law by Governor Ronald Reagan on September 24, 1974.

Meanwhile from April through December of 1974, NAPA focused media attention on the Langley Porter Neuropsychiatric Institute, a medical center within the University of California, San Francisco. This involved picket line demonstrations, public calls on staff there to engage in debates on ECT, and marches to both Langley Porter and the offices of noted ECT therapists, culminating in a San Francisco Mental Health Advisory Board meeting in January 1975. The major point made by NAPA at this hearing concerned the lack of controlled clinical trial data in support of either the efficacy or safety of ECT.[50]

The constitutionality of AB 4481 was challenged by psychiatrist Gary Aden, and on December 31, 1974, one day before it was due to go into effect, it was suspended. Subsequent action resulted in a modified law, AB 1032, which took effect in 1976, but the original spirit of the law remained, and the result was to severely limit the use of ECT in California. ECT stopped completely in San Francisco. The precedent and the publicity that went with it had a worldwide impact.

"Damn It, I Hate It When They Don't Breathe"

John Pippard worked within the British National Health Service as a psychotherapist for his entire career. His medical experience began in the army in World War II, where he saw ECT delivered for the first time to a young soldier brought into the hospital. The young man lay on the floor with electrodes applied to his head, and when the current button was pressed, his body arched in a full convulsion. For Pippard the experience was both extraordinary and dispiriting.[51] On returning from the war, along with many other soldier-physicians in both the U.S. and the British armies, he turned to psychiatry. Although most people assume medical care is about treating heart attacks and tumors, military service for Pippard and others had opened another window on illness, diagnosis, and treatment. They witnessed a pattern unfolding among many of the soldiers, who denied their illness when granted a leave, but complained adamantly of symptoms with little physical basis when there was no prospect of leave or discharge. In this system, the doctor was a passport to freedom, but one who first needed to be fooled, whether consciously or not. Physicians coming back from the war noticed exactly the same vague and inconsistent symptoms in many of the patients presenting to them, and they began to think in terms of psychosomatic illness. This led many of these physicians to psychiatry, even though the psychiatry of the day was essentially asylum-based.

Although initially repelled by ECT, Pippard came to understand that it delivered results where nothing else could. After the war, he learned to administer unmodified shock treatment without anyone to teach him. When the first report of curare to modify shock treatments appeared, he, along with colleagues, "experimented" with the new approach. Modification made a difference, but it was clear that these new methods required anesthesia. Therefore, Pippard and his colleagues began to give anesthesia—on their own, without anesthetists. So Pippard was by no means hostile to physical treatments, but his experience in the war had led to an appreciation of how psychological factors can color presentations and responses to treatment, even physical treatments. For most of his career, Pippard practiced as a psychotherapist. As he neared retirement in 1979, looking for something else to do, he spotted an advertisement in the *British Journal of Psychiatry* for research on the use of ECT in Britain. The interviewers from the Royal College of Psychiatrists were astonished to find that among the junior doctors they had expected to be interested in the project was this older, recently retired consultant, but Pippard's balanced reasonableness and prior experience with ECT won the day.

What Pippard found was a world in which ECT patients were wheeled into a communal room for treatment, perhaps with curtains between the beds, perhaps not. The anesthetist and a junior doctor delivering the treatment rolled their trolleys through the room, leaving a trail of subdued patients behind them and generating a number of increasingly apprehensive patients ahead of them. These patients witnessed the underbelly of ECT practice, down to anesthetists swearing: "Damn it, I hate it when they don't breathe." If the patient next in line was not frightened at the simple prospect of ECT before coming along to treatment, this kind of scenario was almost designed to induce fear.

This state of affairs is likely to have been the norm for ECT practice in Britain, the United States, and elsewhere from the mid-1950s to mid-1980s, but what did it matter, if the treatment worked? Yet in such a lax environment, the treatment often did not work, because patients were not receiving ECT as it was intended. The junior doctors, who were often primary-care trainees without any formal training in ECT, were commonly called in to press the button after a night on-call. The patient responded with a twitch or a small spasm, and this was taken for a grand mal seizure. Against a background of modified ECT, which was supposed to almost abolish convulsions, the lack of EEG recording facilities on 1980s ECT machines in Britain meant that it took experience to know if the patient actually had had a fit or not. Vignettes like this, indicating that patients might get better on nonexistent ECT, added to a sense of crisis about ECT as a treatment. Did it work, or were people just deluding themselves into thinking it worked?

Pippard concluded that in 40 percent of the British hospitals he visited, he would have been happy to be a patient and receive ECT; in a further 30 percent, the standards were unsatisfactory, and he would only reluctantly have submitted to ECT; in another 30 percent he would, under no account, have agreed to the treatment. He documented problems with obsolete machinery, unsuitable premises, low standards of care, local hospital protocols for ECT that bore little relationship to any science base, and physicians who followed an inner drummer even when the nursing staff clearly told them there were problems.[52] In addition, there was enormous variation in ECT use across the country, with certain hospitals administering it frequently and other hospitals never employing it. Such variation existed even within the same unit: some consultants referred patients often whereas others never did.

The Pippard study highlighted the fact that ECT was the therapy with the greatest variation in all of medicine. At a time when the medical profession was heading into an era of "evidence-based medicine" such disparities seemed insupportable. Either ECT worked, and there should be no hospitals that were "ECT-free zones" and no psychiatrist who would refuse to ever use it; or ECT did not work, and those who were using it enthusiastically needed to have their practices investigated. And to whom were they giving ECT? Was it personality disordered patients? Was it the kind of treatment-resistant depression that manifested in young women in their late teens or early twenties, linked to possible sexual abuse? And if so, did the use of ECT in these circumstances reflect a further abuse?

Pippard's findings led to a working group, which advised on replacement of obsolete ECT equipment. The Royal College of Psychiatrists considered instituting a requirement for training and the appointment of regional advisers on ECT, but in the end decided, just as the APA in the United States had done, that standardization was not called for and that it was the responsibility of individual hospitals to look after their ECT services. Services in Britain did move toward nominating an individual consultant to assume responsibility for ECT and distributing informational booklets for patients. But essentially little else happened.

Following the British lead under Pippard, the APA considered undertaking such an audit, but the feasibility of doing a comparable survey across a range of institutions, private and public, in fifty states seemed too daunting a prospect. Though no audit was ever undertaken, the informal view was that the United States was likely to show even greater variation. Comparing the state of American and British psychiatry around the time of Pippard's survey revealed striking differences. A much higher proportion of British psychiatrists had a recognized qualification in psychiatry, but only 5 percent of them, compared with 50 percent of their American counterparts, worked mainly in private practice. However, 71 percent of American psychiatrists who prescribed ECT administered it themselves, whereas in Britain, this only happened in private practice. In public hospital settings, junior doctors administered the treatment. Twenty-two percent of U.S. psychiatrists were then using ECT, whereas in Britain 45 percent of psychiatrists at least referred patients for ECT.[53]

That there was a perceived need for a comprehensive study of ECT at the national level was evident, as both Sweden and Canada undertook comparable surveys. In Sweden, a questionnaire was sent to seventy-four Swedish hospitals with 100 percent compliance. As in Britain and America, there was a marked variation in the use of ECT from hospital to hospital and consultant to consultant; the most significant difference between Sweden and both Britain and the United States was that in Sweden, three-quarters of the ECT delivered was unilateral.[54]

The Canadian report arose following public controversy surrounding ECT in the province of Ontario. The committee members who wrote it, with one exception, favored continuing the availability of ECT on the basis that banning the treatment for those who freely elect to have it would be equivalent to denying them the opportunity for a better and more useful life. The Canadians also emphasized that informed consent was a prerequisite for treatment; where patients were incompetent to make a decision, there should be impartial procedures in place for determining whether treatment was appropriate or not. The committee encouraged the medical profession to look at the standards of practice for ECT as well as the quality of the machinery and recommended that all ECT outcomes should be reported to a national database, so that variations in practice could be monitored.[55]

For an organization such as the Royal College of Psychiatrists, faced with a report like Pippard's in 1980, the politics were simple. Little needed to be done by the College. The notion of continuing to audit conditions at these institutions was never considered. But Pippard did more than establish the facts of ECT: he helped create the concept of audit. His 1991 follow-up study was a first example of a profession's collecting concrete facts about a particular therapy and setting standards to which practitioners should aspire. He found that his recommendation that ECT be given in a dedicated suite had been implemented. ECT was no longer being carried out on open wards. The general anesthetic and recovery equipment were also broadly speaking up to standard. But he still found that seizures were missed regularly and that no clinic had an EEG facility linked to its ECT machine. Most ECT was still delivered by junior doctors who had no training. He maintained reservations about providing ECT in half of the clinics that he audited, because the machinery could not be depended on to deliver a convulsion reliably, and the medical personnel giving the treatment were untrained and had no idea what to do should things go wrong. Whereas his first report had been cautiously phrased, the second, which was now explicitly an audit, was far more scathing about the failure of practitioners to recognize problems and to institute change.[56] This was not a case of ECT failing the profession, as he saw it, but rather of the profession failing ECT.

Over the period between Pippard's first and second audits, the use of ECT had dropped by a third in Britain. However, there were still huge variations, with some regions having more than halved the ECT they delivered, while others increased the number of treatments. Overall there was a twelvefold variation between the two regions that he looked at. In Greater London, for example, some units used ECT so infrequently that administrative difficulties in getting it done meant that the therapy had been almost completely abandoned by the late 1980s. A third audit in 1996 showed some improvements.[57] Private ECT suites were more common, and the practice of wheeling an ECT machine from one patient to the next had stopped. Most old ECT machines had been replaced, and a slightly higher proportion of senior psychiatrists were involved in clinics. But for the most part ECT was still being given by untrained junior doctors in the absence of any consultant staff.

Memory Wars

As we have seen, from early on complaints about memory problems following ECT had been common. Although these problems had long been recognized, concerns about memory became widespread only during the 1960s. In response, clinicians attributed such problems to the lack of oxygenation that happened in the course of the fit. Anesthetic cover and oxygenation became more common, and concerns over memory deficit were alleviated; patients no longer turned blue in the course of treatment.

With the advancement of Jan-Otto Ottosson's theory that the seizure itself was the therapeutic agent in ECT, clinicians suggested that excess electrical current was responsible for memory problems. This led during the 1970s and 1980s to a widespread replacement of the sine wave machine with an apparatus capable of delivering brief pulses of treatment (see chapter 6). In the late 1980s, under the influence of Harold Sackeim, a professor of psychiatry at Columbia Psychiatric Institute, it became the norm to limit the amount of electricity used to doses only marginally in excess of the seizure threshold (see chapter 10). With these developments, the clinical script changed, and memory problems attributed to ECT were ascribed to the use of old-fashioned machinery delivering excess doses. Still other clinicians argued that the illness itself—depression—was the source of the memory problems. Depression is undoubtedly linked to some memory and concentration problems,[58] but recovered patients found themselves being told by therapists and experts that any lingering memory-related difficulties must be the result of depression expressed in some latent fashion.

A huge range of issues are at play here. Foremost are a patient's concerns about the nature of the material that has been lost. Individuals whose jobs required memory skills and who prior to ECT relied on extensively learned and utilized mnemonic retrieval systems sometimes found that after treatment these systems did not work as reliably and often had to be relearned. Of greater concern to patients, however, was the loss of personal, biographical memories. For example, Diana Rose, the lead author in a review of consumers' perspectives on electroconvulsive therapy, reported taking a vacation with her husband to a place of great significance to both of them, a place they had gone to before, and discovering that she had no memory of things that he told her they had done there previously.[59]

One of the most vivid descriptions of the phenomenon was given by Anne Donahue from Vermont, later a congressional representative for the state, in 2000.[60] Donahue described how she was given thirty-three treatments in the fall of 1995 and spring of 1996, which she credits with saving her life, but how as the weeks went by after treatment, she found ever more areas of her life affected by memory loss. She had complete recollection in some areas of her life, total loss in others, and suspected she had created memories through external information in yet other areas. She reported enduring memory loss for events as significant as hosting Mother Theresa for a day in 1989 and sitting beside Colin Powell while they both received the National Jefferson Award in 1990, and the loss of events like these led her to lament the "aura of dishonesty" about this side effect. This article appeared twenty-five years after the memory wars kicked off.

On September 9, 1974, the *New Yorker* magazine featured a piece titled "As Empty as Eve" by Berton Roueché.[61] The article presented the case of Marilyn Rice, under the pseudonym Natalie Parker, a forty-four-year-old economist in the U.S. Department of Commerce who, in June 1972, had been referred to an orthodontist to get her front teeth straightened. Her treatment went wrong, and she became depressed. She was prescribed an antidepressant, which did not suit her, and she was then hospitalized. She was keen to have psychotherapy, but when ECT was raised, she refused it and dismissed her doctor, John Nardini (an electrotherapist at NIMH). Her new doctor, Peter Mendelis, when learning that she was the financial supporter of her artist-husband, argued that psychotherapy, being a long-term and expensive option, was not the appropriate treatment for her and that ECT would be a better bet, and she was referred back to Dr. Nardini for the therapy. She was told there might be a temporary loss of memory, but that, except for the period just prior to and immediately after the shocks were delivered, it would return fully in about three weeks. As she recounts her story, the memories did return, but it was her memories of things that she did not want to remember that returned first. In July 1973, she went back to work, and it was then she became aware of the real problems with her memory. "I could feel. I felt as if I could think. But the fuel of thinking wasn't there. And it didn't come back."[62]

By September, she submitted a disability application. In February 1974, she filed a malpractice complaint against the treating psychiatrist.[63] In answer to questions related to the case, Rice stated: "I have lost the vast edifice of specialized knowledge that I had been adding to almost every day of my adult life. I've lost the pride and self-confidence, and income that go with being an expert in one's field. I've lost the intellectual joy of utilizing my mental capital. I've lost my value to society in that the work in which I was engaged was dependent on my unique assemblage of knowledge. I've lost much of my general education. I've lost personal memories that I would never willingly have

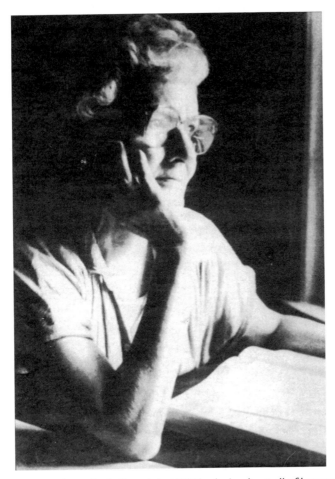

Marilyn Rice, a patient who believed that ECT had wiped out all of her memories; she became an iconic figure in the anti-ECT movement. *San Francisco Bay Guardian,* April 18, 1990.

given up—people I have met, places I have been, books I have read, plays I have seen."

She was asked: "What was your area?" Her reply:

Mine was to pull everybody else's together. . . . In the twenty some years I had been there I had worked on a number of areas. . . . I had the broadest knowledge. Any one person working on a particular thing knew more about that thing than I did, but I knew the connections between the work of the various individuals. . . . I had worked on the federal government, personal income, consumer expenditures, savings and investments, input, output analysis. . . . I was working on an investigation of the structure of the security industry and how we used statistics concerning security transactions in our estimates of corporate profits. . . . Nobody [is working in my position now]. This is not nice for my office. One of the chiefs, when I was telling him the situation in the summer said "but you're the only one who has the knowledge and the patience" and I said "what I am trying to tell you is, where I had that knowledge I have just a great big blank."

After a twelve-day trial in January 1977, a Washington, D.C., jury decided Rice's suit in favor of John Nardini. Rice went on to found the Committee for Truth in Psychiatry (CTIP), whose mission was to campaign for proper informed consent regarding ECT. Following Rice's death in 1992, Linda Andre became the most active force in CTIP.[64] Andre had been given ECT in her twenties and claimed that her cognitive function had been severely compromised as a result.

An unbroken series of verdicts against patients and in favor of the treating doctor followed for the next twenty-five years. Then in 2005, *Salters v. Palmetto Health Alliance, Inc.* hit the headlines.[65] Peggy Salters, a former nurse, was successfully treated for depression with ECT but was maintained on a further course of daily treatments delivered on an outpatient basis. Memory difficulties plagued her, and she took legal action. The resulting verdict in her favor was hailed by critics as a first-ever verdict against ECT. This verdict was extraordinary in a number of respects. It was returned against her referring doctor rather than the doctors who administered ECT, and it appears to have been primarily motivated by jury concerns that a woman as actively suicidal as Salters should not have been receiving daily ECT on an outpatient basis. For many Americans in the early years of the twenty-first century, managed-care systems made it effectively impossible to hospitalize patients like Salters for treatment.

Rice, Andre, and Salters had engaged Peter Breggin, a former student of Thomas Szasz, as a psychiatric expert in their cases. Based on his involvement in Rice's case, and as an invited critic of ECT to the APA Task Force, Breggin wrote a book on the brain-disabling effects of ECT, which articulated the emerging battleground.[66] ECT caused brain damage, not just as a side effect, but as its core mode of action. If patients were properly informed of this, its use in clinical psychiatry would come to an end. To be sure, Breggin loudly and widely took this message to the streets.

From Fear to Damage

The mechanism of ECT's therapeutic effect is still not fully understood. But the first theories of what happened in ECT were psychoanalytic. These focused on the convulsion, and the mental confusion and amnesia following ECT, as manifestations of the repressive process;[67] as such ECT was almost antithetical to psychoanalysis[68] (see chapter 5). But some psychoanalysts were prepared to see the tonic-clonic movements of a convulsion as expression of in utero movements, indicating a literal regression to the fetal level of functioning. Some even could see in the gasping of breath, in the sucking movements, or in occasional fecal smearing following ECT, the stages of Freudian psychosexual development and posited that Oedipal conflicts had been reactivated. Against this background, the real therapeutic agent was the quality of the relationship the patient had with his or her therapist or primary caregiver.[69] ECT was the mother, in the sense of an agent of rebirth, as another theory put it.[70]

Behaviorism, a school of thought in psychology advanced by John B. Watson, B. F. Skinner, and others, had its own theories about ECT.[71] Noting the level of fear that treatment could induce in patients, they argued that this was the effective therapeutic agent.[72] This may well have seemed to be the case when Metrazol was used to induce convulsions rather than ECT. However, deliberate attempts to induce fear without convulsions or to verify that the element of fear corresponded to the degree of improvement afterward proved negative.[73] An analytic variation on the fear hypothesis was that ECT was seen as a punishment, which when undergone allowed atonement and delivery from evil.[74]

Behaviorists also recognized that electroconvulsive shock (ECS) delivered to animals was a new tool with which to explore behavior through their stimulus-response paradigm.[75] This research generated an interest in learning and memory, and theories based on fear were put aside.[76] The expectation was that memory loss was greatest for the period immediately prior to ECT; extrapolating to humans, the memories most likely to be forgotten arose in periods of greatest psychosis. One possibility was that patients actually learned a protective amnesia, as opposed to having amnesia directly caused by the treatment.[77] Taking this notion one step further led to the idea of using ECT for depatterning, or what was later termed regressive ECT (see chapter 6).[78] This involved giving ECT at a rate of one or more treatments per day until patients became totally amnesic, confused, and even doubly incontinent. As they recovered, new and more appropriate patterns of behavior could be instituted.

Another concept postulated by the behaviorist school was the competing-response theory. According to this hypothesis, the coma following the seizure produces a protective inhibition, and this becomes conditioned to surrounding stimuli. If this theory is correct, ECS given at the same location as the original learning took place should not disrupt learning as much as treatment given in dissimilar situations. Learning here is assumed to involve a neural consolidation process in which the formation of new memories occurs through the conversion of temporary memory traces into a more permanent form. ECS appeared to interrupt this process, leading to a retroactive or retrograde amnesia.[79] But efforts to test this premise in animals have produced some surprises. ECS, it appears, can lead to a proactive effect: material learned after treatment is stored better than would ordinarily be the case.[80] Moreover, in 1954, Joseph Brady, a leading behavioral psychologist, and his colleagues showed that material that had been learned before ECT, and which was apparently lost following the treatment, could sometimes be recovered. This finding caused problems not just for many theories about ECT but for theories of memory in general at that time.[81]

A completely different set of proposals about the mechanism of ECT became the focus of controversy in the 1970s and 1980s. In the 1950s, Max Fink and others outlined a series of organic changes following ECT. Fink's theory of the mechanism of action of ECT was a neurophysiologic-adaptive view that stemmed from studies of the interaction of brain function, personality research, and the use of barbiturates in patients with cerebral damage put forward by Edwin Weinstein and Robert Kahn.[82] After ECT, there was evidence that EEG slow-wave activity increases with each seizure, and these EEG changes persist during the interseizure periods. This is a signature for an organic change state: patterns of neural activity have been altered as a result of convulsion. One way to interpret this is that the brain has been traumatized, but this view is not necessarily correct. The intriguing thing about the EEG response for Fink was that the effect could be inhibited by anticholinergic drugs, such as scopolamine or procyclidine, and enhanced by

barbiturates. Anticholinergic drugs block the action of the neurotransmitter acetylcholine and are not thought to either cause or reverse
brain damage. Similarly barbiturates, which act as central nervous system depressants, do not aggravate or ameliorate brain damage.

What Fink described were some of first efforts to map the effects
of both psychotropic drugs and ECT on the electroencephalograph,
which is a quantitative surface recording of overall patterns of brain
activity.[83] All physical treatments, including the antipsychotics and antidepressants, turn out to have an EEG signature, or as it might otherwise be put, a distinctive set of organic changes. The organic effects
of antidepressants on the EEG can, in fact, be demonstrated several
months after the last intake of drug. But as EEGs have been replaced
by brain scanning techniques, there has been an almost complete loss
of awareness of this fact. Brain scans do not reveal the effect and thus
ignore an important measure of overall electrical activity apparent
across the surface of the brain.

There is a world of rhetorical difference between ECT-induced organic changes and ECT-induced brain damage, but these early findings
showing organic changes in patients after ECT[84] were later put forward
as evidence of brain damage.[85] Another feature of both organic changes
and brain damage can be denial of illness. In the hands of ECT critics
in the 1980s, the fact that patients might deny the existence or extent
of their problems became, in its own right, an indicator of brain damage in the person treated. The bottom line was that consent to treatment could never be informed. Breggin's 1979 book on ECT introduced
the claim that it was a brain-disabling treatment comparable to the effects of lobotomy (which is self-evidently brain damaging), referring to
ECT as electro-lobotomy. He and other critics argued that authorities
on ECT, such as Lothar Kalinowsky and later Max Fink, quite openly
and frankly conceded the damage caused by ECT in a more innocent
time, the 1950s, but following the criticism of ECT in the 1970s, these
same authorities became more guarded in their language. This new
guardedness was portrayed as evidence that the advocates of ECT and
professional organizations such as APA were conspiring to defend the
treatment against its critics.

Strictly following the brain-disabling hypothesis would mean elimi-
nating not only ECT but also antidepressants, tranquilizers, and antipsychotics, for each of these agents causes changes in the brain.
Although many critics of psychiatry would readily throw out the pharmaceuticals along with ECT, that position, taken one step further but

with the same logic, would mean that alcohol, tea, and coffee should be restricted as well. In their more pragmatic moments, most people who think that brain disabling does not sound like a good idea, when presented in the abstract, concede that they readily seek disablement at moments of crisis. Ironically, a good case can be made that the entire consciousness-altering movement of the 1960s, which did so much to fuel antipsychiatry, explicitly aimed at brain disablement, whether for oblivion or enlightenment. However, the idea that we should be in the business of providing humanistic rather than brain-disabling treatments is a powerful rhetorical position to take, and one that retains force even when the inconsistencies are pointed out.

Compared with ECT, where no neurological sequelae to treatment can be demonstrated, antipsychotic drug treatment can readily be shown to produce neurological syndromes such as Parkinsonism, dystonias, or dyskinesias, and patients not infrequently develop permanent neurological syndromes such as tardive dyskinesia. Indeed, brain scan research shows that one dose of an antipsychotic can alter the brain forever. It is almost certainly the case that the SSRI group of drugs, for example, can inhibit growth in children, reduce bone density, and cause bleeding into the gut, womb, skin, and brain. This risk is greatly increased when the SSRIs are combined with commonly used drugs such as aspirin or other anti-inflammatory agents. There is evidence that SSRIs, and probably antipsychotics also, can cause testicular shrinkage, which in the case of pubertal boys is clearly not inconsequential. Compared with ECT, these drugs act on all bodily systems and leave a trail of significant and permanent organic changes behind them.

But a major difference between Prozac and Zoloft compared with ECT is that these drugs come with the stamp of familiarity, whereas ECT for most people is quite alien. ECT is treated as a stranger; Prozac is treated as a neighbor. A critique of brain disablement works well when the treatment is one that the public is not familiar with, but it would have much less impact if it was centered on a treatment like Prozac, which people feel comfortable with. There are hazards associated with Prozac, but rightly or wrongly, we feel we can get these into perspective and thus continue to support its widespread use. This point goes directly to the question of consent. Early studies on informed consent by Louis Lasagna demonstrated that volunteers in a trial of a new drug, when presented with a list of side effects, would frequently decide to withhold consent. But when later informed that these were the side effects of aspirin, their willingness to take aspirin remained unchanged.[86]

A further angle on the conspiracy theories, and one reason to write history, is that meanings change. It is simply not possible now, for instance, for most people to read works of early-nineteenth-century psychiatrists and understand them the way they were written: a word like *neurosis* has changed its meaning completely, so that it now indicates quite the opposite of what it once meant. Typically, clinicians and others coming into the field, when they read old literature and are perhaps not sympathetic to the points being made, fail to appreciate that the material cannot be taken at face value.

In much the same way, the early use of the antipsychotic group of drugs, such as chlorpromazine, was accompanied by statements from its proponents that it offered, in effect, a chemical lobotomy. These efforts to describe the drug's effects were made by practitioners not operating in contested situations. They were comfortable with the idea that medicine often involves a trade-off between effects that may counterbalance (rather than cure) the changes brought about by an underlying illness. This was a generation of clinicians who infected patients with malaria to cure neurosyphilis, who collapsed a lung to control tuberculosis, or removed most of a stomach in order to treat ulcers. For them, trade-offs of this sort were the medical norm. There was no pressure to believe that antipsychotics represented a true cure for the disorders for which they were being used—only that they improved a patient's quality of life to a degree. The pressure to provide cures without consequences emerged in the 1970s and 1980s and was arguably less rational and more mythical than the earlier view of what these drugs did.

What occurred was a shift in thinking comparable to others in the course of history. In the West, cultivated gardens were once viewed as the pinnacle of natural beauty, and wilderness was seen as ugly and something to be tamed. With a change in our collective consciousness, prompted by Romanticism, we now see wilderness in all its wildness as beautiful. Similarly, we have also seen a cultural shift in medicine from an emphasis on the heroic effort to fight the scourge of disease to a view that is more likely to accentuate the wisdom of the body and to extol efforts to work in concert with it—a more Romantic view of medicine, perhaps. And although this approach has its place, it can stand in the way of practical thinking about devastating illness. Romance is fine for spring breezes, but not so good for hurricanes.

Ironically, one of the best symbols of the shifting terrain lies in *One Flew over the Cuckoo's Nest,* the book that later caused ECT so many problems. Kesey's idea for the book came from his work as a night orderly at a VA hospital, but the inspiration came from the world of diverse mental states he encountered in Leo Hollister's experiments with psychedelic drugs.[87] Kesey seems to have viewed ECT as not dissimilar to LSD—another means to alter consciousness. In a way that will seem scarcely credible to an ECT "survivor" or to those whose views of ECT have been shaped by *One Flew over the Cuckoo's Nest,* before writing the ECT scenes in the book, Kesey had a friend rig up an electrical apparatus at home, aimed at delivering a convulsion, and "took a treatment" to explore what was involved.[88]

But Why Memory?

This is a history, not a chapter in a task force report, and hence it is not our goal to establish whether ECT causes memory problems beyond the relatively short-term difficulties that everyone agrees can arise for some people immediately after treatment. But memory losses following treatment emerged as a concern thirty years after ECT had been introduced into medicine. It became one of the central battlegrounds in psychiatry, and an important question for us is to consider why this was the case.

The first point is that the problems that may exist with ECT have been tremendously difficult to bring into focus. Harold Sackeim, after twenty years of research and with more funding than anyone else to look at this issue as well as the resources of Columbia's Psychiatric Institute to support him, has effectively been reduced to saying: many of us think there are problems, but I cannot be more specific than this.[89] The difficulties in assessment stem from many sources. Given the severity of the problems that lead people to ECT, it is likely that they will have been prescribed pharmacological treatment, such as benzodiazepines, in the course of their clinical encounters. Drugs are routinely given in conjunction with ECT, and during ECT itself anesthesia is used.

One of the best established facts in the domain of biological treatments and memory concerns the impact of the benzodiazepines (such as Valium) and barbiturates on anterograde amnesia—that is for memories of events that occur to individuals forward from the time treatment ensues. Classic examples involve people who have taken a pill, perhaps to alleviate the anxiety of air travel, who on arriving at their destination will meet familiar people and then the following day have no recollection of the meeting. This is a phenomenon comparable to alcoholic blackouts. If people have been on benzodiazepines for weeks or months prior to ECT, there is every chance that memories during this entire period will not have been converted for long-term storage. Some individuals are particularly sensitive to these effects and suffer losses of memory for highly significant personal events on what are relatively small amounts of benzodiazepine. Furthermore, almost any investigation of patients receiving anesthesia for surgery will uncover evidence of memory problems linked to the anesthesia. It is not uncommon for patients to report memory problems after ECT, but when probed, such problems are little to no different from the memory problems experienced after anesthesia for other purposes.

And there are a host of other vagaries connected with autobiographical memory, about which we understand very little. One of the best examples can be found in Timothy Garton-Ash's book *The File*, published in 1998.[90] Garton-Ash was a journalist working in Eastern Europe before the fall of the Berlin Wall, tracking the rise of social movements like Solidarity in Poland. In East Germany, where he lived for a considerable period of time, the secret police, or Stasi, kept a close watch on him. As did so many others following the collapse of the East German state, Garton-Ash had the opportunity to look at his own file. A great deal of the drama in his book lies in what he discovered about himself. The Stasi had recorded, for instance, an affair that he had had with an East German woman that he had completely forgotten about. Researching the history of ECT or psychopharmacology, it has been common to find that senior figures, when presented with programs for meetings they attended twenty, thirty, or forty years previously, may have no recollection of these gatherings.

This goes to the heart of what memory is. Great debates persist about whether memory involves the retrieval of almost photographic records of events laid down, in which case the inability to retrieve such events points to the destruction of some archive or the physical degradation of its contents. The alternate view is that memory is a much more constructive process and that the events we retrieve are constructions rather than videotapes of the past. A great deal of research now suggests that these constructions may be open to considerable distortion, and we may, for instance, remember abuse that never happened, as the work of Elizabeth Loftus demonstrates.[91] In fact it seems relatively easy to construct memories in this way, and memories of abuse, constructed or real, have been close to psychiatry's dominant theme for the past century. Memories, constructed or not, are absolutely central to psychotherapy. The question of memory then is not simply a matter of some cognitive function that may or may not be affected by treatment. We live in a period where for various reasons memory is seen as the critical human faculty, the thing that makes us human, and it has a centrality it did not have before. This centrality has been shaped by a variety of forces, and a treatment that might degrade our memories verges on something that is considered a last resort treatment, especially for patients who expect a more psychotherapeutic approach to their disorder.

In addition to treating diseases that at the severe end of the spectrum can seem like categorical disorders, such as obsessive-compulsive disorder, psychotic depression, and schizophrenia, psychiatry cannot avoid personality variations. Huge components of our personalities and our habitual modes of responding have little to do with any memories we may have. It is unquestionably true that many individuals remain very clearly and recognizably themselves even in the face of gross memory difficulties. But these dispositional aspects to personality are not now the focus of our funded research or cultural attention, aside from the occasional debate as to whether it would be a good thing if we were all contented extraverts, managed by Prozac.[92] There is little emphasis on the upbringing of children aimed at managing their dispositions, as there has been in previous eras. For whatever reason, a premium has been placed on memory; this problematizes difficulties in the realm of memory to a greater extent than might have happened in other eras. The question of problems with memory that ECT exposes needs to be seen against this background.

Consider the cognitive consequences of coronary artery bypass surgery.[93] When open-heart surgery began during the late 1950s and early 1960s, many patients postoperatively were left clearly confused. This confusion could extend for weeks or months, and was commonly termed a postoperative psychosis (but according to post-1980s diagnostic nomenclature, this term is inappropriate).[94] The rate of cognitive difficulty following cardiosurgery was considerable, and greatly in excess of that linked to ECT. It was well understood by physicians and other health-care staff that cognitive problems were an accepted feature of such operations, but patients were rarely informed of this. The official explanations given for these postsurgical problems parallel those given for the cognitive problems following ECT. Such patients were often labeled as being depressed, and any cognitive deficits were explained as postoperative depression. However, when efforts were made to control for this by testing cognitive function and levels of depression before and after surgery, it became clear that levels of depression were greater before surgery, while the cognitive problems were quite clearly greater after surgery.[95]

Settling the issue of depression did not prompt surgeons to accept that the surgery or anesthesia was at the root of the problem. An alternative hypothesis was that the cardiovascular difficulties that gave rise to full-blown heart disease affected the entire system, including the blood vessels to the brain, leading to an incipient brain failure in addition to coronary infarction; this, according to the surgeons, was reflected in postoperative confusion. Factors such as this may have played some part, but clearly there appears to be a dynamic at work here in which the proponents of any treatment—whether surgeons treating heart disease, psychiatrists delivering ECT, psychotherapists offering hypnosis, or pharmacologists prescribing SSRIs—are slow to see the harm they are doing or slow to accept any responsibility for that harm.

More to the point, however, is that these problems with cardiac surgery were to some extent swept beneath the carpet, even though many of those suffering were medical professionals with access to the means to investigate the problem. The fact that no one has attempted to ban cardiac surgery speaks volumes about a systematic bolstering of cardiosurgery as a treatment option. The typical cardiac patient is white, middle class, and advantaged, but for the most part those receiving ECT, at least within the United States, are of a similar profile—of European ancestry treated in private hospitals.

But research from the patient point of view on the efficacy and side effects of ECT brings to light issues that are important for all of health care. In 2003, the *Lancet* carried a review of the efficacy of ECT, which concluded that it was more effective than drug treatment for depression.[96] The patients' organization, Mind, objected, not so much to the findings as to the one-sidedness of the evidence reviewed.[97] Soon after, a review of patient views of the efficacy of ECT and the problems it might leave in its wake appeared.[98] This demonstrated a divide between clinician and patient perceptions. The recipients of treatment were much less likely to view it as efficacious some months later and were more aware of ongoing cognitive problems than were the physicians. Who was right?

The key question is probably not who was right, but rather should the recipients of a treatment have a place at the research table, deciding the direction and process of medical science? And if that is the question, there can only be one answer. It has been clear for well over a decade that what psychiatry and medicine need is research directly involving the patient population.[99] Some patients experience enduring problems after ECT, but compared with postcardiac complications, these effects are subtle. Only patient involvement is likely to sort out the resultant memory deficits after anesthetic treatment in general from those specific to ECT, and determine whether concomitant drug intake during ECT has contributed to the problem.

But more generally, health care may be driven by arguments made by surgeons, physicians, and psychiatrists for treatments that appear to them to work, where a consideration of the outcomes enjoyed or suffered by the recipients of surgical or medical enthusiasm might lead to a different set of investments. Although ECT appears less effective when judged by patients, it nevertheless still appears effective; by contrast, on patient-rated quality of life scales, the SSRI group of drugs, including Prozac, Paxil, and Zoloft, cannot be shown to work.[100] In the case of ECT research, there is no evidence that research has been suppressed, whereas in psychopharmacological research there is abundant evidence that patient ratings have simply not been published.[101]

Good health care almost self-evidently needs good research from both perspectives. As things stand at present within psychiatry, many of the "survivor" movements set up in the 1970s have been deflected from their original mission, but they have probably not been subverted by federal funding—inadvertently or otherwise—into consumer groups, as was once argued, so much as they have been penetrated by pharmaceutical company funding. Where they have been resistant to industry funding, the companies have bypassed them and set up their own patient groups to lobby for reimbursement and media access. When problems happen, companies can parade the representatives of their patient groups in front of FDA panels or at other hearings. This at least does not happen with ECT, whose critics remain passionate, but whose advocates are also distinguished and independent and include deans of Ivy League colleges,[102] leading surgeons who claim they would never have had a career had they not received ECT,[103] and even psychologists who found their preconceptions confounded by successful treatment.[104]

CHAPTER TEN

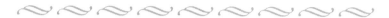

Electrogirl and the New ECT

I n 1965, a patient identified in the court records as "W.S." was hospitalized in 1965 at the Veterans Administration Hospital in Lyons, New Jersey, as dangerous to himself and others. Twelve years later, he experienced a severe exacerbation of his psychosis but did not respond to aggressive courses of antipsychotic drugs, and in fact, he became worse under chemical treatment. W.S. agreed to ECT to "chase the voices away," but the hospital administration deemed him incompetent to give consent, and on May 12, 1977, requested a hearing on his behalf. By then, the patient was on round-the-clock, one-to-one supervision and had assaulted other patients and staff. ECT was recommended, but, without his consent, was he nonetheless entitled to receive it? Four days later, on May 16, a hearing was convened at the hospital. A host of people were present, including the assistant deputy public advocate representing W.S., two attorneys for the VA, an attorney for Essex County (where the hospital was located), a judge from the county juvenile and domestic relations court, the patient, his parents, an independent psychiatrist for W.S. chosen by his lawyer, the hospital's chief of psychiatry, and a court stenographer. The court ruled in favor of treating W.S. with ECT.[1]

By the late 1970s, ECT had been transformed from a routine medical procedure, administered as matter-of-factly as penicillin, to a fearsome last-ditch remedy to be used only under extraordinary conditions and under the most elaborate legal safeguards. A lifesaving procedure once accessible to outpatients was available only to patients behind institutional walls for desperate emergencies. Only an outright legislative ban could have made ECT less accessible than these well-meaning but preposterous restrictions. Before long, the procedure would become a historical footnote to twentieth-century medicine.

Then ECT experienced a revival. By the advent of the twenty-first century, convulsive therapy passed from a highly stigmatized procedure obtainable only in extreme circumstances to a helpful treatment available as a matter of course in many centers, and no more alarming to many patients than the trip to the dentist with which English researchers had once compared it. The rate of ECT use in the Medicare population increased from 4.2 per 10,000 beneficiaries in 1987 to 5.1 in 1992.[2] During this period, psychiatric hospitals began offering ECT services once more, though a 1988 poll by the American Psychiatric Association determined that it was still not available in one-third of American cities.[3] Rockland State in Orangeburg, New York—now called Rockland Psychiatric Center—restored ECT in 2000. Srinivasa Reddy, director of convulsive therapy there, noted a changed attitude among the patients: "What I have observed is that some people really take ECT over the medications and they prefer their family members also take ECT."[4]

"Treatment-Resistant" Cases

In 2003, the *Journal of the American Academy of Physician Assistants* ran an article on "treatment-resistant depression." The article was sixteen pages long and showed a complicated treatment "algorithm" (what to do if your patients do not respond to the first drug) that heavily featured the SSRI (Prozac-style) drug class at every turn. The advice to the assistants was, in short, if your patients do not respond to Prozac, give them Zoloft. ECT was not part of the algorithm at all, yet a brief paragraph at the end of the piece mentioned convulsive therapy, calling it "the most effective treatment of depression."[5] No doubt the nation's many physician assistants would have paged right by this loaded paragraph because ECT was simply not on their radar.

Although ECT did not exist as a treatment option for physician assistants in the United States, it continued to flash on the scope for most psychiatrists, precisely because of the problem of treatment-resistant depression. In the face of legislative restrictions or psychopharmacologic skepticism, this one circumstance kept ECT alive. It was the realization that the new drugs did not work for many patients, and only convulsive therapy could produce clinical results in this population. If the drugs had been as successful as the psychopharmacologists first believed, there would have been no need for ECT. But they were not. On the whole, perhaps a third of all patients treated with antidepressants and antipsychotics failed to get better. There are several reasons for nonresponsiveness in these patients: the drugs simply did not work, patients prematurely discontinued the drugs on account of side effects, or the diagnosis was incorrect (for example, treating psychotic depression with drugs better suited for nonpsychotic depression). It was the phenomenon of nonresponsiveness that launched the revival of ECT, yet this time around, it was a last-choice treatment.

Historically, the first recognition of a special population of psychotic patients nonresponsive to medication was East German psychiatrist Karl Leonhard's distinction between "systematic" and "nonsystematic" schizophrenias. It was a distinction he had long worked out, but he offered it to the public as a massive scholarly synthesis only as he took the psychiatry chair at the Charité Hospital in East Berlin in 1957.[6] "Systematic" for Leonhard meant that only a single neuronal system was affected, but badly so, worsening the impact on the brain; these patients had a poor prognosis and were typically unresponsive to treatment. The nonsystematic schizophrenias, on the other hand, displayed a variety of symptoms that might change often (in contrast to the starkly etched symptom picture of the systematic variety); the nonsystematic patients were treatable and had better prognoses. The differential responsiveness of the Leonhard diagnoses to ECT has never been studied. Yet it was Leonhard and his followers who inserted into psychiatry the notion that there were well-defined groups of patients whose treatment-responsiveness might differ.

Leonhard's ideas were published on the cusp of the pharmacological revolution in psychiatry, and it was only with the first drug trials that Christian Astrup at Gaustad Hospital in Oslo, using a modified version of Leonhard's diagnostic scheme in 1959, discovered large differences in responsiveness. Among the 185 chronic schizophrenic patients whom he treated with chlorpromazine, those with symptoms of Leonhard's nonsystematic psychoses responded well: forty of forty-eight of those with "slight paranoid defects" improved; among those with "periodic catatonias," ten of sixteen improved. By contrast, few of Astrup's "systematic" schizophrenics responded to medication: of sixty-seven patients with "systematic catatonias," none did well; of thirty-one patients with "hebephrenic defects," only three showed considerable improvement.[7] Clearly, those categories individuated well-defined groups of schizophrenics who were differentially responsive to medication.

Five years later, in 1964, Frank Fish, then at the University of Edinburgh, analyzed the same group he had studied with Astrup in 1959, plus a few more patients. This time, Fish used actual Leonhard categories. Of 285 chronic schizophrenics, those with nonsystematic illness responded well to phenothiazines: 84 percent of those with "affect-laden paraphrenia" showed considerable improvement, as did 78 percent of those with "cataphasia" (both major Leonhard diagnoses). Those with "systematic schizophrenia" responded poorly: of the 107 patients with "systematic catatonia," none showed considerable improvement; results for the other two systematic categories were only slightly more favorable.[8] These findings are important because they showed that the drug-treatment responders in schizophrenia could be predicted. Yet Fish and Astrup's work also pointed clearly to entire groups unresponsive to medication, which might, perhaps, do well with other treatments.

Astrup's and Fish's research remained almost entirely unknown in the United States and had little impact in Europe. Kurt Witton, an émigré psychiatrist at the VA hospital in Fort Meade, South Dakota, found in 1962 that ECT produced a striking improvement in the thought processes of patients who had done poorly on neuroleptic drugs: "I have noted that in many cases refractory to drugs but following a rather prolonged use of phenothiazine derivatives a series of ECT (usually 20 treatments) will obtain a striking unexpected improvement or remission of the active psychotic, mainly schizophrenic, process."[9]

What characterized the psychotic patients who didn't respond to drugs? Since the late 1950s, Fritz Flügel at the University of Erlangen in Germany, and students of his such as Turan Itil, had been interested in the notion of treatment-resistant psychoses. Max Fink knew Itil through his work with the electroencephalograph, and when Fink became director of the Missouri Psychiatric Institute in 1962, he invited Itil to come over from Erlangen. In 1966 Itil, Ali Keskiner, and Fink attempted to define the characteristics of "therapy-resistant" schizophrenia. Of thirty female patients who had failed to respond to the customary phenothiazines, they treated twenty-two with a phenothiazine marketed as Repoise (butaperazine) and maintained eight on the customary phenothiazines. Thirty-two percent of the butaperazine patients and 25 percent of the controls responded well enough to be discharged.[10] The trial is important not because it highlighted the wonders of butaperazine but because it got Max Fink asking questions. When Fink returned to New York, he once again became interested in ECT and wondered whether it was effective in such nonresponsive patients. "What were we to do with persistently psychotic, manic, and depressed patients that required so much attention?" he later asked. "For some practitioners with experience in ECT, the answer was to recall its use."[11]

Meanwhile, treatment-resistant depression was also being documented. In 1965, Ole Bratfos and John Otto Haug at the university psychiatric clinic in Oslo discovered that ECT was an effective treatment for those who did not respond to antidepressant drugs. In the years 1952 to 1957, before the arrival of the tricyclic antidepressants, they had treated their manic-depressive patients with ECT. Of those 127 patients, 61 percent were discharged as recovered. Yet from 1958 to 1963, of the 170 patients treated with antidepressants, only 25 percent were discharged as recovered. The drug nonresponders in this group were then treated with ECT: 56 percent of them were subsequently discharged as recovered. The relapse rate for the ECT-responders and the antidepressant-responders was about the same.[12] A large group of depressed patients was clearly unresponsive to psychopharmacology. As Georgia psychiatrist Corbett Thigpen observed in 1963, "Frankly, I have not been greatly impressed with either tranquilizers [phenothiazines] or anti-depressant drugs in private practice. Only occasionally do these drugs seem to help. As a rule, acutely disturbed patients . . . must be hospitalized and/or given electroconvulsive therapy."[13]

In 1975, just as ECT was being phased out in most hospitals, Alexander Glassman at the New York State Psychiatric Institute acknowledged that most patients with psychotic depression who were unresponsive to antidepressants did well on ECT. Glassman studied blood levels of the tricyclic antidepressant imipramine (Tofranil) to determine whether patients with high blood levels had a better clinical outcome. As he reviewed the patients who were not getting better on imipramine, he realized that most of them had psychotic thinking. Psychotic depression is not clinically unusual; about a third of the inpatients on a depression service are so depressed that they experience delusional thinking and suicidal ideation. Wanting to do something for them, Glassman put them on ECT—and they rapidly improved.[14] (This was the beginning of the realization that psychotic depression might be a separate disease from other kinds of depression.) Glassman commented later: "There are clearly people who don't get better with drugs but do get better with ECT. There may be a few examples of patients who don't get better with ECT, and do get better with some crazy combination of drugs, but there are not many."[15]

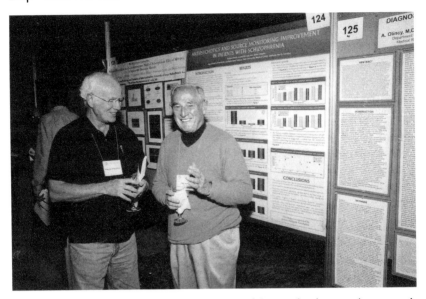

Alexander Glassman and Max Fink at a meeting of the psychopharmacology organization CINP in 2003. In 1975 Glassman, a psychiatrist at Columbia University, put the spotlight on psychotic depression as highly responsive to ECT. Courtesy of Max Fink.

Thus, treatment unresponsiveness became widely noted among both schizophrenic and depressive populations. In 1984, a scholarly journal asked Rich Weiner at Duke University to prepare a major article on memory and ECT, then invited a number of authorities to comment, in effect creating a kind of "symposium" on ECT. At the time, the air was thick with talk about the neuroleptics and antidepressants failing to make patients better and causing forbidding side effects. In the symposium, Conrad Swartz, in the department of psychiatry of the Chicago Medical School, noted that the "tranquilization" of the neuroleptics "blunts fine details of personality, including initiative, emotional reactivity, enthusiasm, sexiness, alertness, and insight. Such effects would render most professionals ineffective." In indications such as psychotic depression and manic agitation, he said, ECT offered a plausible alternative.[16] Trevor Price, a psychiatrist at Dartmouth Medical School in Hanover, New Hampshire, told the symposium that "a *very* substantial proportion, ranging from 50–90% of medication-resistant depressed patients, respond well to ECT." This was especially true of those with delusional symptoms: "For the majority of patients ECT achieves dramatic clinical improvement with otherwise treatment-refractory and often profoundly disabling affective illnesses."[17]

Indeed, as the years passed, clinicians' awareness of nonresponsiveness grew ever greater. In 2004, a group of researchers at the RAND Corporation in Santa Monica, California, found that fully half of patients in primary care with a diagnosis of depression remained depressed after two courses of drug treatment.[18] The authors did not comment on ECT, but statistics such as these grab physicians' attention: what options could they offer to this half of the patient population? It was against this background of rising consciousness of patients' nonresponsiveness to pharmacotherapy that the road was reopened for ECT.

The Road Back Begins

The revival of ECT occurred via two routes. One was defined by the struggle against crippling legislation, and was focused on California and Massachusetts. The other route featured science more than organizational and legal activity and began in New York, led by Max Fink, Richard Abrams, and others in an effort to demonstrate with new standards of evidence that ECT was safe and effective. They also aimed to enlarge the indications for ECT from a last-ditch treatment for depression to an application for a variety of psychiatric illnesses.

Returning to our discussion in chapter 9 of the legal cases against ECT in the early 1970s, ECT advocates entered the ensuing battle by locking arms against California's 1974 anti-ECT law. But even the modified legislation, in effect from 1975 until 1987, remained highly restrictive. Voluntary, competent patients who requested ECT were required to pay for a second psychiatric opinion and to undergo a mandatory delay before treatment. The families of more disturbed patients had to hire a lawyer and pay for extra medical consultations; a public defender would be assigned and a court hearing held, even when the patient did not want such a hearing. As one medical journalist noted: "The court process often delays treatment for weeks or months. Families are not allowed to provide consent on behalf of seriously ill loved ones, and the law makes no exception for life-threatening emergencies such as self-starvation or unrelenting suicide attempts."[19] There were deaths as a result of delays in treatment imposed by the 1974 law.

The situation moved Gary Aden, a San Diego psychiatrist, to file suit to have the law suspended, and to ask the American Psychiatric Association for help. The APA's interest in convulsive therapy went back at least to the days of the Group for the Advancement of Psychiatry and the presidency of William Menninger in the late 1940s (see chapter 5).

In 1953, the APA issued some guidelines for the practice of electrotherapy (see chapter 6), which were then withdrawn in 1959. At the time
of the Eagleton affair in 1972, the APA delivered another statement in
support of ECT.[20]

In the Aden court case leading to the first judicial reversal in 1975,
the APA filed an amicus curiae brief. In response to a wave of anti-ECT
legislation looming in a number of state legislatures, the APA formed a
task force to study ECT in 1975. Although the task force's report in 1978
was one of the central events initiating the comeback of ECT, it would
not come soon enough for Aden and his followers. At the 1975 national
meeting of the APA in Anaheim, California, they decided to organize
to oppose a further state clamp-down on ECT. They called their group
the International Psychiatric Association for the Advancement of Electrotherapy (IPAAE) and held their first meeting in 1976 in Miami.[21]

Efforts to build the APA task force began with Boston psychiatrist
Lester Grinspoon, who managed the research council at APA. He recruited Fred Frankel, a psychiatrist involved in the ECT controversy
in Massachusetts (see chapter 9), to chair the new task force. Frankel
conferred with Max Fink, who in 1972 had left the New York Medical
College for the State University of New York campus at Stony Brook. In
that same year, Fink had organized a symposium on ECT's mechanism
of action and was known for his activity in the field. Frankel, not at the
time an ECT specialist, later said: "Max should really have been Chair,
but I know why they didn't pick him," an allusion to Fink's partisanship.[22] Indeed, from the 1970s on, Fink committed himself wholeheart-
edly to the struggle for ECT.

Frankel also asked Michel Mandel at Harvard and Iver Small at the
University of Indiana to serve on the task force. Alan Stone, professor
of psychiatry and law at Harvard, functioned as a consultant early on,
but did not stay to the end.[23] By October 1975, two additional mem-
bers were named: George J. Wayne, a Los Angeles psychoanalyst, and
T. George Bidder, an ECT specialist at the VA Hospital in Sepulveda,
California; later, neuropsychologist and memory expert Larry Squire,
at the University of California at San Diego, and ECT-researcher Paul
Blachly, at the University of Oregon, would join the task force as well.
(Blachly died in 1977 before the report was published.)

The task force went about its work and in 1976 circulated a questionnaire to a one-fifth sample of the APA's national membership, receiving
back about three thousand responses. In May 1976, it held hearings at
the association's national meeting in Miami. Karliner and Kalinowsky

were both in attendance. As Max Fink recalled the meeting: "People got up, came before the committee and said ECT is the most horrible thing in the world. I remember sitting there. I was still a young man at that time, and heard what these people were saying about me, and about people like me. They were throwing mud. It was really horrible."[24] Nonetheless, the task force pressed on, and by the end of 1977, had a draft ready for circulation to selected members.

Mindful of the vociferous public attacks on ECT in those years, the task force had been cautious in the extreme. The members agonized at length about informed consent, bending over backward to make sure that all current ethical precepts about consent were satisfied. They had originally recommended that even for voluntary, competent patients, the consent session be videotaped, possibly in the presence of a lawyer.[25] As the draft was circulated, New York psychiatrist Leonard Cammer blew up when he saw this: "The recommendation to videotape or tape-record the consent session, or to have an attorney present where consent has to be obtained, violates the entire sense and fabric of the doctor-patient rapport. . . . Incidentally, where does one store all these tapes? Office rentals cost $11.00 a square foot."[26] That particular recommendation was deleted from the final version, but it illustrates the defensive crouch in which the members were squatting as they contemplated the enemies of ECT.

With the exception of Max Fink's irritation at the willingness of his colleagues to countenance restrictions, the task force's discussions had been relatively free of acrimony. The animosity came on December 9, 1977, when Frankel approached the APA's board of trustees. The board generally felt that the task force had been much too defensive about ECT and overly cautious in its approach. Louis Linn opened the discussion with, as Frankel said: "a broadside that led me to expect the Red Queen to appear and shout 'Off with their heads.'" Linn told Frankel: "If we think that the California legislation has done damage to ECT, this Report will bury ECT." Linn argued for a stronger affirmation of ECT for elderly patients, and the task force's elaborate precautions about informed consent drew general condemnation. The task force, said the board, had been far too specific about treatment techniques, opening up psychiatrists who did not follow the guidelines exactly to the threat of litigation.[27]

The final report of the ECT task force, published in September 1978, was more audacious than earlier drafts, though not overly so. For what conditions was ECT appropriate? "Severe depression," said the report, where suicide loomed; "severe psychoses," where the safety of the patient or others is at stake; "severe catatonia," where the patient has not responded to drugs; and "severe mania," where likewise drug treatment has failed or is deemed unsuitable. By contrast, ECT was only "probably effective" for endogenous depression (though this was the classic indication for ECT for forty years) where drug treatment has failed; also it was only of doubted value in psychoses where drug treatment has not availed. Was it useful for schizophrenia? Nobody knows, said the task force.[28]

Frankel's own remoteness from the ECT world (although he had prescribed it as a young doctor in Johannesburg) doubtless contributed to the conservative tone of the report. His main research interest was hypnosis, and he had been quite sympathetic to such anti-ECT proposals as requiring the court's permission to be renewed every month.[29] At task force meetings, Fink found himself constantly butting heads with Frankel and others. Fink later expressed his exasperation at this whole approach of making scientific policy by consensus: "I did not like voting on science at the Task Force. It drove me nutty to vote on RUL vs. BT, on atropine or glycopyrrolate, on training. That is why I took a year off and wrote my 1979 textbook."[30] (RUL is an acronym for right unilateral placement of electrodes, BT is for bitemporal placement; atropine and glycopyrrolate are intended to lessen the autonomic effects of ECT.) Fink's *Convulsive Therapy: Theory and Practice* was the first ECT textbook since Lothar Kalinowsky and Paul Hoch's in 1946, and it helped put the field on a modern, scientific basis by distilling the most useful information from the enormous literature that had appeared over the course of forty years.[31] Said Richard Abrams of the book: "Max's Magnum Opus . . . really had a very powerful effect. . . . [It] was the earliest objective scientific assessment."[32]

One positive effect of the task force was that it served as a catalyst for this more scientific approach to understanding ECT and managing its clinical practice. More important, the report placed the influential American Psychiatric Association firmly in support of ECT. The official organization of scientific psychiatry entertained no questions of "brains being fried" or "lifetimes of memory lost." The report supported doctors in their briefs to hospitals to establish ECT services. Task force members were invited to hospitals to advise medical boards and hospital directors in this undertaking.

On the negative side, the report put a definitive end to office-based or outpatient ECT, which over the years had established itself as a safe and effective way to extend electrotherapy to the many individuals who could not afford hospitalization or who shunned the stigma associated with a "psychiatric institution." The report stipulated that "ECT [should] only be administered in a location, and under circumstances, where there is immediate (i.e. within 2–3 minutes) availability or an access to . . . [technology] to manage complications which can occur unpredictably. . . . In general, this will necessitate that the treatment be administered in a hospital."[33] As one critic of the report, Iverson Brownell, head of psychiatry at Greenville Hospital System in South Carolina, said to the APA board: "Here it is spelled out quite plainly that [ECT] should be given only in a hospital setting with considerable back-up with all life-saving equipment. I feel this in itself makes the procedure seem much more dangerous than it actually is." Brownell felt that this would also increase costs for the patient. "Having used Electric Shock treatment in an office setting for the past thirty years with minimal complications, I would hate to lose this flexibility of treatment plan because of rigid guidelines."[34] These guidelines would guarantee a punishing settlement in court against any psychiatrist who violated them in the future. The William Karliners of psychiatry, their offices full of working parents on Saturday mornings, would be no more.[35]

The Road Back: The New York Scene

Coupled to the APA's activities in resuscitating ECT were the efforts of research-physicians like Max Fink. He began the 1970s as the principal ECT grant-holder in the United States, and in 1971 he organized a conference on the treatment at the behest of the National Institute of Mental Health. He ended the decade as the author of the definitive medical text on electroconvulsive shock. Fink was born in Vienna in 1923. His parents, citizens of Austria-Hungary, were both in medicine. His father, Julius, was a general practitioner, and his mother, born Broniaslawa ("Bronia") Lowenthal, had been admitted to the University of Vienna medical school in 1920 as one of the first women to study medicine there. (She did not complete her training because of pregnancy but would later graduate from Columbia University's School of Social Work.) In 1924, the family emigrated to the United States, and Fink grew up in the Bronx. In 1945, he graduated with a medical degree from New York University College of Medicine, the youngest member of his class, and interned at Morrisania City Hospital in the Bronx. As an intern, he studied under a series of eminent psychiatrists and neurologists, and was inspired to embark on a research career in medicine.

After internship, Fink served two years in the army, training in the spring of 1946 at the School of Military Neuropsychiatry at Fort Sam Houston in Texas. Psychiatry held a fascination for Fink. When he was growing up in New York, the family home had been full of guests from the field of medicine; many were fellow Austrian émigrés fleeing Hitler, including such eminent psychiatrists as Paul Schilder, Bernard Dattner, and Josef Gerstmann. These were internationally known members of the University of Vienna's psychiatric clinic, and young Fink, a high school student, found contact with them awe-inspiring. At Fort Sam Houston, Fink learned the somatic therapies, particularly insulin coma and ECT, but at the time had no particular interest in them. He applied them routinely at the army hospital in Fort Knox, Kentucky, where he was in charge of three psychiatry wards. In 1948, after being discharged, Fink trained in neuropsychiatry at New York's Montefiore Hospital and Bellevue Psychiatric Hospital, qualifying in neurology in 1952. That same year, he began a psychiatry residency at Hillside Hospital, a place populated with some of the great names in psychoanalysis. Fink chose Hillside because he wanted to deepen his knowledge of psychoanalysis. (He had started a training program in analysis after getting out of the army and was certified at the W. A. White Institute of Psychoanalysis in 1953.) Instead, Hillside put him on the ECT-insulin coma service run by Simon Kwalwasser, a former state hospital psychiatrist with little interest in psychoanalysis.

Fink furthered his neuropsychiatry training at the National Foundation for Infantile Paralysis at Mount Sinai Hospital, where he learned electroencephalography under Hans Strauss, who was then lecturing in neurology at Columbia. Fink absorbed the basics of clinical research under Morris Bender, one of the great American neurologists, and under psychiatrist Edwin Weinstein, known for his barbiturate research. When in 1954 Fink received a grant from the newly opened National Institute of Mental Health (NIMH) to work on EEG patterns in convulsive therapy, the hospital established a Department of Experimental Psychiatry with Fink as its director.

Though Fink had aspired to a career in psychoanalysis, he was drawn to practice physical therapies early on. "The remarkable efficacy of ECT, especially when contrasted with the labored and limited efficacy of insulin coma and psychotherapy," he said later, "sparked my interest in how such a gross intervention might work." One could see the improvement in the electroencephalograph. "The more slow waves in the EEG," said Fink, "the more improved the patient! It was illogical that an abnormality produced by the physician was 'good' for the patient. The irrationality of ECT became a challenge."[36] Spurred by the NIMH grant, the experimental psychiatry department at Hillside grew rapidly, and in 1956 Fink published for the first time on ECT.[37]

As psychopharmacology gained ascendancy in the 1950s, support for ECT research began to wane. Fink too lost interest in ECT. In 1962, he accepted an appointment as director of the Missouri Institute of Psychiatry in St. Louis, with a cross-appointment to the biologically oriented psychiatry department of Washington University in St. Louis. Here he was keen on research in psychopharmacology and put ECT aside. Yet things went sour for Fink in Missouri for a strange reason: Eli Robins, head of psychiatry at Washington University, decided to cut the peripheral hospitals from the academic department. This effectively ended the possibility of clinical cooperation at the university and meant that Fink was suddenly isolated, the nearest academic department of psychiatry being in far-away Jefferson City, the Missouri capital.

The separation was emblematic of the shifting terrain in psychiatry. Eli Robins went on to link up with Robert Spitzer, and together they advanced the "Feighner criteria" that began the process of wrenching psychiatric diagnosis away from the analysts and, ultimately, into the hands of the psychopharmacologists.[38] This work culminated in the "research diagnostic criteria"[39] of 1978 that laid the scaffolding for the *DSM-III* and its dramatic reordering of psychiatric diagnoses.[40] Fink was involved in none of these events; his Missouri experience inoculated him against anything coming out of St. Louis and "*DSM*"-style psychiatry. Instead, Fink struck out on the opposing road of physical treatments that stressed such neurohormones as cortisol, rather than neurotransmitters such as serotonin that were, of course, the basis of the psychopharmacology model. The neurohormonal approach became the only standing alternative to psychopharmacology and to the *DSM* approach.

In 1966, Fink, discouraged by his intellectual isolation in Missouri, returned to New York as director of biological psychiatry in Alfred Freedman's department of psychiatry at New York Medical College, a department that hitherto had dozed in silence until Freedman recruited Kalinowsky from the Psychiatric Institute in 1960. At New York Medical College, Fink had a clinical appointment at Metropolitan Hospital,

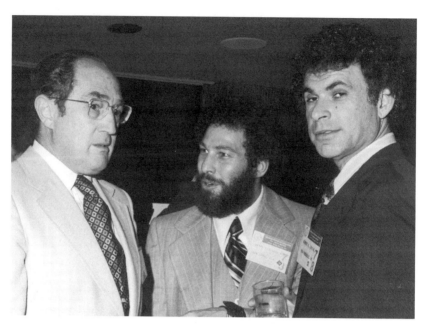

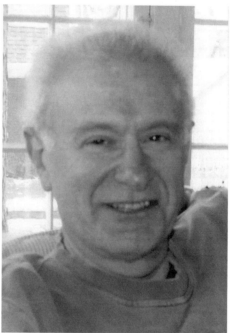

(Top) Max Fink, Barry Reisberg, and Robert Levine at a meeting of the American Psychiatric Association in 1978. At Metropolitan Hospital in New York, Levine and Fink advocated the efficacy of ECT in serious illness as opposed to psychoanalysis. Courtesy of Max Fink. (Above) Michael Alan Taylor who together with Richard Abrams also militated on behalf of ECT at Metropolitan Hospital. Courtesy of Max Fink.

where he ran an addiction service and did research on hallucinogens. Two floors below was a general psychiatry ward, and among the residents on this ward were Richard Abrams and Michael Taylor. "Metropolitan Hospital is really a third-rate place," said Robert Levine later, a fellow resident. "But for a short period of time it had this incredible department of psychiatry. Al Freedman was the chair."[41] Mickey Taylor said of his colleagues then: "We were in a class that was highly critical of psychoanalysis, and all we cared about were 'the data' . . . about what works and is there science to back it up." At rounds, Levine "had his papers sitting on his lap and he would read off a study showing that psychotherapy doesn't work. In front of psychoanalysts, he would discard the paper on the floor—just throw it on the floor, in some disdainful movement. By the end of the hour, he had totally shredded any efficacy [in psychoanalysis]. That was our attitude."[42]

Dick Abrams is best known today for his authoritative text on ECT, now in its fourth edition.[43] He first became interested in ECT during his training in psychiatry at Maimonides Hospital in Brooklyn, where, in 1964, he took part in a journal club that Kalinowsky organized. Abrams's training was interrupted in 1965 when he joined the air force. In charge of a thirty-bed psychiatric ward at a base in Wichita Falls, Texas, he began doing ECT research. His first paper appeared in the *American Journal of Psychiatry* in 1967.[44] With questions about the statistics on a second paper, he corresponded with Max Fink, and in 1967, having finished his military service, Abrams resumed his psychiatric training, this time at Metropolitan Hospital so that he could study with Fink.[45] Having worked with Fink at Metropolitan, and with Kalinowsky, first at Maimonides and later at Gracie Square Hospital in Manhattan, Abrams was influenced by two of the most active practitioners of ECT in the United States.

Gracie Square Hospital on East Seventy-sixth Street opened in 1969 as a 220-bed private, mainly psychiatric hospital. An upscale kind of Bellevue, it cared for patients with serious mental illness. Its large ECT division was supervised by Kalinowsky, who was revered by the hospital's owners, Lawrence and Richard Zirinsky. Alfred Freedman arranged privileges for New York Medical College staff to do research at Gracie Square. "Gracie Square paid a lot of money for research," said Herbert Fox, a staff psychiatrist who came to the hospital in the mid-1970s.[46] Between 1968 and 1974, Abrams was an attending physician at Gracie Square; Mickey Taylor was there from 1971 to 1976 (prior to that he directed the ECT unit at a navy facility in Oakland, California).

Abrams, Fink, and Kalinowsky agreed to undertake research on electrode placement in ECT, with Fink and Abrams going after an NIMH grant for the work and Kalinowsky functioning as a consultant. This was Gracie Square's first NIMH grant. In the early 1970s, the hospital became the center of an intense research effort involving Fink and Abrams on one research project, and Taylor and Abrams on another.[47] Karliner and Kalinowsky supplied the patients. Publications began to emerge from the Abrams-Fink project in 1972, when Milton Greenblatt asked Fink to edit a special issue of *Seminars in Psychiatry* on "Convulsive Therapy." In this issue Fink and Abrams contributed a paper "Answers to Questions about ECT," and Fink wrote separately "The Therapeutic Process in Induced Convulsions (ECT)." [48] Other members of the New York Medical College were also represented: Jan Volavka wrote on EEG in convulsive therapy; Rhea Dornbush on memory.[49] The studies showed that bitemporal placement of the electrodes was better than right unilateral (RUL), and that multiple-monitored ECT (MMECT) was inferior to the standard variety. (Fink said later: "RUL should have died a natural death but it was unnecessarily resurrected by [Harold] Sackeim and [Richard] Weiner.")[50] The publication of this issue of *Seminars in Psychiatry* marked the reemergence of ECT as an academic research subject, showcasing it as a procedure with uses other than last-hope suicide cases that had failed all trials of medication. The mechanism of ECT's action remained to be discovered, but researchers were asking questions based on the new science of the brain and biological psychiatry.

Fink's collaboration with Abrams and Taylor continued at Stony Brook, as the three of them ended up there together in the mid-1970s. This resulted in a wave of what one might think of as anti-*DSM*-type scholarship, finding the nosology of the *DSM* system unconvincing. It also opened up a whole new indication for ECT: as a therapy for treating catatonia. As early as 1966, Fink had become caught up in Abrams and Taylor's interest in catatonia, and in their desire to delineate true psychiatric diseases.[51] Before that, American psychiatrists saw catatonia only as a symptom of schizophrenia. Fink said: "Their challenge to American psychopathology was a spur to me to look askance at DSM. Our challenge to DSM-III, by arguing for a home of its own for catatonia,[52] and the ongoing work with melancholia, offered the message that Robins and the St. Louis school led psychiatry as far astray as did the psychoanalysts." [53] Because many forms of catatonia are highly responsive to ECT, indications for the procedure began to enlarge beyond the last-hope suicide scenario.

A Wave of Support

Interest in ECT at the National Institute for Mental Health went back to 1971 when Thomas Williams, the chief of the "depression section" of NIMH's Clinical Research Branch, proposed a conference "on the use of ECT in the treatment of patients suffering from the depressive illnesses."[54] He asked Fink, who at the time was the principal NIMH grantholder in convulsive therapy, to help put together a planning committee, which also consisted of Seymour Kety at Harvard and James McGaugh at the University of California at Irvine. The conference was held in mid-April 1972 at the Dorado Beach Hotel in Dorado, Puerto Rico. Conference papers were published in a 1974 volume, *Psychobiology of Convulsive Therapy*. Together with the 1972 special issue of *Seminars in Psychiatry*, the two works went far in establishing that ECT had a scientific underpinning, was effective on a statistical basis, and had minimal side effects. Dick Abrams, Jan Volavka, Joyce and Iver Small, and others attended the conference and contributed articles, as did Giacomo d'Elia and Jan-Otto Ottosson from Sweden, and Silvio Garattini, the dean of Italian psychopharmacology, who had traveled from Milan to talk about electroshock and neurotransmitters in mice and rats.[55]

Despite its sponsorship of the conference and the publication of proceedings, NIMH did not show sustained interest in convulsive therapy. By the end of the century, the agency had supported 171 drug trials for depression, 21 trials for acupuncture, and only 4 for ECT.[56] In 1975, Martin Katz, chief of the Clinical Research Branch, considered organizing a follow-up conference to the Dorado Beach meetings.[57] He asked Fink informally to write a proposal for government funding of the conference. Yet at a stormy meeting on January 30, 1976, at NIMH headquarters in Rockville, Maryland, Katz withdrew the invitation because his bosses wanted someone less controversial to be the point man. Fink resigned from the committee in irritation, and the conference never took place.[58] It is telling that NIMH rejected further proposals from Fink throughout the late 1970s.

The clinicians at NIMH themselves had so little interest in ECT that no one could find the ECT device the government had once purchased (see chapter 7). Zigmond Lebensohn said in 1977: "As a consultant, I have seen several patients at the NIMH Clinical Center who have desperately needed ECT. No apparatus for administering ECT was available at NIMH. Someone dimly remembered that there was an ECT machine when NIMH opened many years ago. However, no one could locate it so that we had to import our own equipment in order to give the treatments."[59]

It was in this climate of clinical hostility and bureaucratic indifference that Matthew Rudorfer, who in 1981 came to NIMH to find himself the agency's ECT expert, proposed a "consensus conference" on convulsive therapy to determine if the quarreling about the treatment could somehow be reconciled.[60] Between June 10 and 12, 1985, the Office of Medical Applications of Research of the National Institutes of Health, in conjunction with NIMH, held a Consensus Development Conference on Electroconvulsive Therapy. This notion of consensus development is a kind of NIH specialty: come let us reason together. And it made Max Fink nervous, who felt it was no way to conduct science: "The essence of science is that there is no middle ground. There is a correct ground—the facts that Nature lets you find. You can't have one person saying the speed of light is 186,000 mps and one saying 187,000 mps and they agree on 186,500 mps."[61] The panel itself was heavily weighted toward psychopharmacologists, psychologists, and laypeople, and it concluded rather conservatively that "ECT is demonstrably effective for a narrow range of severe psychiatric disorders in a limited number of diagnostic categories: delusional and severe endogenous depression, and manic and certain schizophrenic syndromes."[62] Glen Peterson, an Oakland psychiatrist and executive director of the IPAAE, commented: "As might be expected from relative 'strangers' to the actual practice of ECT, the tone of the statement suggested even when it is offered in clinically appropriate situations, a good deal of apprehension and foreboding ought to surround the application of ECT."[63] Yet the panel did recommend that ECT be incorporated into the basic training of every psychiatrist and that ECT questions be included on the licensing exams.

The panel also concluded that much additional research was needed, and the American Psychiatric Association took this as a warrant for deepening its own involvement with ECT. Since the Task Force Report of 1978, the APA had maintained a Task Force on the Development of a Safety and Performance Standard for ECT Devices, chaired by Richard Weiner. Weiner, a New Yorker by origin, had studied electrical engineering as an undergraduate at the Massachusetts Institute of Technology, going on to systems engineering in a master's program at the University of Pennsylvania, then had earned a Ph.D. in physiology and an M.D. from Duke University in 1973. He also had a background in EEG research and drifted into the ECT field because, as he later remarked,

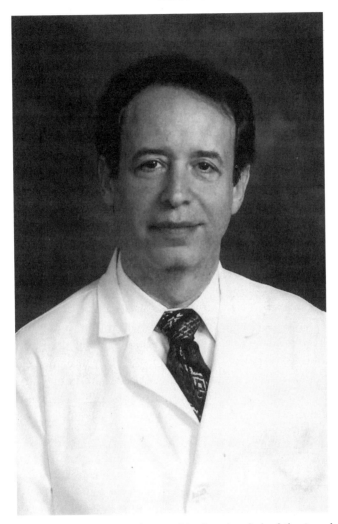

Richard Weiner, the Duke University psychiatrist who chaired the American Psychiatric Association's Task Force on ECT; its report in 1990 helped rehabilitate electroconvulsive therapy. Courtesy of Richard Weiner.

as a resident he had learned electrotherapy via the classic route of "see one, do one, teach one." "I was very disconcerted at the lack of knowledge about providing electrical stimulation to people's brains." When he came to the VA Hospital in Durham, North Carolina (home of Duke University), in 1977, it was with a "research career development award" from NIMH to study how ECT worked.[64]

In December 1986, Weiner responded to the APA board's request to develop some kind of strategy for moving forward from the NIMH consensus conference.[65] The APA then decided to convert Weiner's "devices" committee into a new task force to work out ECT "guidelines."[66] Weiner said: "The Task Force . . . had a specific mandate to develop standards for how ECT should be administered, all aspects of ECT administration, along with training for ECT, and also credentialing of practitioners for ECT."[67] A year later, the ECT task force was up and running and had as members, in addition to Weiner, Max Fink, Donald Hammersley (an APA official), Iver Small, Louis Moench (a Salt Lake City psychiatrist who was the liaison to the APA's "Assembly"), and Harold Sackeim of the New York State Psychiatric Institute, who served as a "consultant." The committee's expenses were paid by an NIMH contract.

By October 1988, the task force devised a set of recommendations intended to expand access to ECT: nurse-anesthetists and psychiatrists themselves might administer anesthesia (waiting for the anesthetist to turn up had become a major burr for many ECT practitioners, yet the final report deleted the recommendation for nurse-anesthetists); outpatient ECT was acceptable (in proper facilities); continuation ECT was fine (to prevent a relapse, patients who had completed an ECT course were maintained on periodic electroshock treatments or on medication); and brief pulse direct current was preferred to alternating current as a wave form. Monitoring ECT treatments with an EEG was encouraged (this was to make sure that a proper grand mal seizure had occurred).

The task force's recommendations were launched at a press conference in December 1989. In a news release, APA president Herb Pardes stated: "The ECT recommendations contained in today's report are, in effect, a 'practice parameter.' . . . A practice parameter outlines the indication for a given treatment, how the treatment works, expected results, possible side-effects, and contraindications. The ECT guidelines published today are a prototype [for other such parameters in the future]."[68] The volume published shortly thereafter was quickly sold out.[69] "It was very well received," said Weiner in an interview. "It was very influential outside the United States, in other countries, setting their standards for ECT; it really set a model for the world."[70]

In this process of routine acceptance, endorsements from the commanding heights of medicine were important. Eight months before the release of the task force's recommendations, the American Medical Association had approved ECT "as an effective treatment modality in selected patient populations."[71] By the end of the 1990s, endorsements began to flock in. In 1998, in a lead editorial in the *American Journal of*

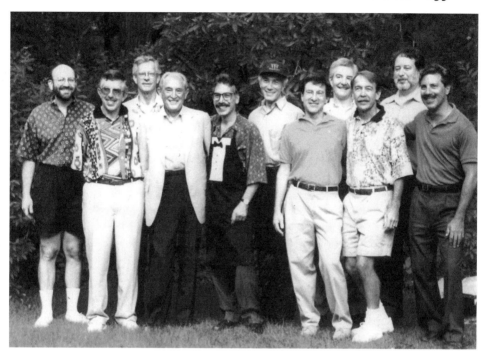

ECT "Victory Party" (1994): Guests at a party thrown by New York psychologist and ECT specialist Harold Sackeim at his home in honor of Max Fink, celebrating the founding of the journal *Convulsive Therapy*. Left to right: Matthew Rudorfer, Benjamin Lerer, Tom Bolwig, Max Fink, Harold Sackeim, John Mann, Charles Kellner, George Alexopoulos, Edward Coffey, Richard Weiner, and Robert Greenberg. Courtesy of Max Fink.

Psychiatry, Harvard's Carl Salzman expressed bewilderment that ECT was not more widely adopted. "Among psychiatric treatments, data for the efficacy of ECT . . . are incontrovertible." Yet there was wide variability in its use. "What is to be done?" he asked. The key, he said, was to "overcome a professional ambivalence toward ECT and ignite the imagination and enthusiasm of our trainees and young research colleagues."[72] The days of cringing in response to images of brains being "fried" were now long gone.

In a 1999 report on the nation's mental health, the United States Surgeon General's office came out in favor of ECT after a trial of medication. The report cited evidence of controlled clinical trials and "sham" ECT (giving the patient anesthesia but not shock, used to rule out a placebo effect). "No controlled study has shown any other treatment to have superior efficacy to ECT in the treatment of depression," the report noted.[73] And in 2001, the deputy editor of the *Journal of the American Medical Association,* Richard M. Glass, argued in an editorial on ECT that it was "time to bring it out of the shadows." The therapy had no long-term effect on memory, he said, and even though many patients relapsed after treatment, they could be successfully maintained on antidepressant medication.[74]

Three years later, in 2004, the World Psychiatric Association endorsed ECT. Noting the comprehensive literature survey of the United Kingdom Review Group of the previous year, the WPA said that "ECT is strongly recommended as a first line acute treatment for severe depressive disorder, particularly depressive disorder with psychotic symptoms . . . depression with high risk of suicide, harm to others, self neglect and physical deterioration." [75] As a "first line treatment," ECT's use would no longer be restricted to a last-ditch effort to save patients who, over the course of many long months, had failed to respond to one antidepressant after another and whose lives, as well as those of everyone around them, had been shattered by the experience.

Ironically, this is what Cerletti believed in the 1940s; it had taken a full sixty years for the rest of the medical community to agree.

Psychologists and ECT

The foregoing account has a triumphant ring. But it was not yet a triumph, because the colossal dispute about memory loss still plagued ECT. In the previous chapter, we saw that memory has a social construction of its own. Here we see that it also has a politics.

David Levy was an important pediatric psychoanalyst in New York in the 1950s, known for coining the term *sibling rivalry.* He used ECT in both children and adults. One day, in the recollection of colleague Arthur Zitrin, a "Mrs. Gruenstein" came to him, worried about memory loss. He said: "Mrs. Gruenstein, I have some bad news for you. You're going to remember everything."[76] That you would remember everything was more or less the classic view at that time: the problem was trivial to nonexistent. When in 1963 Milton Greenblatt, then superintendent of Boston State Hospital, undertook a survey of side effects of ECT compared with antidepressants in three state hospitals in the Greater Boston area, memory loss was not even on the list![77]

Yet over the years, concerns about memory loss multiplied rather than subsiding in the manner that worry about broken bones had been assuaged by the introduction of succinylcholine. By 2000, Sackeim would write: "Virtually all patients experience some degree of persistent and, likely, permanent retrograde amnesia."[78] He later said in an interview: "There are some people, we don't know how many, going to lose five years of their life."[79] Loss of retrograde, or past, memories—the stuff of one's autobiography—is potentially terrifying. For Sackeim and his researchers at PI, memory loss was a grave enough problem to justify the introduction of experimental alternatives to ECT, possibly less effective but certainly more sparing of cognition, in the event that cognition needed sparing (see chapter 11).

Was Sackeim's work an aberrant deviation from the mainline of ECT thinking? Or did it represent the triumph of reason in a field sundered by partisanship? Sackeim was a psychologist, and psychologists had taken an interest in memory questions from the very beginning of ECT. In 1941, Joseph Zubin, a psychologist, and psychiatrist Eugene Barrera at the New York State Psychiatric Institute, had done tests and found that "one of the most striking psychological concomitants of this treatment is the characteristic impairment of the patient's memory." Yet they believed that the loss affected mainly "recent memory."[80] When more than forty years later, in 1984, Zubin, now at the University of Pittsburgh, revisited the memory question as part of Richard Weiner's write-in symposium on memory loss and brain damage, he was quite skeptical of claims of devastating memory loss: "There is little evidence that the loss is permanent."[81]

Yet by the 1980s, many psychologists supported the opposing viewpoint: ECT was a harmful procedure precisely because of such huge losses of memory. In 2001, a survey of psychiatrists and psychologists, among other professionals in the North London hospitals, asked whether it might be appropriate for a patient to have ECT: of the psychiatrists, 75 percent thought that it would be all right (although 33 percent said only as a last resort). Of the psychologists, the vast majority thought it would harm the patient and cause brain damage. Half claimed it was a "cruel treatment," and 27 percent thought it should be banned.[82]

Digging through the professional literature of psychology on ECT is like boring into a steam tunnel. At the Weiner symposium in 1984, psychologist Donald Templer at the California School of Professional Psychology in Fresno likened the damage of ECT to that experienced by boxers.[83] And psychologist John Pinel at the University of British Columbia in Vancouver volunteered that there was little evidence of the value of ECT: "Do the possibilities of a brief remission of depression justify the risks of interfering with a patient's memory?"[84] he asked. These comments are typical of psychologists in those years.

In 1970, at Hawthornden State Hospital in Ohio, the staff psychiatrists had ordered ECT for five patients "who had become destructive." The four psychologists on staff at Hawthornden sent letters to the patients' relatives and to the governor of Ohio alleging that "the shock treatments were administered as 'punishment' or 'torture' of the mental patients." The psychologists were removed from office, and when one of them subsequently died, his widow appealed his dismissal to the courts. The hospital board described the ECT situation as a "pitched battle" between psychologists and psychiatrists.[85]

Many psychologists began styling themselves as the patients' protectors against the brutal psychiatrists with their ECT electrodes. A psychologist at the VA Hospital in Portland, Oregon, felt that the duty of psychologists in team treatment was to defend the patients against ECT: "If ECT is recommended, the psychologist should assist the patient in deciding whether to receive ECT."[86] In 1997, an official document of the American Psychological Association said that "ECT continues to be controversial." Quoting anti-ECT activists, the APA-sponsored brief maintained that "the most serious and disturbing side effects, confusion and loss of memory, occur in virtually all cases."[87] Irreversible brain damage was indeed to be feared.

The psychology profession's sudden solicitousness about memory in ECT is a bit of a mystery. Perhaps it was political: psychologists may have used memory loss as a wedge in battering down the citadel of medical authority. The other great treatment method of psychiatry, prescribing psychopharmaceuticals, was a privilege that psychologists had hungered after for years. So opposing ECT by raising memory loss issues would have made sense as a tactic in professional rivalry: destroying the one treatment that psychologists could not provide.[88]

There is, of course, the possibility that the psychologists were correct. Within psychology, there was no greater friend of ECT than Harold Sackeim. Yet it was Sackeim who waved the red flag of memory loss in front of a generation of neuroscientists and endeavored to displace ECT with other supposedly more memory-sparing techniques. (See the next chapter on these alternatives.) Sackeim was born in Hackensack, New Jersey, in 1951, and studied psychology at Columbia University in New York, then, after a year at Oxford, earned in 1977 a Ph.D. in clinical psychology at the University of Pennsylvania. His first post was as research associate at the New York State Psychiatric Institute, and it was at PI that he remained for the rest of his career, becoming in 1991 chief of the department of biological psychiatry. Over the years, he gained an extraordinary record of research support, especially from NIMH, in cutting-edge neuroscience. "Harold Sackeim is really the top researcher in ECT," said Weiner, "both clinically and in terms of basic science. He's a psychologist, who actually knows more clinically about ECT and technique of ECT than just about any psychiatrist does. He's sort of the renaissance man of ECT."[89]

Sackeim's first publication on ECT was in 1983,[90] and in 1985 he joined the editorial board of the *Journal of ECT (Convulsive Therapy)*. "In psychiatry, ECT was extraordinary to me," said Sackeim in an interview, "because you took the sickest patients and you got them the most well."[91] From the outset, Sackeim was convinced that unilateral electrode placement was considerably more memory-sparing than bilateral (this was long known) and at high doses of electricity, virtually as effective.[92] This revived the unilateral-bilateral debate that Abrams and Fink at New York Medical College thought they had settled (to the advantage of bilateral) in their publication in 1972 in *Seminars in Psychiatry* and elsewhere (see above). In subsequent years, Sackeim and his team at PI published much in favor of unilateral ECT, and excused its generally lesser efficacy on the grounds that memory effects in ECT could be awesome and must somehow be countered. Though the question of electrode placement is still not definitively resolved, the point is that the psychologists as a group had fanned patients' worries about memory and, rightly or wrongly, that one of the nation's premier neuroscientists had judged these concerns fully justified.[93]

Meanwhile, the psychiatrists stood aside flabbergasted. First of all, none of the veteran ECT-specialists had ever seen anything like the devastating, permanent abolition of memory of which some anti-ECT activists complained. Kalinowsky just scoffed at the notion,[94] and Rich Weiner said: "If someone comes in and says, 'I can't remember anything, going back to when I was a child'—can't happen, at least biologically it can't happen."[95] As Leonard Cammer told the APA's task force in 1976: "Of 1,125 patients two developed severe confusion, one after the fourth treatment, the other after the second treatment. Both recovered with no loss of memory." He underlined the following sentence: "*Complaints of memory difficulties of any significance after 4 to 6 weeks are non existent in patients who show clearcut recovery from a depressive episode, who have long remissions or who are much improved to the extent that they are not dysfunctional in their usual activities.*"

By contrast, patients who remain symptomatic, who demonstrate psychosomatic symptoms "and other evidence of a continued disaffection with life," continue to complain of memory difficulties. He concluded that memory loss "appears to be a functional complaint of the persons who do not get better."[96] Today, a majority of psychiatrists who occupy themselves with convulsive treatment would probably stand behind this statement.

There was also some empirical evidence on behalf of the psychiatrists' views. Weiner noted that patients who are getting maintenance ECT—maybe once a month, "tend not to be bothered by their memory."[97] In 1963, two Swedish researchers, Börje Cronholm and Jan-Otto Ottosson, discovered that depressed patients successfully treated with ECT believed their memory *improved*.[98] Psychologist Larry Squire at UCLA spent years of his career chasing memory losses of various kinds. In 1984, he finally concluded: "It is already rather clear that memory functions substantially improve after ECT, except for memory of events near the time of treatment, and despite repeated efforts it has not yet been possible to demonstrate persisting memory impairment following a standard course of treatment."[99] It would be hard to imagine a more definitive statement. Several years later he seemed to have lost patience even further with the memory-loss proponents. Squire's comments as an expert witness in a bribery-conspiracy trial involving television personality Bess Myerson among others, were summarized by the *New York Times*: "Several months after the treatments [Squire said] patients remember new events perfectly, as shown on psychological tests. They are left with a gap covering a few weeks before, during, and after their treatments. Some patients will also have 'some spotty memory loss going back months' before their treatment, Dr. Squire said, 'but that's it.'"[100]

What could account for the rising frenzy about memory loss in the absence of any evidence of actual long-term impairment? In dealing with a culture that lives on a diet of media-induced sensation, one can never discount the impact of suggestion: people believe that something will happen to them because the notion has been implanted in them by suggestion. One sees this in the epidemic spread of such illness attributions as "chronic fatigue syndrome." Could "memory loss" be a similar phenomenon? If earnest psychologists suggest that you, as a patient, will lose large tracts of memory, post-ECT you might well be alarmed to discover that you cannot recall, in fact, what happened to you in 1985. "Anyone attending the twenty-fifth reunion of his college class can readily gather convincing evidence of the normal memory gaps that aging leaves behind," said University of Vermont psychiatrist Lelon Weaver in 1984.[101] How easy to become hypervigilant about these normal losses and to attribute them to ECT.

In preparing patients for ECT, Harold Sackeim said of his procedures: "For decades I've discussed with patients—things like encouraging their family members to go over with them photographs or review before the treatment important events, or diaries."[102] Although this demonstrates a very humane and endearing concern for one's patients and their lives, nonetheless, reviewing photographs and diaries before the treatment at the recommendation of a professional conveys a certain expectation that one's memories of these events would be obliterated afterward. What better way is there to suggest one's patients into the belief of memory loss?

It is possible that in the memory loss wars we are dealing with a conflict of cultures, a difference in ways of knowing, rather than with a scientific debate. Psychologists and social workers are acculturated into the view that the sheer act of talking with patients, of counseling them, will make them better. The ECT specialist arrives with a machine, and the press of a red button often makes the patient's condition dramatically better. As one observer speculated of the psychologists' reactions under these circumstances: "Feelings of impotence, of being unable to help the patient are experienced as the staff sees . . . a powerful and mysterious treatment." Defeated self-esteem, resentment, and envy often follow.[103]

Thus, within psychology and social work, a professional culture hostile to ECT developed. Zigmond Lebensohn, who treated many government bureaucrats and high officials, and those who dealt with them, recounted the following case: "A 51 year old Jewish housewife from one of the mid-Atlantic states who developed a clear-cut, middle-aged depression with suicidal thoughts and psychomotor retardation" was admitted, he said, to the depression unit of NIMH. "One of the patient's daughters was a psychiatric social worker in Washington, who was undergoing psychoanalysis. She told her mother under no circumstances, to agree to ECT." The mother stayed on the depression unit for nine months, "during which time a wide variety of antidepressant drugs were used. . . . Unfortunately, she had adverse reactions to all of them and became infinitely worse." Finally, by the time the mother was emaciated, ripping off her clothes, and "wandering about the ward in a mute, disheveled manner" beyond the ken of meaningful conversation—and incontinent in addition to suffering from a terrible psoriasis that covered her entire body—the decision was made to transfer her to Lebensohn's ECT service at Sibley Memorial Hospital in D.C., where Lebensohn gave her twenty-seven ECT treatments. "She made a striking improvement. After the twentieth treatment she began to talk slightly, she began eating and became passively cooperative. Her psoriasis cleared up entirely, and she regained her normal body weight. Eventually she was able to talk quite freely and clearly about herself, and went on to make a complete and spectacular recovery." She returned home and, as far as Lebensohn knew, received no further psychiatric treatment.[104]

Reverse Spin!

"The electrical current throbs from one side of the skull to the other," began an ECT story in the *Los Angeles Times* in November 2003, "scrambling circuits along the way." The piece said there was no "scientifically rigorous evidence establishing the treatment's safety or effectiveness." It also mentioned the possibility that the procedure could result in "mossy fibers" growing out of the brain cells.[105] Yuck! Who would want such an awful therapy! Yet since the late 1980s, negative media spin such as this began to reverse direction. Especially in the quality broadsheets such as the *New York Times* and the *Washington Post,* writers decided that they liked ECT after all. Rather than representing "getting your brains fried," ECT held out the promise of an effective and safe treatment for some terrible illnesses.

The *Cleveland Plain Dealer* is one of the quality papers in the Midwest. In 1986, an Ohio hospital contacted its medical editor, Bob Becker, inviting him to see for himself what ECT was really about. As one of the staff psychiatrists then reported to Dr. Glen Peterson, who was director of an ECT-provider group at the hospital: "[Becker] observed the administration of an ECT, talked to a number of our patients, who had received ECT's in the past, and had a lengthy interview with us. . . . He was so engrossed in watching the treatment that he did not describe it quite correctly, probably expecting something horrible to happen. We, of course, do not use straps for patients . . . and nobody else does to my knowledge."[106] Becker's story ran on page one.

For this book, we analyzed all articles in the United States daily press making substantial mention of ECT between 1994 and 2004. Of these ninety-three articles, 58 percent made positive mention of ECT, in the sense that if you were a patient, you might feel comfortable agreeing to the procedure after reading the article. Another 34 percent were hostile, and 8 percent were neutral.[107] It is clear from other sources that coverage in the quality press for the 1970s and 1980s was overwhelmingly negative (see chapter 7). So a 58 percent positive reporting record represents a real change in attitudes.

Of newspaper comments on ECT in the 1994–2004 period, much came from the *New York Times,* if only because of its extensive book reviews. Of the negative comments, most occurred in those reviews. The intellectual class clung to its discouraging views of ECT far longer than the science writers. A reviewer of a 1997 novel about rural life tells us that "Nora's husband, Neal, quickly destroys the horse, subjects his despairing wife to electroshock treatment and tries to force her to sell the farm."[108] This is, of course, a discussion of a work of fiction, yet readers form impressions from book reviews too, and the impression of ECT leaping from these book-review pages was that you would not want to choose it for yourself nor for your loved ones.

By contrast, the science writers at the *New York Times* in the 1990s and after were almost uniformly enthusiastic. A former patient at Silver Hill Hospital in New Canaan, Connecticut, is quoted as saying: "The great thing about psychiatry today is that there are new drugs and electroconvulsive therapy, which today is safe. Drugs did not work for me and I underwent a series of electro-convulsive shock treatments. I have been my old self since."[109] In another issue, science writer John Horgan says that even though "no one has any idea why shock therapy works . . . for severe depression, shock therapy is the most effective treatment we have."[110] Whether these powerful endorsements overrode the negative assessments of the littérateurs would be decided at the breakfast tables of the *New York Times*'s readers. But the era of newspaper negativism toward ECT was ending.

Television's negativism had done even more to reinforce the stigma, given the indelible nature of the images. It was therefore an important step when on Monday, February 16, 1987, Peter Jennings presented on ABC a largely positive version of ECT, balancing it, to be sure, with Scientology claims that it caused brain damage.[111] In 1993, Dan Rather of CBS featured the "return" of shock therapy, balancing the account with clips from *One Flew over the Cuckoo's Nest* and an interview with Peter Breggin, psychiatrist and antipsychiatric activist.[112] Again in 1996, *ABC Evening News* returned to an encouraging account of "shock therapy," balanced as usual by a Scientology spokesperson claiming "brain damage."[113] However tentative these positive accounts might have been, in comparison with ABC's savaging of ECT in 1977 (see chapter 7), this represented great public enlightenment.

In this and the following manner the media began to convey to the public the great human drama of an ECT recovery. At 9:30 in the morning of July 4, 1999, Stacey Patton was in her bed at St. Vincent's Hospital in New York, "wearing only a hospital gown and a pair of ankle socks thinking independence was about to have new meaning for me. I was going to become free from psychotropic medications, manic episodes, recurrent hospital stays, severe depression and the recurring, passionate desire to end my own life."[114] Her mother, who also had manic-depressive illness, had committed suicide while Stacey was a sophomore at a boarding school near Princeton, New Jersey. As graduation approached in her senior year, it turned out that "my bed became the only place I wanted to be." She daydreamed that it was the bottom of the ocean, or that she had been buried in a casket and a grave. A local psychiatrist put her on the antidepressant drug Paxil. A series of hospitalizations followed until, finally, she ended up at St. Vincent's.

"Okay, Ms. Patton, you're gonna take a little nap," said the anesthetist as he inserted the IV into her right hand. The room began to spin, then she felt nothing until she woke up, a bit disoriented and with a headache. She had five more treatments. "As my release from the hospital neared, the symptoms eased. Each treatment was a little easier to weather. When I left St. Vincent's, I had a smile on my face; I felt relaxed and renewed." She had some memory loss. "Why did I have so many pairs of brown shoes?" But eight weeks later her memory returned. "The pain has stayed away. I know it is too early to celebrate," she wrote in the *Washington Post* in September 1999, "but I no longer feel depressed or suicidal."

As her new e-mail name she chose "Electrogirl."

The International Scene

It is ironic that in Europe and the United Kingdom, where the new somatic therapies began in the 1930s, ECT remained much more heavily stigmatized than in the United States. There probably was little difference until the 1960s in the use of convulsive therapy on either side of the Atlantic. But the revolutionary cultural movements that swept Europe in the sixties aspired to put ECT right out of business. And they succeeded in a number of countries.

In the United Kingdom, as we have seen, ECT was readily accepted after its origination in 1938. British psychiatry pioneered several techniques, as leading academic institutions such as the Maudsley Hospital used it widely. Influential psychiatrists such as Michael Shepherd at the Maudsley and Max Hamilton in Leeds were great fans of convulsive therapy, and Shepherd thought highly of ECT in mania, while looking at lithium, the drug treatment of choice for bipolar illness, with a jaundiced eye.

Then ECT fell into disfavor among the English academic elite, who vastly preferred psychopharmacology and thought of convulsive therapy as an antiquated procedure that might be apt for the desperate in the back ward, but certainly not for patients who sought out consulting rooms in London's chic Harley Street. The procedure had been in decline at the Maudsley since 1956, when 34 percent of admissions were treated with it. The rate dropped to 5 percent in 1987, and to less than 1 percent by 1993.[115]

The media elite stigmatized ECT in the United Kingdom even more strongly than in the United States, so that favorable articles about it were rare in the 1980s and 1990s. According to a ProQuest search, of twenty-one articles giving substantial mention to ECT between 1994 and 2004, 57 percent were negative (as opposed to 34 percent in the United States), and only 19 percent were positive. In quality broadsheets such as the *Guardian* and the *Observer,* one would have thought that bloodletting and leeching were under discussion rather than a modern lifesaving procedure. As we learn in the lead paragraph of an ECT story in the *Observer:* "Up to 400 volts of electricity [is] pumped into the brains of the mentally ill, often against their will."[116] The lead paragraph in a *Guardian* ECT story quoted former patient Jean Taylor as saying: "It was the most dreadful, frightening experience of my life. I had no idea what was going to happen to me and I was petrified." She said that if she ever had to have the procedure again, "she would kill herself."[117]

One reason for the stronger stigmatization in the United Kingdom than in the United States was the ferocity against ECT of the British former patients' movement, who refer to themselves as "survivors" (not of the illness but of the treatment), and who claim a place at the table in scientific discussions of ECT. As noted in the previous chapter, it is right that patient-driven research should occur. Yet the line between research and advocacy can be a thin one.

When in 2003 the National Institute for Clinical Excellence (NICE) in the United Kingdom issued a report on ECT, it rather grudgingly admitted that the procedure could be effective in some circumstances. But the report was highly ambivalent, at a time when internationally the former cautionary remarks about only-in-desperate-cases were falling away. ECT use in England and Wales was not to be increased above current levels and preferably reduced, the report said; it was to be used only for "severe depressive illness," catatonia, and last-ditch mania—and after the patient had failed to be helped by multiple rounds of drug treatment. The report frowned on maintenance ECT, and as for the patients' "quality of life," the report said we know so little about it that we had better cut back on electric treatments.[118] It is interesting that on the committee that produced this tepid recommendation sat several members of the militant patients' organization Mind. It is not inconceivable that, committee dynamics being what they are, the Mind representatives heavily influenced the document. Mind certainly beamed about the report afterward: "MIND has congratulated NICE on their decision and the way they gave new credibility to the evidence submitted on behalf of people who had been given ECT treatments, and who want tighter controls."[119] (In fairness, Mind emphasizes that it is pro-patient rather than antipsychiatric; yet the effect of these doubtless well-meant efforts was to restrict access to an important treatment.)

Despite negative press and a pro-patient advocacy movement, ECT was still being performed in the United Kingdom. In Italy, though, after the cultural revolution of the 1960s and the rise of an antipsychiatric political movement, Psichiatria Democratica, with advocates in parliament, ECT was dead. The great antipsychiatry wave began to engulf Italy in 1978 with a law called Bill 180, closing all of the country's mental hospitals, where ECT had commonly been available to average citizens (expensive private sanatoriums offered it to the well-to-do). On February 15, 1999, the Italian Minister of Health Rosy Bindi issued a "white paper" (*circolare*) mandating "special precautions" to be taken with ECT. Indications were henceforth tightly limited and excluded schizophrenia.[120] ECT was banned in private hospitals. Said English psychiatrist Harold Bourne, then resident in Rome: "Henceforth ECT is only permissible in cases of psychotic depression with psychomotor retardation, unresponsive to drug therapy, and in cases of malignant catatonia—provided the patient gives informed consent. It is not explained how informed consent can be obtained from persons in the grip of such extreme conditions."[121] In a further move, on December 30, 1999, the province of Piedmont abolished all convulsive therapy, as had the province of Marche (the Marches) on November 13, 2001. As a special kind of feel-good gesture, psychosurgery was also abolished despite having come to an end about forty years previously.[122] Thus in this country of 60 million people, ECT remained available only in several university psychiatric clinics, such as Pisa. In the land of its birth, ECT had been virtually outlawed.

In Switzerland, according to a public opinion poll in 2005, 56.9 percent of the population felt ECT was harmful; only 1.2 percent believed it might be a good idea.[123] In Slovenia, ECT was actually forbidden in 2002, one of the few countries formally to outlaw convulsive therapy in legislation.[124] Yet in other countries, ECT managed to maintain itself quite well despite the antipsychiatric assault of the 1970s and 1980s. In Denmark all thirty-five departments of psychiatry "use ECT on a regular basis," according to Copenhagen professor of psychiatry Tom Bolwig.[125] Fifty-seven percent of the psychiatry departments in Hungary were said to "use" ECT on a regular basis, though in most quite infrequently.[126]

The comeback of ECT, however, was the big international story. In Israel, for example, it coincided with the arrival in the 1980s of the Russian Jews, who bore with them that classic East European optimism about physical therapies and matching unfamiliarity with psychotherapy. It is a fitting bookend to the history of ECT in Israel that one of the treatment's earliest sites worldwide was Haifa Mental Hospital in Palestine in the late 1930s.[127] In 2005, the active Russian ECT scene saw the publication of a comprehensive textbook that called attention to convulsive therapy in addiction medicine, among other indications unfamiliar in Western psychiatry.[128]

The way back for ECT in Italy began in February 2006, with the founding of the Italian Association for Electroconvulsive Therapy (Associazione Italiana per la Terapia Elettroconvulsivante, or AITEC), under the leadership of Athanasios Koukopoulos, director of the Lucio Bini Center in Rome. There were 115 founding members, among them numerous chiefs of psychiatry. Other Italian colleagues told Koukopoulos "they could not join because they feared negative consequences."[129] Nonetheless, it was a beginning.

Nowhere was the comeback more robust than in Germany and Austria, countries that had once harbored deep enmity against convulsive treatment. In fact, once when Max Fink was lecturing in Munich, members of the audience challenged him: "As a Jew, how could you support such a Nazi treatment?" Hanns Hippius, the host, spoke up to warn the audience that Fink was a guest.[130] In 1992, psychiatrists in Graz, Austria, hosted the First European Symposium on ECT.[131] At the symposium it emerged that 75 percent of Austrian psychiatrists "believe that ECT should be offered by every psychiatric hospital."[132] In the 1990s, German and Austrian psychiatrists began buying "Thymatron" ECT devices, and in 2004 a group of Austrian authors published an ECT textbook.[133] In 2004 as well, the committee on biological procedures of the Austrian Psychiatric Society published a consensus statement on ECT that ranked in the international forefront of progressive guidelines.[134] As a German medical news service noted in November 2003: "In recent years ECT has experienced a boom internationally and in Germany": the German Medical Association had just announced electrotherapy as the treatment of choice for serious, treatment-resistant depression.[135] Under Tom Bolwig's leadership, in February 2006, the European Forum for ECT (EFFECT) was founded in Louvain, Belgium.[136]

The rebirth of ECT was thus not some idiosyncratic American experience, but an international development resulting, finally and after much ardor, in the triumph of science over political passion and prejudice. Bernard Lerer, director of the biological laboratory of Hadassah University Hospital in Ein Karem, Israel, once talked to a journalist from the newspaper *Haaretz* about the effectiveness of ECT in depressed Israeli patients: "Have you ever asked yourself how it is that a treatment with such a terrible stigma, a treatment that the public is afraid of and is said to be primitive and unhelpful—has, despite all this, survived into the twenty-first century, and not in obscure little places but in the world's most advanced medical centers? The answer is simple. Because it works."[137]

CHAPTER ELEVEN

Magnets and Implants
New Therapies for a New Century?

On May 1, 2000, a further chapter in the history of the shock therapies opened. Katherine X, a twenty-year-old depressed woman, was wheeled into a specially prepared room in the university psychiatric clinic in Berne, Switzerland, where she was put to sleep in the way patients have been put to sleep for ECT for decades. But instead of being given ECT, she had a magnetic paddle placed in close proximity to her skull, and with the stimulus delivered in this way she went on to have a seizure. The team looking after her, Thomas Schlaepfer and Sarah H. (Holly) Lisanby, were mightily relieved that the seizure happened uneventfully. And there was a pleasant surprise in store for them. When she awoke, Katherine appeared to have less confusion than sometimes accompanies recovery from ECT. She had three further magnetically induced seizures before finishing her treatment course with conventional ECT, and during these three additional magnetic treatments, the beneficial cognitive profile of the new treatment appeared to be maintained.[1] Magnetic seizure therapy (MST) had been born—or had it?

Katherine had previously been treated with eight different courses of antidepressant drugs with no success. In many countries, despite her age, she would have been a candidate for ECT. In Switzerland, however, the idea of giving her ECT was relatively novel. Only a few years earlier, ECT had all but been banned. Schlaepfer and a small group of younger clinicians had been instrumental in effectively reintroducing it, portraying modern ECT as a treatment in which the writhing of patients was abolished by suxamethonium and the convulsive process was monitored scientifically by simultaneous EEG recording. Schlaepfer had gone as far as bringing patients' relatives or their advocates and antipsychiatry

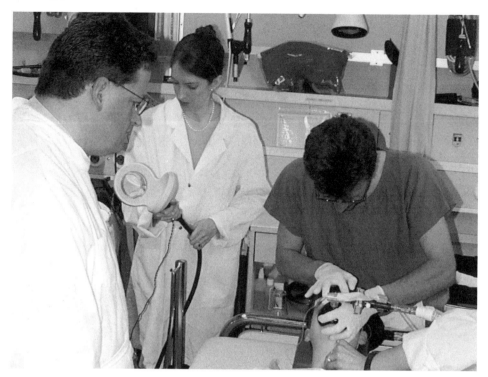

A picture taken at the occasion of the first therapeutic use of Magnetic Seizure Therapy in a patient with resistant major depression on May 1, 2000. From left to right Thomas Schlaepfer (Department of Psychiatry, University of Berne); Sarah H. Lisanby (Columbia University); Martin Luginbühl (Department of Anesthesiology, University of Berne). The patient was twenty years old at the time of treatment and she had suffered from a major depression for three years. She had had a total of eight treatment failures; at that time, she was in university but dropped out due to her depression. After the treatment course she was well and able to pursue a career in physiotherapy. Courtesy of Thomas Schlaepfer.

critics of ECT into the treatment suite to monitor what happened. And there they saw a treatment that much more closely resembled a standard surgical procedure than the stuff of *Cuckoo's Nest* fantasy.

Reintroducing ECT, however, was not something that had to be sanctioned by an ethics committee. But an entirely novel treatment, such as magnetic seizure therapy, would have to be approved by such a committee. Schlaepfer had brought his proposals before the Berne Institutional Review Board and had been knocked back twice. He, Harold Sackeim, and Holly Lisanby were aiming at a proof of concept—demonstrating that a seizure could be safely induced in this way. Their plan was to administer the treatment to four patients, who would each begin a course of convulsive therapy with magnetically induced seizures and finish out their treatment with a proven therapy—ECT. The Berne ethics committee had serious problems with this, wondering what image Schlaepfer and his colleagues must have of human beings if they were prepared to treat people this way. On the third attempt, the new procedure passed. But this was not simply a case of Berne conservatism holding back science; the reason to go to Berne was that Sackeim, Lisanby, and Schlaepfer recognized that there was even less likelihood that Columbia University, Sackeim and Lisanby's parent institution, would pass a protocol for the new treatment.[2]

Years after her treatment, Katherine had not had any relapse of her illness nor any recourse to psychotropic drugs. MST was given to three more patients in Berne and as of the end of 2006 had been given to twelve patients in the United States and fourteen in Europe with broadly similar results.[3] Patients appear to do relatively well, and, according to the advocates of the treatment, its cognitive complications appear quite benign. For some, this has raised the possibility that MST might be a replacement for ECT. But if we pull our focus back from the figure of Katherine to take in the room in which she had treatment, the picture becomes more complex. The suite was specially adapted for the purposes of treatment. Huge orange power cables had to be engineered into the room to feed the magnetic capacitor that made inducing a seizure possible. One estimate was that the amount of power involved would have supplied the needs of two typical Manhattan blocks. So if MST were ever to replace ECT, it would, at the very least, have to wait for technological developments to meet the enormous energy demand. And even then, there still remains the question as to whether it works. It is clearly possible to induce a seizure magnetically—there had in fact been little reason to doubt this, but these seizures are triggered in regions of the cortex near to the surface of the brain, and it is not yet clear that seizures initiated in this way will bring about changes in whatever key brain areas mediate the beneficial effects of ECT. Since Jan-Otto Ottosson's work in the 1960s, it has been a clinical truism that not all seizures are equivalent.[4]

Transcranial Magnetic Stimulation

The developments that brought Katherine to a room in Berne began some twenty-five years earlier in Sheffield, England. While engaged in his doctoral dissertation in the mid-1970s, Anthony (Tony) Barker came to the conclusion that there might be some benefit in altering human electrical fields with magnetic stimulation.[5] Barker wanted to selectively stimulate fibers within a peripheral nerve. Peripheral nerves contain both fast and slow fibers: the fast fibers carry reflex motor actions, while the slow fibers transmit somatic sensations like pain and heat. These have different thresholds of stimulation, so in principle it should be possible to stimulate one set of fibers and not the other. But electrical stimulation applied to the surface of the arms or to the skull activates both fast and slow fibers. It was almost impossible to get selective results with an applied electric field.

Magnetic fields were an alternative, and in 1982, after getting his Ph.D., Tony Barker returned to the topic, which was to selectively stimulate fast nerve fibers while leaving slow fibers untouched. Using a magnetic coil applied to the nerves in the arm, he was able to do just this.[6] Could the same be done for the brain? Approaching the problem as an engineer rather than as a biologist or a physician, this project seemed to have potential pitfalls to Barker. Could magnetic stimulation of the brain wipe out memory, or otherwise interfere with important, intimate functions, and perhaps do so permanently? Barker was unfamiliar with the precedent of ECT, and he was also unaware that eighty years earlier a number of less cautious experimenters had put their heads inside large magnetic coils and reported that switching on the coils could induce the perception of flashes of light, or phosphenes, and other indications of brain stimulation.[7]

Discovering the work of the London neurophysiologists Patrick Merton and Bert Morton on transcranial electrical stimulation, Barker reasoned that it seemed possible to stimulate electrical circuits in the brain directly and produce effects without permanently affecting the memories and personality of a human volunteer.[8] The problem was that the amount of electricity required to get through the bones of the skull was painful to the skin and could lead to burns, if given continuously rather than in the brief fashion used in ECT. In line with his original vision, Barker's new approach offered an ideal way around this problem, in that a magnet held near the scalp can induce changes in the electrical fields of the brain without having to travel through the scalp or skull. There is no pain; there are no burns. Barker and his group tried it out on themselves, and it worked. He arranged to visit Merton and Morton in their department in London, bringing his homemade magnetic stimulator with him in two suitcases. They set their apparatus up in the laboratory in London and, holding a large magnetic coil over the vertex of the head, magnetically stimulated the brain of a volunteer whose hand moved without discomfort.

A series of phone calls brought others from elsewhere in London to the laboratory, and transcranial magnetic stimulation (TMS) was born. Word spread quickly, and Barker and his group did a number of public demonstrations of the new technique during 1985 at the Physiological Society meeting in Oxford and the Eleventh International Congress of EEG and Clinical Neurophysiology in London, at which queues of people lined up to be tested. They went back to base and constructed six machines, one of which went to John Rothwell at the National Hospital for Neurology and Neurosurgery in Queen Square, one of the leading neurological centers in the world.

The first vision for TMS was that it would be used for diagnostic and research purposes. And it still has a place in these areas. Many departments of psychology and neurology have TMS machines to map brain functions. The technology allows researchers to pinpoint where in the brain certain functions are localized, or in some cases what areas of brain or peripheral nerves have been damaged in the case of brain disorders such as motor neuron disease or multiple sclerosis.

Barker formed a company based in Wales, called Magstim, with one of his Ph.D. students, Reza Jalinous.[9] This was one of four companies that began to supply devices for use in the field. The others were Cadwell Laboratories in Washington State; Dantec, a division of the giant medical devices company Medtronic, based in Michigan; and Neotonus in Georgia. By the year 2000, three thousand papers on the use of TMS had appeared, with new papers appearing at a rate of one per day.[10]

TMS in Psychiatry

At no point did it cross Tony Barker's mind that TMS might offer a treatment for any psychiatric disorder. The idea that TMS might have an application in psychiatry seems to have taken root simultaneously in several different settings in the early 1990s. The first published use came from Bonn, Germany, where Gerd Hoflich and colleagues tried TMS in two psychotically depressed patients who were resistant to antidepressants, prior to proceeding to ECT. Neither patient responded, although both later responded to ECT.[11] Another group in Krakow, Poland, linked to Jerzy Vetulani, also saw potential in the new method as a possible replacement for ECT—although no trials in patients were reported.[12]

The first positive results came from Israel, where Robert Belmaker and colleagues at Ben Gurion University in Jerusalem treated a series of patients, after first experimenting with TMS in an animal screening test for antidepressants—the Porsolt swim test.[13] This is a behavioral despair test, rather than a test that explicitly tries to model depression, but a number of antidepressants and electroconvulsive stimulation (ECS) when given to animals, delayed the onset of despair in this test. When TMS produced the same results as antidepressants and ECS in this model, Belmaker was interested. In 1994, he and his group reported the first beneficial effects of TMS in depressed patients at a European College of Neuropsychopharmacology meeting in Jerusalem.[14]

But the main action happened in the United States, in the NIMH/ NIH, where almost unbeknownst to one another there were three sets of players, two of which were linked to Robert Post, who had a long-standing research program looking at the effect of anticonvulsants on mood, and another group that no one was aware of. In 1980, Post reported beneficial effects of carbamazepine, an anticonvulsant drug marketed as Tegretol and prescribed for epilepsy, in treating mania, and he proposed a theoretical model for why anticonvulsants might act as what later came to be called mood-stabilizers.[15] He suggested that recurrent mood disorders and recurrent convulsive disorders might share a common pathophysiology, in that each dysthymic or convulsive episode kindled the next episode. This pointed to the need for a treatment that quenched the risk of future episodes, and this he suggested was what anticonvulsant drugs did.

Post's hypothesis was hugely influential during the late 1980s and early 1990s, particularly following the marketing of semi-sodium valproate by Abbott Laboratories in the United States for bipolar disorder. It became common practice to review all anticonvulsants for possible mood-stabilizing properties and for treating mania in bipolar disorder. Vigabatrin and topiramate, also anticonvulsants, were found not to be effective in stabilizing mood, and their use came at a very high cost in terms of side effects. Other anticonvulsants, such as lamotrigine, may have antidepressant activity but do not have convincing mood-stabilization properties. Nonetheless, there has been little serious questioning of Post's idea. The logical extension of Post's argument is to diagnose patients who are thought to be prone to bipolar disorders early in life before their first episode and to start them on anticonvulsants from their preschool or certainly preteen years.[16] This now happens widely in the United States—but not in Europe—suggesting that there was something peculiarly relevant to that nation in Post's original vision.

Whatever ECT did to get patients well, paradoxically almost, it also raised seizure thresholds just as the anticonvulsants did, making the occurrence of a subsequent clinical episode harder to kindle.[17] Post himself was not a fan of ECT, but it made sense to investigate whether TMS might also make further seizures less likely. Post's team, including a postdoctoral student named Susan Weiss, were interested in how one convulsion kindled the next. They reasoned that if the same thing happened in mood disorders, then what was needed was a treatment that "quenched" the propensity for seizures. Weiss developed an animal model of quenching and found that TMS did, indeed, appear to extinguish that propensity, indicating TMS as a potentially beneficial treatment for mood disorders.[18] There was initial excitement, but efforts to replicate this effect failed. Meanwhile, other developments in NIMH linked to Post were about to steer TMS in a different direction.

Visualizing the Brain

Mark George studied medicine at the University of South Carolina and then secured a place at NIMH. Convinced that most psychological syndromes would turn out to be brain circuit disorders, George was intent on training in both neurology and psychiatry. During a sabbatical year beginning in the summer of 1990, he worked as a fellow at Queen Square Hospital in London with Michael Trimble, a leading British neuropsychiatrist and behavioral neurologist. Trimble's team was based on the eighth floor, one floor below the labs of David Marsden and John Rothwell, both of whom studied movement disorders. One day while taking the elevator down, George met a man who was clearly puzzled, explaining that "some doctors up there put a magnet on my head and caused my hand to move." Taking the elevator back up to the ninth floor, George encountered a team led by Rothwell who were using magnets placed over the top and middle of the head of subjects— corresponding to the site of the motor cortex—to cause hands, arms, or legs to move.[19] Intrigued, George asked them whether they had considered moving the magnetic coil over the prefrontal lobes of the brain. They were surprised that anyone might want to do that. Neurologically, the prefrontal areas of the brain are largely silent. Nothing moves on stimulation, not fingers, arms, legs or toes, and if something does not visibly respond, for most neurologists it does not exist.

But George's early work on neuro-imaging was just then starting to take focus, pointing to a more dynamic and important role for traditionally more quiescent areas of the brain such as the prefrontal cortex. Positron emission tomography (PET) scans and magnetic resonance imagery (MRI) revealed activity in brain tissue in a completely new way, suggesting underactive and overactive brain circuits played a role in conditions from Parkinson's disease to obsessive-compulsive disorder (OCD). One of the images that came into focus was that of the depressed brain, where it seemed there was reduced activity in the prefrontal lobes and an underlying pathology in the frontal lobes themselves or in the basal structures of the brain that interconnected with the frontal areas.[20] If some treatment could be found that stimulated activity in these areas, it might turn out to be a cure for depression. Perhaps this was the mechanism by which ECT had its effect—the current in bilateral ECT is, after all, directed through the prefrontal lobes.

George had to wait until he got back to NIMH to test his ideas. Scheduled to work in Post's unit, George found he had little in common with others in the group. They were primarily interested in neurotransmitters, and for George, the neurotransmitter paradigm, which viewed the brain as a chemical soup, made little sense. In contrast, the motor group in the neurological service at NIH led by Mark Hallett had one of the few TMS facilities outside of Queen Square, and Hallett and Eric Wassermann were using TMS in much the same way that it was being used in London. Nominally supervised by Post, George approached Hallett and Wassermann, armed with brain scans showing prefrontal underactivity in depression. Hallet and Wassermann listened with interest, but their reaction, like that of Post in psychiatry, was that this was an intriguing hypothesis rather than systematic science. George was given the opportunity to use the laboratories early in the morning or late in the evening, when he would not interfere with the real work going on. So all of his early studies were done before 8 A.M. and after 7 P.M.

George ran into problems and delays. Early work on TMS in neurological subjects had shown that it could occasionally induce seizures.[21] Institutional review boards and ethics committees in the NIMH therefore wanted studies of healthy volunteers to establish the safety of the parameters being proposed for his work. No one knew what the effects of prefrontal stimulation might be. No one knew either whether to stimulate the right or the left prefrontal region, or whether it was better to apply high- or low-frequency stimulation. Using healthy volunteer studies to work this out, George found to his surprise that left-sided stimulation seemed if anything to enhance functioning in healthy volunteers, whereas high-frequency right-sided stimulation induced anxiety.[22] In contrast, one person had a noticeable mood change after medial prefrontal stimulation, feeling sad while remembering a funeral scene. This individual also had a kick in his prolactin levels, suggesting that the treatment was having an effect on deeper brain structures and might be close to causing a seizure. In general it appeared that TMS could also change peripheral thyroid hormone levels.[23] This was important in the long run, as it suggested that although the direct effects of TMS are on superficial areas of the motor cortex, these effects can trigger changes deeper in the brain.

It was clear that as part of the development of the new treatment, randomized controlled trials would be needed in which active TMS was compared with a placebo. George and colleagues devised a sham procedure. Active treatment would involve the traditional placement of the magnet in a position parallel to the head so that the magnetic field affected underlying electrical flow in the brain, whereas sham TMS used the very same magnets held in a position perpendicular to the brain so that there would be little effect on the underlying brain circuits. This was quite convincing in that one of the most salient aspects of treatment is the noise the magnets make, and this was the same for both treatments.

George and colleagues then did a within-week crossover study on chronically depressed inpatients who were given repetitive sham TMS, or TMS over the left prefrontal lobes at 1 Hz or 20 Hz, or over the right prefrontal lobes at the same two frequencies. In this single-blind randomized crossover study, active TMS produced no benefits over sham treatment—although it should be noted that convincing effects within a week have not been found with any treatment for depression, except perhaps ECT. Again, they found that patients got more anxious with right-brain stimulation, especially at the higher frequency.[24]

Combined, these results suggested that the best bet for treatment was repetitive high-frequency left-sided stimulation of the prefrontal lobes. A new treatment, rTMS (repetitive TMS), was born. Whereas other investigators in the field held the magnetic paddles over the vertex of the head, just as the neurologists had been doing, or over the midline of the frontal lobes, George and his group were stimulating to the side and the front of the brain, driven by brain imagery of where the problem might lie. At the same time, George and Eric Wassermann began studies in patients who had OCD. Guided by brain images that showed hyperactivity in what appeared to be a discrete brain circuit, they attempted to treat OCD with TMS by interfering with specific circuits rather than stimulating the brain as a whole. In the case of treating OCD, however, rTMS was overtaken by a more direct method of stimulating the same circuits, as we shall see.

In addition to the theoretical issues about where to stimulate, there were practical issues to consider. George at this point was using a Cadwell machine. This had a tendency to "blow up" at six-monthly intervals, which meant the team had to have several machines. Also, the Cadwell was cooled by water, and in earlier models the water was only separated from a considerable electrical charge by a thin rubber ring. As a physicist put it to him at one meeting—he was going to die if he kept on doing TMS with this machine. (Similar exchanges in all probability also played a part in the early history of ECT.) NIMH absolutely refused to support another of his proposals, which was to deliver TMS within an MRI scanner. Who knew what would happen if a powerful magnetic flux were created within a static magnetic field; the radiology department feared for the safety of the very building.[25]

Treating depression with TMS was more problematic than treating OCD. Although decreased activity in the frontal lobes had been described by a number of researchers, the changes in neuronal firing patterns were less clear cut than those reported in OCD. To tackle this issue, they began with an open study of TMS and depression, and soon treated a number of people who would clearly be called "responders." One was a woman from Maine who was a software developer and a pilot, with a ten-year history of treatment-resistant depression. She had previously responded to ECT, and to carbamazepine, but her responses had been transient. On the second week of rTMS, she showed a clear lightening of mood, which in turn, elated the research team. While treating her and others with rTMS, they also ran concurrent PET studies to see whether they could demonstrate actual brain changes that might coincide with any therapeutic response.

For their first real treatment study, George had to justify to the NIMH institutional review board his idea of pitting this new treatment against a sham treatment that clearly would have no effect. There was pressure on them to keep the sham treatment period short, so they opted for a two-week trial, reasoning that this was the minimum schedule needed to see effects with ECT. There seemed to be benefits with rTMS, but these were not dramatic. Yet after all, showing any kind of improvement after two weeks was more than most people might have expected, and these slender benefits provided real grounds for optimism.[26]

Before George and his group could publish their findings, another group, operating outside the constraints of the U.S. system for research in human subjects, reported positive results in treating depression with TMS. Alvaro Pascual-Leone, working at NIH on TMS with Hallett and Wassermann at the same time as George, had returned to his native Spain, and in short order, he recruited a group of psychotically depressed subjects to a study in which high-frequency left prefrontal rTMS was compared to sham TMS. The results reported in the *Lancet* showed that in seventeen patients with medication-resistant psychotic depression—the severest kind of depression—there were dramatic responses after a week of treatment. "Our findings emphasize the role of the left dorsolateral prefrontal cortex in depression and suggest that rTMS of the left dorsolateral prefrontal cortex might become a safe, nonconvulsive alternative to electroconvulsive treatment in depression."[27]

George, Belmaker, and others were stunned. Someone working in their midst had managed to pull off a study like this without any of them aware that it was being undertaken. The outside world was electrified, expressing intense interest in the new treatment. Within three or four years, most departments of psychiatry in Germany, for instance, a country that had traditionally been hostile to ECT, were engaged in TMS research. When a chair in psychiatry in Berne fell vacant, half the applicants listed TMS as their research area of interest. Countries like Holland, Belgium, Germany, and Japan, in which ECT was banned or restricted, saw an upsurge of interest in TMS. In these countries, which were often heavily oriented toward either psychotherapy or psychopharmacology, and in which the traditional physical treatments in psychiatry were often linked to the horrors of World War II, physical treatments once more appeared to offer possibilities.

If triggering activity in the frontal lobes of the brain mediated the therapeutic effect of ECT, it seemed reasonable that a method to induce focal changes in the brain, such as TMS, might do so much more selectively and without producing the contentious side effects of ECT. The arena of physical treatments was thus transformed from one in which all the key theoretical breakthroughs were thought to have been made forty years beforehand (and the only innovations came from minor modifications in the machinery), into a playing field for new conceptualizations. It seemed possible to develop new treatments that might avoid the seizures and stigma of ECT; research seemed driven by theoretical questions that excited psychiatrists and neuroscientists alike in a way that psychopharmacology had long since failed to do.

Comparing the two procedures, TMS was less problematic than ECT. In the case of ECT, the bones of the skull and the oiliness of the scalp and hair obstructed the effective transmission of an electrical signal. It was impossible to judge how much electricity was needed to trigger a seizure other than by trial and error and rules of thumb, such as the fact that older people, in general, need a higher dose than younger people owing to a thickening of the skull that occurs with age. Within the skull itself are fissures where the bones connect, and these sutures provide sinks through which electricity can readily pass. The precise location of these fissures varies from person to person, and thus, so does the distribution of electricity within the skulls of individual patients. With TMS, on the other hand, the skull is effectively transparent. The reversing magnetic fields alter the current in the brain cells underneath it with no need for the signal to travel through the skull.

The big drawback to TMS, however, was that it did not penetrate the brain to any great depth. If the effects of ECT are mediated through some action of the induced seizures or the electrical current on deeper brain structures such as the thalamus, hippocampus, or other components within the neuroendocrine system, then TMS was at a competitive disadvantage. To combat this, TMS therapy could attempt to change cortical circuits that, in turn, modified deeper cell networks, but in the late 1990s, this remained at the level of aspiration. The only possibility left was to reach deeper into the brain by using TMS to produce a seizure. It was this latter possibility that led Harold Sackeim, allied with Holly Lisanby at Columbia, and Thomas Schlaepfer in Berne, to take the approach opposite to Mark George's: instead of avoiding rTMS-induced seizures, they would crank up the intensity of the stimulation in order to trigger them.

Left or Right?

TMS arrived on scene with a natural ally: its development coincided with the emergence and diffusion of brain-imaging techniques. Researchers could look at what was happening in the brains of patients during TMS application. Did the reduced blood flow to the frontal lobe found in depression reverse itself with ECT or TMS? Did left-sided

TMS produce benefits that right-sided TMS did not? Mark George's thinking may have propelled questions in this direction, but Harold Sackeim had launched the debates in the 1980s and 1990s.

Sackeim trained in psychology in Philadelphia before moving to Columbia in 1977, where he split his time between the Psychiatric Institute at Columbia and New York University's new clinical psychology training program. One of his main interests was in the neuropsychology of affect, and in particular its lateralization—which half of the brain dominated mood-based and emotional-social behaviors. In 1980, he cowrote a grant application with Sidney Malitz to look at the affective and cognitive consequences of ECT. In the midst of an administrative crisis, PI asked Malitz to be its director, and this left Sackeim holding a funded grant on ECT, never having witnessed its actual clinical use.

Completely new to the field, Sackeim posed a number of questions aimed at controlling the research parameters. What was the right dose? It turned out there was no consensus on this issue, partly because the seizure, or the response, was seen as the mediator of benefits, and the electrical current, or the stimulus to that response, was viewed as almost incidental. This was the central tenet of ECT's mechanism of action, since it had been articulated by Jan-Otto Ottosson in 1960. But for a study of the cognitive effects of ECT, there was clearly a premium on standardizing the dose of electricity. As part of their research, Sackeim and colleagues devised a protocol that involved titrating the dose of ECT so that patients received stimulation sufficient to induce a seizure, but not so high as to cause cognitive problems.[28]

Another strategy for managing the cognitive effects of ECT was to use right unilateral rather than bilateral ECT. The rationale here was based on hemispheric lateralization: the right side of the brain is the nondominant one (in most individuals), so passing current through this hemisphere should lead to a generalized convulsion with electrically induced side effects localized to the right hemisphere only. As this is the nonverbal hemisphere of the brain, the hope was that verbal or memory-related capacity would be spared. A series of research programs starting with Richard Abrams in the 1970s had suggested that this might be the case, but successive projects and later clinical practice indicated that patients treated with right unilateral ECT were less likely to recover or were slower to respond to treatment than were patients treated bilaterally (see chapter 6).

One explanation for the different responses to bilateral and unilateral ECT was that the point in the brain through which the current passed might be critically important to the therapeutic response. If this was the case, it might be possible, by targeting the locus of stimulation in each patient, to produce a therapeutic response using electrical current without inducing seizures. An alternative theory was that the effects of ECT were not mediated through some generalized consequence of a seizure, such as a neuroendocrine change, but rather, that there was something more localized or focal about its effect. Either way there seemed to be a premium on localization.

As it happened, owing to his position at PI, Sackeim's group was among the first to produce brain images of altered frontal lobe functioning in depression. Imaging the brain after therapeutically effective, bilateral ECT showed a shut-down of function in the frontal lobes, which Sackeim interpreted as a regional inhibition, whereas unilateral ECT showed inhibition of the motor strip only but not the frontal lobes.[29] These findings suggested that one reason for the failure of right unilateral ECT to produce the benefits of bilateral ECT was that right unilateral stimulation did not trigger a seizure in the frontal lobes to the same extent as bilateral, and thus was ineffective at inducing postictal inhibition of some key brain activity. If this were the case, one possibility was to increase the dose of the stimulating current used in unilateral therapy. A higher dose would ensure current flowed to the right frontal lobe and triggered a seizure there.

At this point Sackeim's work began to converge with the emerging field of TMS, and specifically with the work of Mark George. This was reflected in an editorial debate between George and Sackeim in 1994 in *Convulsive Therapy,* where George proposed that subconvulsive brain stimulation might produce a cure in depression, while Sackeim argued that the new field of magnetic stimulation might be better off aiming to trigger seizures rather than trying to avoid them.[30] This was a first proposal of the idea of magnetic seizure therapy. At this point, Sackeim was joined by Holly Lisanby from Duke University, and her brief within the group was to help develop MST. George's contribution offered the first articulation of the idea that a seizure might not be necessary for ECT.[31] This was a heretical idea for some and simply not worth taking seriously for others. The battle lines were most clearly drawn between George and Max Fink. Sackeim was initially in the middle, but the developing logic of the Sackeim position eventually drew him closer to George.

The next step for Sackeim was to see what happened with right unilateral treatment delivered at a higher dose. In a series of studies

Sackeim suggested that right unilateral ECT at higher doses produced comparable benefits to bilateral ECT while at the same time sparing cognitive capacities. Fink and Abrams responded that right unilateral ECT, no matter how high the dose, remained less effective than bilateral ECT and that at higher doses the adverse cognitive effects of right unilateral ECT were as obvious as any following bilateral ECT.

The issues developed a generational flavor. On one side was an old guard denying there was any problem with the standard treatment. On the other was a group of younger researchers armed with a battery of new technologies. The ability to visualize the brain almost forced new questions, and certainly created new grant-getting opportunities. A series of new therapies also began to hover on the horizon—vagus nerve stimulation (VNS) and deep brain stimulation (DBS). Money and influence began to drift toward the younger generation and the newer technologies. The journals and organizations within the field document the shift as well.

In 1945, a new organization, the Society of Biological Psychiatry (SBP) was inaugurated, with its journal, *Biological Psychiatry*, at about the same time that the Electroshock Research Association (ESRA) was organized by David Impastato, William Holt, and Zigmond Lebensohn. ESRA published its proceedings in a Swiss journal, *Confinia Neurologica*. In the late 1950s, a carbon dioxide therapy association formed around Ladislaus Meduna, and this group published their proceedings in yet another new periodical—the *Journal of Neuropsychiatry*. By 1960, the three societies recognized that they had similar interests, and SBP absorbed the other two in 1963. But the resulting society was plagued by a dynamic that has been common to psychiatric and psychopharmacological societies ever since—it became polarized between a group of clinicians who saw themselves as trying to advance therapy (those who had formerly been in ESRA and the Carbon Dioxide Association), while the SBP wing saw themselves as "scientists."[32] With the decline of ECT in the 1960s, the SBP faction won out.

When the California legislature passed anti-ECT legislation in 1974, Gary Aden of San Diego organized a group to oppose these developments (see chapter 10). It first met in May 1975 in conjunction with the annual APA meeting. In May 1976, this became the International Association for the Advancement of Electrotherapy (IPAAE). At first, IPAAE was largely a political organization composed exclusively of clinicians, but in the late 1970s, it began inviting attendees from the main APA meetings, such as Max Fink and Dick Abrams, to contribute. By

1984, IPAAE meetings were organized around invited speakers on ECT topics.

In 1984, Fink established a new journal, *Convulsive Therapy,* which published its first issue in early 1985. Looking for a membership organization that would support the journal, he turned to IPAAE, which made *CT* its official journal in 1986. IPAAE then changed its name to the Association for Convulsive Therapy (ACT), and membership included a subscription to *CT.* Fink served as journal editor from 1985 to 1994, when Charles Kellner took over, who in turn was succeeded by Vaughn McCall in 2004. In 1997, a number of new members were suggested for the editorial board of *CT,* who were distinguished by their interest in TMS rather than in ECT. By 1999, these new board members pushed through a change in the name of the periodical to the *Journal of ECT: Dedicated to the Science of Electroconvulsive Therapy and Related Treatments* (*JECT*). The journal continues to publish under this name, even though few papers on TMS have actually appeared in it. Also in 1999, TMS featured prominently in symposia at ACT's annual meeting, and since then VNS, and more recently MST, have been highlighted. Meanwhile, the APA Task Force on ECT also had its name changed to Corresponding Committee on ECT and other Electromagnetic Therapies, and, as of 2004, the task force has been chaired by Holly Lisanby, whose primary background was in TMS rather than ECT.

The split between the new and the old guard was portrayed by Sackeim in 2004 in an editorial written for *JECT,* in which he viewed himself and other like-minded researchers as occupying a middle ground, under assault from the Church of Scientology on the left and from the old guard in ECT on the right. The old guard, according to Sackeim, believed that ECT properly used was almost universally effective and never caused problems, and this obviated the need for any further research.[33]

In contrast, rTMS, for instance, appeared to be as rational a treatment as could be wished for. George had linked TMS usage to an effort to alter blood flow through the prefrontal cortex in a manner that would reverse psychiatric symptoms ascribed to this area. Increasing the dose appeared to have a bigger effect on changes in blood flow, opening up the possibility of establishing TMS as a highly rational and predictable treatment option. Investigators looking at the therapy's effects on the biochemistry of the brain, such as alterations in neurotransmitter activity like dopamine or in terms of changes in the level of gene transcription, as evidenced by activation of immediate early genes, found that TMS produces effects that mapped onto those previously reported for antidepressants.[34]

When in Doubt, Electrify: The Lure of Electromagnetism

But all was not as it seemed. The first problem was that Pascual-Leone's research, rushed to publication in the *Lancet* in 1996, turned out to be mysteriously unreplicable. No one else has been able to show a comparable response in psychotic depression, especially on the time-scale of a week. Although researchers from Germany to Japan and from Brazil to Canada attempted to reproduce the results of this study, all have achieved negative results. The negative findings could be explained to some extent on the basis that trial protocols were still limited to two-week studies for the most part, and by the fact that the dose of treatment and the best site for stimulation had still not been worked out. There were even doubts as to the best shape of the electromagnetic coil. Combined with different intensities of stimulation, differently sized and shaped coils might produce a broader effect on the brain with greater biological and therapeutic consequences.

The bubble burst, however, when from within the field of rTMS research, Thomas Schlaepfer and others meta-analyzed the body of published studies as of 2003 (limiting their analysis to those studies with reasonable protocols and where results were adequately reported), and concluded that "current trials are of low quality and provide insufficient evidence to support the use of rTMS in the treatment of depression."[35] TMS appeared to have some effect on mood, but it was not significant enough to replace anything in the therapeutic armamentarium, and certainly not ECT. Some within the field all but accused Schlaepfer of attempting to sabotage developments, but in one sense, this simply restored rTMS as a tool for researchers. It produced clear changes in brain function that could be used to map out further interactions between brain circuits, and it held some promise as a therapy in that it had a distinct, if minor, effect on mood. This reasonable stance, which was the position Mark George had adopted prior to the fuss generated by the Pascual-Leone findings, was not the message of support the field was looking for, and interest in rTMS began to ebb away.

The Pascual-Leone episode, however, was not an aberration within an otherwise rationally developing field. Within the new guard the competition was intense, with different parties jockeying for priority on treatments from TMS, MST, VNS, and DBS. At one point, one of the early movers in the emerging field, about to deliver an invited lecture, found himself handed a written statement to sign renouncing priority in the development of one of the new treatments that might have interfered with the patent application of his host: fail to sign and the lecture would be cancelled.[36]

But there was an even deeper problem. Efforts to come to grips with the history of ECT have often subsumed the subject into the history of medical electricity. The opening chapter of Timothy Kneeland and Carol Warren's *Pushbutton Psychiatry* details the origins of medical and therapeutic interest in electricity in Hippocratic medicine.[37] Part of our fascination with the fossil resin amber supposedly comes from a recognition by the ancients that amber could be electrified by friction, and the term *electricity* itself comes from *electron,* the Greek word for amber. Our focus in this book is on ECT in terms of the convulsion produced, rather than as another episode in the history of medical electricity. Electricity is incidental to the story of ECT as told here, but the history of medical electricity is highly germane to the TMS story.

Belmaker, George, Post, Lisanby, Weiss, and Pascual-Leone met in December 1996 at a workshop on rTMS in Puerto Rico.[38] The first question for the workshop was: what are the differences and similarities between electrical and magnetic stimulation of the scalp, particularly on the depth and magnitude of neuronal excitement? None of the participants appeared to be aware of the prior existence of transcranial electrical stimulation, or of the history of electrotherapeutics dating back a hundred years or more. An awareness of this history might have led to much greater skepticism regarding what they might have been seeing, but the notion that they might be reinventing the wheel was not welcomed.

Just as Tony Barker initiated the history of TMS by using magnets to trigger selective movements in the digits of the hand, so too the discovery of animal electricity by Luigi Galvani involved demonstrations that the limbs of even dead animals could be made to move by the application of an electric charge to nerve endings.[39] This gave rise to a bitter dispute between Galvani, who proposed the existence of animal electricity, and Alessandro Volta who denied this possibility.[40] Galvani's position effectively won out within medicine, and efforts to follow his lead by seeing what happened when electrical charges were applied to the brain, in due course gave rise to a new therapy, galvanism, and, it can be claimed, to neurology as a medical discipline.

The outlines of galvanism as a therapy had existed before Galvani. Earlier in the eighteenth century, John Wesley, an Anglican minister and leader in the Methodist movement, for instance, used a machine to deliver electric shocks to his congregation.[41] The first record of a patient with a clear mental disorder being treated with electric current applied to the head stems from John Birch, a surgeon at St. Thomas's Hospital in London in November 1787. The patient, who had many of the classic features of melancholia, had his head covered with a flannel by Birch who "rubbed the electric sparks all over the cranium; he seemed to feel it disagreeable but said nothing. On the second visit, finding no inconvenience that ensued, I passed six small shocks through the brain in different directions. As soon as he got into an adjoining room, and saw his wife, he spoke to her and in the evening was cheerful, expressing himself as if he thought he should soon go to his work again."[42] When seen three months later this man apparently remained perfectly well.

Galvani's breakthrough lay in his recognition of what happened when electricity was applied directly to nerve endings. He saw electricity as the agent of nervous action. But stimulating nerve endings directly was not necessary for the new therapists, in that most people understood electricity to be in essence a fluid of some sort, like ether, whose application to any part of the body could have tonic effects.[43] The issue was much more a case of devising methods to deliver this field, and an industry developed to meet the new need.[44] By the early nineteenth century, the potentially invigorating effects of electricity had become sufficiently established to feature prominently in Mary Shelley's *Frankenstein,* whose creation was, of course, brought to life by electricity.

There was a steady pace of electrical developments through the nineteenth century. In 1831, Michael Faraday discovered the interaction between electrical currents and magnetic fields and how to convert mechanical energy into electrical currents. James Clerk Maxwell linked electricity and magnetism in one of the first great unifying theories of physics. In 1875, Alexander Graham Bell invented the telephone, and in 1878, Joseph Swan in Britain developed the filament lamp. Thomas Edison developed, improved on, and mass-produced many electrical devices, and by the 1880s, cities were illuminated, and tramways began service as a result of electrical technology.[45]

Against this background, electrotherapeutics flourished. French, German, and English asylum doctors (alienists) published on the topic. In 1855, Guillaume Duchenne wrote *A Treatise on Localized Electrization and Its Application to Pathology and Therapeutics.*[46] Emil Du Bois-Reymond had also published a treatise titled *Investigations on Animal Electricity.*[47] The study of galvanism and electrotherapeutics pulled the discipline of neurology into existence and established a role for neurologists in the management of patients who would later be regarded as having psychosomatic problems.

In the 1870s, a series of British hospitals set up dedicated rooms in which electricity was used to treat patients. Very early on, medical practitioners from the most prestigious hospitals complained about the use of electricity by quack-physicians or healers.[48] As might be expected, the medical view was that only those specialized in the use of electricity and capable of understanding clinical pictures should be permitted to use these methods for therapeutic purposes. Allan Beveridge has argued that asylum doctors were particularly motivated to take up the use of electricity, as the notion of physical treatments endorsed their claims that insanity was a medical disease appropriately treated by medical practitioners rather than by moral or other means in asylums or other institutions run by nonmedical personnel.[49]

The forms of treatment were continuous current treatment—galvanism—or treatment with induced currents—faradism. These were both extensions of the methods used by Wesley and others previously, which had involved the delivery of a shock by means of frictional or static electricity. An alternate approach had been to insulate the patients, electrify them, and draw sparks from them.[50] The course of the new galvanic and faradic treatments ranged from a few days to several months, with therapy being applied in daily or alternate daily sessions, lasting for anything from ten to twenty minutes. In the midnineteenth century, electrodes were often placed on the patient's hands, but as the century went on they migrated to the head. Patients treated in this way, especially within the asylums, appear to have been predominantly depressive.[51] Occasionally, electrical treatments were linked with the induction of epileptic convulsions, but convulsions were thought to be undesirable, and for the most part, physicians preferred weaker currents to strong ones.[52]

Toward the end of the nineteenth century, however, electricity began to fall out of favor in the asylums. Even though dramatic responses had been reported in patients who had been considered insane for seven years or more, the treatment within the asylum did not have the same general degree of success that physicians treating patients with fashionable nervous complaints in office practice settings were reporting.

Among those treating psychosomatic patients with electricity were some of the most famous names of the day, such as George Miller Beard, who described a new syndrome—neurasthenia—that might have been conjured into existence for the purpose of response to electrotherapy.[53]

A range of theories developed to supplant the early idea that electricity provided a fluid that entered the body and exercised a tonic effect. Some thought electricity was stimulating, whereas others believed it to be sedative.[54] In a distinct echo of later TMS research, some thought it increased the blood flow to the brain,[55] while others argued that it decreased blood flow.[56] Poor results with electricity were put down to the fact that doctors or quack-healers had not followed guidelines, had not understood the nature of electricity, or had not chosen the correct patients. As Beard put it: "There is a vulgar error abroad, both in England and the United States, that any 'Old Granny' can make applications of electricity. . . . No man can apply electricity with a higher success until the details of the application had become to him a matter of routine, so that he can use any one of the methods on any kind of patient without fear or doubt. Skill of this sort in any art, cometh not of observations, it is acquired only by careful, studious and repeated experience."[57]

Interest in electrotherapeutics began to wane at the turn of the century, even in neurology. A 1901 review caught many of the issues:

> The employment of electricity in medicine has passed through many vicissitudes, being at one time recognized and employed at the hospitals, and again being neglected, and left for the most part in the hands of ignorant persons, who continue to perpetrate the grossest impositions in the name of electricity. As each fresh important discovery in electric science has been reached, men's minds have been turned anew to the subject, and interest in its therapeutic properties has been stimulated. Then after extravagant hopes and promises of cure, there have followed failures, which have thrown the employment of this agent into disrepute, to be again after time revived and brought into popular favor.[58]

As the neuroses became psychoneuroses, the possibility opened up that the effects of such an unquestionably physical therapy as electrotherapy might stem primarily from suggestion. A London physician, Hector A. Colwell, struck a more skeptical note in 1922: "On the occurrence of cases which refused to yield to any ordinary remedy, the mandate 'Let them be electrified' has often been issued, too frequently, rather with a vague hope of obtaining relief from an extraordinary remedy than from any well defined view of its real influence."[59] In this case, though, Colwell's skepticism was also a vivid demonstration of the ebb and flow of fashions in medicine, in that he was, in fact, citing the 1841 words of another physician, Golding Bird.

By 1922, electrotherapeutics was dead. But it came back in two forms. One was in the form of transcranial electrical stimulation (TES). TES was essentially a derivative of galvanism and goes back at least to Stéphane Armand Nicolas Leduc in 1902 and possibly before, depending on the definition.[60] Patrick Merton and Bert Morton from London had been using TES as an investigative tool when Tony Barker began his TMS experiments in 1982, but they thought its use was limited, as a continuous electrical current was painful. For several decades previously, however, TES had flourished within the Soviet Union as a therapy, apparently without causing pain, with clinicians claiming benefits in a range of psychoneurotic conditions. And there is strong evidence that TES can modify most of the cortical circuits that TMS can modify, leading researchers in Boston and elsewhere to suggest it might be as effective a therapy as TMS, but a much cheaper option for countries in the developing world.[61]

The difficulty in distinguishing between fast and slow nerve fibers in the spinal cord that Barker had sought to solve by introducing TMS, in fact also produced another therapy that everyone conceded works, albeit with a modest effect—transcutaneous electrical nerve stimulation (TENS). The easiest nerve fibers to stimulate electrically are the slow, small-diameter fibers that conduct pain sensation: increased firing in these fibers activates neurons that project to the brain and blocks a gate-mechanism that would otherwise let pain signals through to the brain. This is the basis for the gate-control theory of pain put forward by Ronald Melzack and Patrick Wall in the 1960s. In the 1970s, this phenomenon was utilized as a therapeutic procedure in chronic pain syndromes and in childbirth.[62] Although TENS is now widely employed in hospital settings, there is also a thriving undergrowth of companies offering variations on TENS, such as Alpha-Stim, which purport to be treatments for anxiety, depression, and stress. Companies like Alpha-Stim offer FDA-"registered" devices that aim to restore harmony to the electrical balance of cells, organs, and whole bodies.[63] Although TENS unquestionably works, many of these related devices resemble the electrotherapeutic apparatus of a previous century and appear targeted at a vulnerable, desperate, or psychosomatic marketplace.

The group that included Belmaker, George, Post, Lisanby, Weiss, and Pascual-Leone assembled at the ACNP workshop in Puerto Rico in 1996 were largely ignorant of this backdrop. Given the dramatic findings of Pascual-Leone and the visible changes in brain blood flow in response to rTMS, there seemed every reason for them to disregard history and continue to believe that what they were seeing represented a radical break with the past. Yet historical cycles have a way of re-asserting themselves, and the results from blind trials suggest that a good deal of the TMS craze to date has represented a further chapter in the history of electrotherapeutics rather than anything else. There are in fact companies delivering rTMS therapies in Canada and elsewhere that seem indistinguishable from Alpha-Stim. These companies and their glossy brochures seem to be feeding on the same population of patients that visited neurologists at the turn of the nineteenth century for the latest electrotherapy. This is a therapy in which small gains are being made, but which is open to gross exploitation, as the story of an-other electrotherapy—VNS—seems to illustrate.

Vagus Nerve Stimulation

Beginning with the discovery of a possible mood-enhancing or stabi-lizing effect of valpromide, a drug first used as an anticonvulsant in epileptic patients in Lyon, France, in the mid-1960s, interest had been growing in a possible relationship between anticonvulsants and mood stabilization. Carbamazepine (Tegretol), another anticonvulsant, was shown by researchers in Japan in the early 1970s to also balance mood. This correspondence led Bob Post to propose his kindling hypothesis of mood-stabilization.

A zeal for anticonvulsants developed on the assumption that almost any anticonvulsant would act as a mood stabilizer. This produced, for instance, an explosion in the use of gabapentin (Neurontin) in the late 1990s, fueled, it appears, by a series of ghostwritten articles, planted in a series of journals by the drug's manufacturer, Warner Lambert, that suggested gabapentin would be effective for mood disorders.[64] At one point gabapentin was grossing $1.3 billion a year, a very large proportion of which came from its off-label use as a mood stabilizer. The bubble was punctured when a randomized controlled trial demonstrated that gabapentin had little if any mood-stabilizing property.[65]

This background set the scene for the discovery or creation of an-other mood stabilizer. In the late 1980s, a new treatment was introduced for refractory epilepsy—vagus nerve stimulation (VNS). The vagus, or tenth cranial, nerve is unique in that linking heart, lungs, and other major organs with the brain, it is composed primarily of ascending fibers that run from these organs to the brain rather than, as in the case of the other cranial nerves, descending fibers running from the brain to innervate muscles or organs. This fact about the vagus was known from the 1930s.[66] And indeed there are good grounds to think the brain is more concerned about events happening inside the body that anything happening in the environment. A full bladder or bowel tends to grab our attention just as much as any threat in the environment does. Because these bodily functions happen so easily, we tend to forget about what might be called the visceral brain and think only of our auditory or visual brain sensations.

Jake Zabara, an electrophysiologist at Temple University in Philadelphia, seized on the idea that stimulating the vagus nerve influences those brain areas receiving input from vagal nerve fibers to investigate in the mid-1980s whether stimulation delivered in this way might be anticonvulsant.[67] Zabara found that vagal stimulation in dogs suppressed epileptic activity. He trailed his idea around device companies but got nowhere until Reese Terry at Intermedics responded. But this was outside Intermedics's core area, which was cardiac rhythm management, and the company stalled on the project. Terry remained enthusiastic, however, and set up his own firm in Houston in 1987, Cyberonics, having obtained the rights to the idea from Zabara.

Kiffin Penry and Christine Dean in Salem, North Carolina, treated the first patient with VNS in 1988 as part of a pilot study with patients who had treatment-resistant partial seizures and who were not appropriate for surgery.[68] This work was done in conjunction with Cyberonics, which by this stage had developed a repetitive mechanical stimulator, effectively a modified cardiac pacemaker for further studies.[69] (The technique involves implanting a pulse generator about the size of a pocket watch in the left chest wall to deliver electrical signals to the left vagus nerve through an electrode wrapped about the vagus nerve in the neck.) Using the Cyberonics stimulator, two open trials and then two randomized trials were undertaken. In the randomized trials, patients were assigned for a twelve- to sixteen-week period to either low- or high-stimulation conditions, with the low-stimulation intervention serving as a placebo. These patients had on average a more than twenty-year history of seizures and were taking at least two anticonvulsants. Overall, the high-stimulation group showed a 24.5 percent reduction in seizure frequency compared with 6.1 percent for the low-stimulation group.[70]

These results are not dramatic. But interest in the treatment developed on the back of results from follow-up studies. Seizure frequency seemed to diminish to an even greater extent over the subsequent year. VNS turned out to be quite different from other anticonvulsant treatments. It is not an acute treatment for convulsions, and although early trials demonstrated some anticonvulsant effect, VNS showed a developing anticonvulsant effect over time.[71] On the basis of these findings, VNS devices were approved in 1997 by the FDA for the adjunctive treatment of resistant partial and complex seizure disorders. As of 2004, approximately twenty thousand people had received implants.

Researchers using VNS to treat epilepsy became aware of "mood changes" in their patients, just as had happened with other anticonvulsants. Among the first to point this out was Gerda Elger, a neurologist from Bonn married to a psychiatrist, who claimed that there were positive mood changes in patients undergoing VNS that could not simply be explained in terms of improvement in the patients' epilepsy.[72] This finding was quickly picked up by Mark George and research groups active in TMS, for whom VNS appeared to offer another nonseizure-based physical therapy, and in addition a possible new research tool.[73] The first person explicitly given a VNS implant for a resistant mood disorder was treated in July 1998 at Mark George's unit in the Medical University of South Carolina.[74] As George would later show, the vagus nerve stimulates areas of the brain that can be termed the visceral brain and brings about changes in the orbital cortex and other limbic areas that are quite significant—at least as great as the changes occurring elsewhere in the brain in response, for example, to loud noise.

Cyberonics saw a much larger market—the same market being chased by Alpha-Stim and others. Panels of consultants were invited to explore the possibility that VNS might have a role in alleviating anxiety disorders, depression, obesity, Alzheimer's disease, and a myriad of psychiatric complaints. Satellite symposia, journal supplements, and glossy reprints of early articles were sponsored and supported by corporate interests. Company representatives enticed clinicians to learn about the new breakthrough and adopt the technology in their practice. Investigators brandished PET-scan evidence that VNS treatment affected the metabolism of limbic structures in the brain; neurochemical studies in both animals and humans were said to show VNS effects on concentrations of monoamine neurotransmitters within the central nervous system. Partisans conceded that controlled trials were still needed, and that animal and other studies were also required to support the claims of the treatment. Yet confident that the more rigorously tested results would confirm VNS as a revolutionary tool in biological psychiatry, a number of senior figures launched ahead to recommend the use of VNS in selected patients with treatment-resistant affective disorders.[75] Cyberonics brought the kind of muscle to this previously staid corner of the psychiatry world that a major pharmaceutical company would.

Using the very same techniques as in epilepsy, a first depression trial, the D01 study, involved Lauren Marangell at Baylor College of Medicine in Texas, Mark George at the Medical University of South Carolina, Harold Sackeim at the New York State Psychiatric Institute, and John Rush at the University of Texas Southwestern Medical Center at Dallas. Thirty patients were recruited in the first instance, followed by another set of thirty. The patients were an unusual group with an average of ten years of unmitigated depression before they entered the study, a very high depression score on the Hamilton Rating Scale, and on average, a failure to respond to sixteen distinct prior psychiatric interventions, including in two-thirds of the patients, ECT. Approximately one-third of the patients in this open trial showed some positive effect from VNS, yet only 15 percent could be considered actual responders.[76] But just as in earlier studies on epilepsy, where only 30 percent of the original group showed some response, this positive response rate increased to 45 percent over the course of the year.[77] Furthermore, the best predictor of a failure to respond to VNS was prior treatment resistance—the most treatment-resistant patients proved treatment-resistant to VNS also. This opened the door to considering what effect VNS might have in a less severely disturbed group.

A second trial, the D02 study, was planned as a controlled trial, designed to get FDA approval for the treatment of depression. Even though the group was much less severely ill, the response rate to VNS remained at 15 percent, while patients on sham VNS showed a 10 percent response. There was no significant statistical difference between these two groups. After ten weeks of sham treatment, patients in that arm of the trial were switched to active treatment, and as in the previous trial, a year later more had responded, with up to 30 percent of patients showing benefit.[78] The results, however, remained unpublished.

A third open study, D03, was undertaken. The results were mixed, though similar trials in Europe showed a somewhat better response profile, leading, in 2003, to European approval and licensing of VNS for the treatment of depression despite the weak data.[79] This occurred because medical device registration in Europe requires only that a manufacturer demonstrate safety; it does not have to show the device works in a clinical setting. The initial argument for registration of VNS in the United States was that it was already registered for use in Europe. The company pushed for an expedited review, and at an FDA advisory meeting on June 15, 2004, the panel, in a split vote, recommended approval for marketing. Stock prices for Cyberonics, a publicly traded company, jumped. On August 12, however, the FDA made it clear that the trial results were unconvincing, and it did not intend to follow the panel's recommendation.[80] Cyberonics's stock fell. At the start of February 2005, the FDA reopened the possibility of a future approval for VNS, and this time, stock zoomed 30 percent.[81] Finally, on July 15, 2005, it approved VNS for treatment-resistant depression, despite considerable skepticism on the part of some of the panelists regarding whether clinical benefits had been demonstrated.

The large amounts of money invested in Cyberonics stock brought a commercialism previously found only in psychopharmacology to the heart of the physical treatment of psychiatric disorders. The pitch to the press by the company was that there were up to four million Americans with treatment-resistant, or hard-to-treat depression, who might be candidates for VNS—a number well over 1 percent of the population.[82] The VNS market for epilepsy is considerably smaller. Currently, American psychiatrists are being flooded with brochures for VNS, and Cyberonics sponsors a Web site on VNS therapy for practitioners and prospective patients. Only time will tell what the cost of this treatment is for patients: VNS is a surgical procedure requiring general anesthesia to install an electronic device, which once inserted cannot ever be fully removed.

After a decade of VNS treatment for epilepsy, the therapy has been linked to a number of deaths. The FDA dismissed these fatalities as not yet replicated in the case of depression treatment. More to the point, the notion of mood stabilization—the idea that anticonvulsant treatments act by quenching kindling in both mood and convulsive disorders—rests on shaky ground. In June 2005, a controlled trial including more than 1,800 epilepsy patients showed there was little reason to think anticonvulsants diminished the risk of subsequent seizures. Patients who were not given anticonvulsants immediately after their first convulsion were as likely to be seizure-free as those given immediate treatment. Those in whom treatment was delayed or forestalled had a better quality of life than those who had been given immediate treatment.[83] This suggests the entire theoretical framework for a common treatment pathway for epilepsy and depression is flawed, raising problems and concerns with the whole approach.

Deep Brain Stimulation

VNS is far from being the only problematic new treatment on the block, however. The late 1990s also saw the emergence of deep brain stimulation (DBS), a treatment linked to what may be potentially even greater problems than those related to VNS. From the 1940s onward, there had been evidence that cutting pathways in the globus pallidus or the thalamus, both subcortical brain structures, could in some cases relieve severe tremors and other treatment-resistant aspects of Parkinson's disease,[84] and could also be beneficial in chronic pain syndromes.[85] The development of neurosurgery for Parkinson's disease ran parallel to the development of psychosurgery for psychiatric disorders during the 1950s. When psychosurgery came under a cloud in the late 1950s, neurosurgery continued, although the focus of treatment in Parkinson's disease switched to the new pharmacological possibilities following the discovery of dopamine depletion in the subcortical nuclei of these patients. This led to breakthrough treatments such as l-dopa. But although the new pharmacological treatments, aimed at replacing dopamine or stimulating the dopamine system, produced miraculous cures in some, they did not put things right for everyone, and a small number of patients continued to be candidates for surgery.

Thus, even though surgery for Parkinson's disease was a rarely used option, the need to intervene in chronic pain syndromes remained, as there were no comparable developments in the pharmacological management of pain. In the 1950s, reports of brain stimulation as a means to manage pain began to appear.[86] Then in the 1970s, based in part on the success of TENS, a surge of interest occurred in brain stimulation techniques as an alternative to surgery, and the procedure known as deep brain stimulation (DBS) emerged.[87] This approach was encouraged by the discovery of endogenous opiate pathways in the brain.

In the 1980s, stimulated by developments in pain management, neurosurgeons interested in Parkinson's disease began to experiment with DBS as an alternative to the irreversible effects of surgical interventions in this patient group. The method aimed to knock out brain circuits by stimulation from implanted electrodes and gave the neurosurgeon the ability to turn the stimulus on and off in order to track the effects of treatment. The benefits seemed dramatic in many cases, and the treatment was publicized with videos of advanced Parkinson's patients once unable to budge now able to move about freely; moreover, their requirements for ongoing drug medication were dramatically slashed.

As with TMS, DBS depends on neuro-imaging technology. In order to implant the electrodes in the correct location, it is necessary to be able to map each patient's brain in great detail using both MRI and CT scans, fusing these with computer programs to get a precise fix on the path of nerve tracts and blood vessels. A misplaced electrode can cause hemorrhage and death. The 2004 remake of *The Manchurian Candidate* gives a reasonably accurate image of what the procedure looks like. When the electrodes are in place, a battery operated device produces a stimulation that can be increased or decreased in frequency based on feedback from the patient. This stimulation can theoretically work by either overstimulating nerve cells, leading to somatic fatigue, or jamming the nerve cells so signals do not get through, in either case producing a functional lesion.

Awareness of the possible use of this technique in psychiatry grew following observations in Parkinson's disease that some electrode placements could trigger dysphoria, raising the possibility that the surgeons had tapped into a depression center.[88] These observations were reported widely in both the academic and lay media as dramatic new developments. As interest rose in the possible use of DBS in psychiatry, several groups had already made progress, with a team in Belgium, for example, reporting in the *Lancet* on DBS as a treatment for OCD.[89]

OCD was the most likely candidate for the first studies of DBS, having shown the best response rate to psychosurgery when that approach was still practiced. When the more general use of psychosurgery fell into disfavor, a number of centers in Sweden, Britain, and elsewhere continued to undertake operations for refractory cases of OCD. Another reason OCD was most amenable to psychosurgery and later, DBS, was that it is, unlike depression, less of a reactive condition: the death of a disliked spouse, for instance, does not trigger a dramatic improvement in treatment-refractory OCD in the way it can do in depression. OCD is one of the most sharply defined syndromes, and the arrival of brain imaging in psychiatry in the 1980s provided clear-cut and discrete findings for OCD of increased glucose metabolism or blood flow in the medial and orbital frontal cortex and anterior cingulate gyrus, as well as in the caudate nucleus and the hypothalamus of the subcortical midbrain. Successful treatment, furthermore, whether with pharmacotherapy or behavior therapy, appeared to normalize these overactive circuits. It seemed that there was a clear target at which to aim, and DBS promised to offer a way to test things out without producing irreversible changes.

Working separately but at the same time, Bart Nuttin in Leuven, Belgium, and George Curtis in Ann Arbor, Michigan, began to experiment with DBS. Aware of emerging work in managing Parkinson's disease and pain syndromes, Nuttin spent years considering the possibility of DBS, aware that psychosurgery was viewed dimly and concerned that stimulation approaches, although reversible, might be viewed similarly. But the ethics committee at his hospital gave the go-ahead, as did a few years later, an ethics committee in Paris where psychosurgery had been stopped for years.[90] Many people seemed disposed to view this treatment in a very different light from psychosurgery, though both Nuttin and Curtis had to interact closely with neurosurgeons in order to work out appropriate sites for implants and were dependent on psycho- or neurosurgeons for the technical expertise to implant the stimulating electrodes.

Having graduated from Vanderbilt University, George Curtis did a residency at McGill University in Montreal, where he engaged in research with prominent figures such as Heinz Lehmann and Donald Hebb, and trained clinically with Robert Cleghorn at a time when Ewen Cameron was the department head. Later in Philadelphia, Curtis took up neuroendocrine research in the late 1960s, when stress hormones were coming into vogue and the dexamethasone suppression test (DST) was about to become a symbol of the new biological psychiatry. In the course of this research, Curtis heard a lecture by Isaac Marks on behavior therapy for phobias and thought that exposure of phobics to threatening material would be a provocative challenge to the endocrine system. Little came out of the biological research that he undertook after moving to Ann Arbor, the home of the DST. Yet impressed by the response of phobic and, later, obsessive patients to exposure therapy, Curtis became a behavior therapist. This in due course left him with a cadre of therapy- and drug-resistant OCD patients; in 1995, looking for some treatment to benefit them, and aware of the work on DBS for pain and tremor, Curtis wondered whether deep brain stimulation might be the answer.[91]

The major firm in the field of making electrodes for the treatment of Parkinson's disease and pain syndromes was Medtronic, which supplied both Nuttin and Curtis with electrodes, but otherwise showed almost no interest in developing this new line of therapy. Curtis and his colleagues were held back by the fact that Ann Arbor was a small town and patient recruitment was painfully slow. But Nuttin was at a larger center in Leuven, leading, in 1989, to his group's reporting benefits of DBS for OCD and a show of interest from Medtronic.[92] A short while later, Luc Mallet and a group in Paris also reported that obsessive features appeared to improve in patients otherwise receiving DBS for Parkinson's disease.[93] Medtronic, sensing opportunity, convened a meeting of interested groups.

One of these was a collaboration based at Brown University in Rhode Island and the Cleveland Clinic in Ohio, which had an active psychosurgery program for OCD. This group, led by Benjamin Greenberg, who worked with Mark George and others on TMS at NIH, and Steve Rasmussen, who was integral in establishing the credentials of selective psychosurgery for OCD,[94] became interested in DBS and within a short time had developed the largest patient series for its study.[95] The smaller series studied by Curtis and his colleagues was eclipsed by the Greenberg and Rasmussen effort.[96]

But the more lucrative application for DBS is as a treatment for refractory depression rather than OCD. As of late 2006, a number of groups are chasing success in this area. Unlike OCD, however, there is no consensus on what brain circuitry is affected in depression, and without such accord, many question whether the hazards of this treatment are worth pursuing for a condition that can often clear up miraculously without treatment. DBS may well offer benefits, but efforts to develop it, at least for depression, have the potential to inflict the kind of damage on psychiatry's current stock of physical therapies that psychosurgery inflicted in the 1950s, bringing the whole field to a standstill once more.

The first claims of DBS's success in treating depression came from a group based at the University of Toronto and Emory University in Atlanta, Georgia. On March 1, 2005, the *Toronto Globe and Mail* told the dramatic story of Jeanne Harris, a former psychiatric nurse, who sobbed through an entire summer, spent six months in bed, and shunned food and friends. She had been so depressed for ten years, she was "willing to let doctors drill two holes in her head and implant electrodes in her brain, in one of the most radical mood-altering experiments on the medical books. . . . 'It is an unbelievable, dramatic change for me,' said the 50-year-old Harris after DBS therapy. 'For the first time in ten years, I feel alive, I have energy, it's like a light bulb being turned on.'"[97] In uncontrolled trials of DBS, not reported in the press, three of six patients demonstrated an apparent response to DBS.[98] Although many of these patients had prior episodes of depression and prior treatments, there was little about the patients' symptoms that would have categorized this as a severely depressed group. Two had to withdraw from treatment because of complications. None of the six patients responded to the degree Jeanne Harris reported in newspaper accounts of the research.

The account in the *Globe and Mail* is quite telling:

> Unlike ECT, which shocks the entire brain with electricity to induce brain seizures . . . , DBS is designed to electrically stimulate only the brain region known to be overactive in people [who are depressed]. . . . It is part of an expanding field known as brain pacemakers. . . . DBS is less painful than ECT. . . . However researchers could not first test their hunch in any animal model, and there were risks: a small chance of brain hemorrhage or seizure. But when Ms Harris read through all the information, she didn't hesitate to sign up: "It seemed to make sense to me. At that point, I didn't care. I didn't even care if it killed me." . . . For Ms Harris, who now shops, throws dinner parties, and visits the library, the effects of the new implants were immediate: "When I first came home, I was out with a hat covering the staples on my head and cutting back the hedges that had overgrown for so long . . . I felt that good."

Slipped into the midst of this account was a brief mention that even Jeanne Harris had to have the stimulus frequency of her implanted neurostimulator unit adjusted after several months in response to continuing bouts of depression—although these relapses were reported as being briefer and milder.

The Toronto/Emory group worked with Advanced Neuromodulation Systems to develop and market the new therapy.[99] They applied for an unusual patent for developing the stimulation of a particular brain area, known as area 25, using the cyoarchitectonic system of Korbinian Brodmann. This area identified from brain scan studies by Helen Mayberg, the lead investigator, was not widely accepted as the obvious target for depression-related DBS. But what to make of Mayberg's reported findings that patients with leads inserted into this area often reported an almost instantaneous lifting of mood once the stimulation was turned on?

What may be going on, and the potential for harm, can perhaps best be brought out by the fact that DBS is far from being a novel treatment in psychiatry. DBS was first undertaken at Tulane University in New Orleans in the early 1950s by Robert Heath.[100] This was before the era of chlorpromazine and the development of a neurotransmitter paradigm in psychiatry. Heath and his colleagues were focused on brain circuits, and in the course of this work, they stumbled onto the fact that the brain has pleasure centers and punishment centers. Depressed patients with electrodes inserted into such pleasure zones in the 1950s described strikingly similar changes in mood to those reported by Mayberg and colleagues that have seemed to many to all but prove the validity of DBS.

Although some of those within the field of DBS are aware of the Tulane research, there is a more general amnesia surrounding that precedent, reflecting perhaps a desire to distance the current program from what was viewed, following the antipsychiatry movement, as more problematic ethically than anything else in the domain of physical treatments in psychiatry. In particular, there were two problems with the experiments at Tulane. First is the fact that patients were operated on for research purposes, and not for therapy as the patients themselves had understood. And second, Heath and colleagues did not shrink from their discovery of pleasure and punishment centers, but rather inflicted aversive stimulation on many subjects to explore the consequences. They adopted these methods, for instance, in an attempt to change behaviors such as homosexuality. Both purpose and image are close to the use of DBS to brainwash people depicted in the remake of *The Manchurian Candidate*.

On the Brink of a New Era?

The sometimes not-so-civil war within the shock therapy field has perhaps in its own way delivered outcomes that neither side expected, but that both can celebrate. While none of the new therapies appears remotely as effective as ECT, in recent years, the language of depression and indeed, of psychiatry has changed. Where once there was talk of serotonin levels, now researchers and clinicians alike think and discuss in terms of brain circuits and neural plasticity. Serotonin levels and the brain as a chemical soup still dominates popular debate, but in academic journals, this language has been relegated to the level of advertising copy. This change seems attributable to the efforts of both camps in the shock therapy field: those that see the seizure itself as the primary therapeutic event and those who claim some other mechanism.

In 2004, George reported on the outcome of setting up a magnetic flux within an MRI scanner, a technical maneuver that the NIH balked at out of concern for their building. Simultaneously imaging the active brain during the course of TMS therapy demonstrated that prefrontal TMS could, in fact, activate subcortical circuits. The feat opens up new vistas for research of this type.[101] George was also able to activate VNS devices within the MRI scanner—a nontrivial achievement, because pacemaker devices are highly susceptible to operational failure within a field of magnetic resonance. Together, these studies demonstrate the first visualizations of real-time functioning of what can be termed the visceral brain.[102]

These are substantial scientific developments, whether they have a therapeutic application or not. Although the work of George and Sackeim has clearly played a part, research on seizures has had a key role in changing how mood disorders are understood. In 2000, Tom Bolwig and his colleagues were one of three groups to report that ECT produces neurogenesis—the growth of new nerve cells—in the hippocampus, a region thought to be involved in memory and spatial navigation.[103] It had been thought for a century that nerve cells uniquely could neither replicate nor regenerate after birth. Bolwig's finding turned this wisdom on its head and led to a scramble to see whether antidepressants and other therapies such as TMS might do something similar, with claims for success when these therapies give hints that they might reproduce some of the effects of ECT. Within a year, reviews began to appear in major journals changing the language of depression and psychiatry from a language of neurochemical soups to a language of circuitry and neural plasticity. It seems clear that psychiatry—or at least its clinical neuroscience division—is in the midst of a paradigm change.

Where Sackeim and George have focused on stimulating specific circuits, Fink and others argued that seizures are necessary and that these probably act through the release or inhibition of some endocrine factor, such as cortisol. Such thinking was almost openly derided at one point, but recent clinical trials of mifepristone, a steroid drug, have thrown the spotlight back on the dynamics of cortisol. Mifepristone was developed by Roussel, a French pharmaceutical firm as an abortifacient; it is more commonly known as the morning-after pill, RU-486. In addition to terminating an early pregnancy, it acts to cut cortisol output in the brain, an effect reported in early 2002 to be potentially effective in psychotic depression.[104]

It is far from clear that the results of ongoing trials with mifepristone will be sufficiently robust to warrant its development as a treatment, but this hint of efficacy from "an ECT in pill form" is intriguing for the light it sheds on the field. Were mifepristone successful for psychotic depression, its marketing would make it clear that melancholic or endogenous depressive disorders of this type are, in fact, a different illness from what commonly passes as depression today. Most Prozac-, Zoloft-, or Paxil-responsive depressions, which in the 1980s would have been regarded as anxious or neurotic depressions, would respond neither to mifepristone nor ECT. Conversely, none of the SSRIs has ever been shown to be effective in true melancholia. If mifepristone were licensed for depression, what then would happen to the range of other conditions currently treated with SSRIs?

Would mifepristone transform these states into mythical mental illnesses? Or rather, would psychiatry continue to broaden its working criteria for defining mental illness? And what role would TMS and VNS play in a field differentiating between SSRI-responsive illness and ECT/mifepristone-responsive depressions? Clearly, the range of disorders called "anxiety" or "depression" in the past decades often have psychosomatic features and sometimes are determined entirely by social factors. Yet the disorders in this range almost certainly have more biological roots than is typically recognized. The channeling of TMS and VNS down a "depression" route no doubt owes a great deal to pharmaceutical company efforts to make depression the cash cow it became in the 1990s.[105] It may well be that these treatments are better suited to anxiety than to depression.

The mifepristone, DBS, and VNS stories, however, also expose some disturbing aspects of the new commercialism in the physical therapies of depression. Whereas antipsychiatry activists once railed against what they claimed was an establishment conspiracy to defend ECT, both academics and patients are now facing a world in which there is no incentive for the proponents of new therapies to concede that their procedures entail any risks, and there is every chance that only selective data will be published in ghostwritten articles.

It may not be possible to lift the academic gaze above the new commercialism to ask questions such as whether the real split is between seizures and stimulation, or between efforts at harmonization or enhancement on the one side and therapeutics on the other. When physical treatments like DBS were initially applied to Parkinson's disease, clear and relatively discrete brain circuits were sought as sites for stimulation.

But this did not necessarily mean that those involved in the field were seeking to attack the root of the illness. Many researchers readily conceded that all they may be doing is to produce compensatory responses, or indeed inducing further brain dysfunction, in order to balance out the original disturbance, whatever that might be. For instance in Parkinson's disease, the stimulation of the subthalamic nucleus produces therapeutic effects but does not do so by correcting the initial abnormality. The effect is to produce a compensatory lesion that, as it were, rebalances the system rather than corrects the problem. A preparedness to induce a therapeutic disturbance is also at the heart of treatment with ECT. But this medical perspective is entirely alien to the mind-set of electrotherapeutics, which from galvanism in the nineteenth century to Alpha-Stim in the twenty-first, has been all about trying to restore or induce harmony in the electrical fields of the body.[106] In this, electrotherapeutics, old and new, resembles nothing so much as magnetism and Franz Mesmer's Society of Harmony.

In the case of DBS for depression, the language hitherto has been all about correcting the problem through the induction of an immediate pleasurable response, rather than inflicting a therapeutic disturbance. In so far as this is the case, recent developments in brain scanning open up new intriguing prospects for treatment. If turning brain areas on and off by direct stimulation can produce benefits, it is quite likely that with new functional imaging (fMRI scans), subjects could be trained to turn these same brain areas on and off by means of neurofeedback.[107] It seems increasingly clear that subjects who can see areas of their brains light up on brain scans in real time can learn to activate or deactivate these same areas, just as we can learn to increase or decrease our heart rates based on feedback.

Neurofeedback seems to have just as much likelihood of working as invasive DBS. But history is not reassuring that we will take the less invasive route. After all, biofeedback was a demonstrable success in the 1960s, but we opted instead for treatment with pharmacotherapy and psychotherapies for a range of conditions from anxiety to hypertension. But if neurofeedback can produce equivalent effects to DBS, this perhaps indicates a fundamental divide between the convulsive therapies and other electrotherapies, because seizure induction by neurofeedback is not an option. For the foreseeable future, although these new therapies may secure a place for themselves, they will not be a replacement for ECT.

There have been efforts from the start of the convulsive therapy era to replace ECT. Even Cerletti hoped to isolate a hormone changed by ECT, which could be given instead the electrical shocks. Fluorothyl-induced seizures and then multiple monitored ECT (MMECT) had their day in the clinics. The literature on TMS, VNS, and DBS since then often explicitly positions these approaches as a means to replace ECT. The worry has to be that in the new medical marketplace, dominated by either pharmaceutical or medical device corporations, the marketing power of the megacompanies has created a situation in which less-effective treatments can drive out better treatments—as the story of the SSRIs perhaps demonstrates.

Time will tell whether another chapter in the history of shock therapy is being written today or not. The history of the past sixty years has been a history of successive attempts to improve ECT. All have failed, even if individual lives were helped along the way. The treatment that Cerletti described in 1938, plus a few modifications involving muscle relaxation and wave form, is still with us today, and a row of bright ideas about magnets, nonconvulsive applications of electricity, and the like have not succeeded in making patient care better or safer. It remains to be seen if the current therapies will provide more convincing alternatives.

CHAPTER TWELVE

Epilogue
Irrational Science

I n 1944, John Whitehorn was asked to review the therapeutic scene within psychiatry for the American Psychiatric Association's one hundredth anniversary. ECT had just exploded onto the scene, and shock treatments dominated the sessions on therapy at the APA meetings. Nevertheless, Whitehorn had difficulties writing his review. ECT was not derived from a theoretical framework; it simply worked, and no one knew exactly why. "The shock treatments remain essentially empirical," he wrote. "We are without adequate rational understanding of their mode of helpfulness: the empiricists have posed a formidable problem for rational research. In addition the shock therapies have stimulated further researches regarding prognosis in the more severe type of psychosis, with the result that there has been a better validation regarding the personality assets long known by the experienced psychiatrist to be important in individual prognosis."[1]

Two decades later, during the 1960s, when the practice of ECT had begun to fall under a cloud in the West, a series of epidemiological studies looking at the incidence and outcome of schizophrenia in both the developed and the developing world was carried out. The study reported that outcomes were significantly better in places such as India than they were in the West. The most common explanation was the role of cultural factors, such as extended family networks supporting patients returning to their community after treatment.

None of these studies commented on the fact that ECT continued to be used in India much more freely than it was in the West at that time. The standard practice in many hospitals and units in India was for patients who had been hospitalized for more than two weeks to receive

ECT almost regardless of diagnosis.[2] As of the 1980s, three-quarters of Indian patients given ECT had diagnoses of schizophrenia, and up to 20 percent of those admitted were treated with ECT. The impression of many Indian psychiatrists and observers was that shock treatment facilitated the discharge of many patients who would not otherwise have been released. In Western psychiatric facilities, practice had meanwhile moved to a world in which patients might be treated with multiple, different psychotropic drugs or combinations of drugs before ECT was ever considered.

This history of ECT has focused very heavily on its use in the West, and in particular on the United States. The story, however, needs to be seen in a global context. In recent years, the use of ECT in India has declined. There are no good figures on this trend, but Indian psychiatrists talk about a substantial decline. When questioned about the reasons for the drop, they note that when Indian movies, made in Bollywood, tackle psychiatric issues, they all too often resort to ECT in unmodified form to convey the horrors of psychiatry. In addition to the influence of the movies, spiritual leaders and others, concerned about the encroachment of psychiatry on their domains, have been critical of the use of treatments like ECT. Finally, driven by psychopharmacology, Indian psychiatry has become industrialized and commercialized, and there is increasing pressure on psychiatrists to opt for drug treatments rather than ECT and to conform in their clinical practice to algorithms and protocols drawn up in the West, which typically place ECT as a final option in any treatment hierarchy.[3] Thus our story, although situated in the West, is replaying itself systematically in other cultures. Does it matter if the story repeats itself?

In 1999, I (David Healy) was involved in a project comparing the prevalence of catatonic features in India and in the West, as part of an effort to replicate the work of Max Fink and colleagues, who using a catatonia rating scale had found a prevalence of 5 to 10 percent of such features among patients admitted to psychiatric facilities in the United States.[4] A number of other studies reported similar findings from the same period.[5] Such a figure seemed extraordinarily high, given the prevailing wisdom that catatonia as a diagnostic category had all but died out in the West.[6] Cases just did not seem to happen any more. The supposed disappearance of catatonia has typically been attributed to improvements in the nutrition of patients since the 1950s and 1960s. It also seemed possible that better health in general and the prevalent use of antibiotics in medicine made a difference. The advent of psychopharmacology led to claims that treatment with psychotropic drugs aborted the development of a full-blown syndrome.[7]

It seemed possible, however, that catatonia might still be present in India at much the same frequency as before the advent of the pharmacological era. Older hospital records pointed to frequencies of 10 percent or more among patients. This led to a project aimed at comparing catatonic features in a hundred consecutively admitted patients in Wales and in Hyderabad. It turned out that up to 10 percent of both Welsh and Indian patients had catatonic features.[8] The implications of this are startling. Highly trained Western physicians, it seems, are systematically missing very clear clinical presentations. If they are missing such dramatic aspects of the mental state of their patients, how can anyone have confidence in the theories or treatments that are being put forward at this point in psychiatry? It is difficult to accept that we are making progress, and we may even have gone backward.

The curious history of catatonia gives some insight to why this might happen. In retrospect, it is clear that when Ladislaus Meduna initially induced convulsions with Metrazol, it was a fortuitous coincidence that many of his first patients were catatonic. This was at a time when catatonia was a hallmark diagnostic feature of schizophrenia. Had Meduna tried Metrazol therapy on noncatatonic patients, the initial results might have been less clear cut.

However, this was not the first discovery of a cure for catatonia. The catatonic patients who responded favorably to Metrazol were, in fact, patients left over from an earlier and forgotten breakthrough. From the late 1920s onward, it was recognized that catatonic patients, if treated with barbiturates before symptoms had progressed too far, could respond fully and be discharged shortly afterward.[9] A subgroup of patients failed to respond, but nevertheless these patients also showed a dramatic response to barbiturate. After injection, these patients woke up from their stupor and were able to converse normally, read, draw, and engage in other activities, before they slipped back into a stupor as the barbiturate wore off. Following the advent of the antipsychotics, these earlier pharmacological dramas became crystallized in the psychiatry of the late 1950s and 1960s as evidence that barbiturates were not a cure for catatonia. They produced only brief responses in schizophrenia compared with the outcomes that more specific antipsychotic drugs delivered.

But there was little reason to think that the antipsychotics would be a treatment for catatonic schizophrenia or to believe that the early use of antipsychotics in the 1950s would lead to a demise of catatonic syndromes. In those days, catatonia was a syndrome that featured heavily in psychiatric theorizing and research. And from the perspective of the key researchers in this area such as Henri Baruk, the exciting thing about the new phenothiazine antipsychotics was that, along with bulbocapnine and a limited number of other drugs, they could *produce* an experimental catatonia in animals.[10] By the end of the 1950s, experimental catatonia was widely used by pharmaceutical companies as a screening method to identify potential antipsychotics. Clearly, substances that induce catatonia would not ordinarily act as effective agents against it.

In 1960, a new side effect of antipsychotics was described by Jean Delay and colleagues in their first clinical trial of haloperidol, which they later termed "syndrome malin des neuroleptiques" because it could be lethal.[11] A smattering of case reports in English-language journals appeared in the following two decades, until in 1980, Stanley Caroff wrote the first systematic paper on neuroleptic malignant syndrome (NMS), an end-stage condition resulting from the use of antipsychotics in certain patients.[12] This registered widely and struck fear into the heart of psychiatrists in the United States, probably because from the mid-1970s these clinicians had found themselves the subjects of lawsuits for antipsychotic-induced tardive dyskinesia.[13] Along with ECT, tardive dyskinesia had become a lightning rod for antipsychiatry. Putting patients afflicted with this highly visible condition on the witness stand or in front of television cameras was almost as potent a weapon as Jack Nicholson playing the patient Randle McMurphy receiving unmodified ECT. Tardive dyskinesia spread a chill over the pharmacotherapy of severe mental illness. But at least patients with tardive dyskinesia stayed alive. Neuroleptic malignant syndrome killed. Up to 50 percent of the patients affected were at risk of fatality, and there were claims that as much as 1 percent of patients prescribed antipsychotics were at risk for NMS.

This was the background in 1983, when a young patient at Massachusetts General Hospital was given haloperidol postoperatively for a confusional state and appeared to develop NMS. The patient was the son of a wealthy foreigner. The attending doctor on call, Gregory Fricchione, called in the head of department, Edward (Ned) Cassem, the professor of psychiatry, to help. Cassem, a drinking, smoking, Catholic priest, popular with the nursing staff, faced a patient rigid in his bed; he searched the medicine cabinet, fished out a drug, and gave it to the patient, who responded dramatically. Emerging from his mute stupor, the patient was able to look after himself. After a further dose of the "magic" medicine the following day, the patient was restored, and his care continued uneventfully thereafter. When the nursing staff asked Cassem what he had given, they were told "holy water." In fact it was lorazepam, a benzodiazepine from the same class as diazepam (Valium), and Cassem and Fricchione subsequently gave lorazepam with benefit to a number of other patients with NMS and reported the results in 1985.[14]

Fricchione later worked with Max Fink in New York. There, as they became more aware of the history of catatonia and similarities between malignant catatonia and NMS, Fink wondered whether ECT might be a helpful treatment for NMS. Faced with a patient unresponsive to lorazepam, they tried ECT, which produced a complete recovery.[15] In the course of the following ten years, the great majority of patients given ECT for NMS showed a positive response.[16] This points to a number of possibilities. One is that NMS is a variant of catatonia. Another is the possibility that the primary effects of ECT are on the motor system, given that it works for NMS and Parkinson's disease as well as catatonia.

But the essential historical point here is that Fink and Fricchione had rediscovered something known for a long time: catatonia responds to pharmacotherapy and convulsive therapy.[17] That this information had been unacknowledged to the point of forgetting indicates that, far from current psychiatric practice being evidence-based and rational, it is as ideological as it has ever been, with most clinicians cut off from vast swathes of data and knowledge that do not suit the interests of the dominant paradigm.

Part of the problem lies in the fact that the drug companies were no longer promoting benzodiazepines, as these were all off patent, and by the 1980s, without the kind of support that comes with pharmaceutical company interest it was nearly impossible to raise the profile of catatonia. From the large pool of signs and symptoms that patients present to clinicians, pharmaceutical company promotion emphasizes those that lead to drug-selling diagnoses or profiles. In other words, the pill names the illness.

The psychiatric and psychopharmacological marketplace is now structured to sell SSRI antidepressants and atypical antipsychotics; each specific brand in these drug categories essentially duplicates a compound held by a competitor company. Far from there being a plethora of agents on the market, as the profusion of brand names might suggest, there are only a limited number of truly distinct drugs—fewer in fact than there were in the 1960s. Without diversity in drug-treatment options, companies have little incentive to support different constructions of psychiatric illness or to emphasize the problems following the use of rival treatments. Although commercially motivated, this might at least stimulate thinking, which in turn, would benefit the consumer. But where all companies are essentially trying to achieve the same end, their combined marketing weight drowns out the possibility of noticing discrepant observations. Psychiatric thought, far from having developed since the 1960s, has arguably atrophied. The number of ideas in play is increasingly limited. The only treatment modality that challenges the dominant paradigm is ECT.

Does this matter? There are several issues here. In the first place, there is probably no other branch of medicine where the outcomes for a core disease are steadily worsening. Bacteriologists eliminate diseases. Duodenal ulcers are a thing of the past. The life expectancy of cancer patients is steadily improving. Fatal heart attacks are much less common than they once were. But in the West, patients with schizophrenia are dying younger than they were in previous decades, and furthermore their mortality can be correlated with the number of antipsychotic drugs prescribed.[18] Where is the radical assessment of modern practice that this scandal calls for?

There are good grounds for considering that some of these patients might have benefited from a course of ECT. Patients with schizophrenia display distinct motor features, such as mannerisms, perseveration, or stereotypes, and many cases of thought disorder can be reframed as motor problems. Given the direct motor effects of ECT visible in the response of depression with psychomotor retardation, catatonia, NMS, Parkinson's disease, and mania, there is a therapeutic foundation for thinking ECT may help such patients.

Another basis stems from the response of catatonia, which may well be best described as a disorder where there is a split between will and action. In this case the efficacy of ECT on motor functions might be seen as a form of cerebroversion, aimed at restoring normal signaling sequences in the brain, in just the way that cardioversion resets comparable disturbances in signal sequencing that give rise to heart block or fibrillation.[19] The visual attributes of cardioversion are not pleasant, and yet placing paddles on the chest is celebrated as heroic and lifesaving in television's medical dramas, in contrast to ECT, which is still shown in its unmodified form whenever it is portrayed in film.

Antipsychotic drugs can also in their own right trigger profound motor problems, from Parkinsonism to NMS and tardive dyskinesia. Would these patients benefit from ECT? No one asks that question because when patients fail to respond to one set of drugs, clinicians proceed down a checklist to the next combination of drugs without stopping to examine the specific profile of a drug's effect. Looking for the magic bullet that will clear thought and produce calm, no one notices the onset or offset of motor symptoms inherent in the individual's presentation or as part of a drug-treatment response. The possibility of piecing together the jigsaw that is schizophrenia has been all but obliterated by the removal of key pieces from the clinical board. We are left hoping that the hunt for a gene in a haystack will turn up some answers, and in the meantime the gears of psychiatric theorizing have been shifted into neutral.

It is not important whether this cerebroversion hypothesis is correct; the point is to highlight modern psychiatry's failure of imagination. At the start of the twenty-first century, thinking has been dominated by "bio-babble," a discourse characterized by jargon and an emphasis on the monoamines, dopamine, serotonin, and norepinephrine. Within a few years, this will almost certainly seem as vacuous as Freudian notions about libido. The problem, in the meantime, is that just as psychoanalysis once inhibited a generation from making progress in understanding what mental disorders are, so too psychopharmacology has held back development in theoretical aspects of psychiatry, at the expense of patients. What incentives are there to work out how clinical features and syndromes relate when such efforts are unlikely to be recognized, publicized, or funded in a field so beholden to the pharmaceutical industry? We have reached a situation in psychiatry that is almost the diametric opposite to Whitehorn's 1944 jibe about the shock therapies being entirely empirical. ECT, and its related procedures, rTMS, VNS, DBS, and MST, are the only therapeutic approaches that keep alive the possibility that clinicians might someday understand how the major psychological syndromes cohere.

There have been enormous benefits from research on basic psychopathology, and ECT and the other physical treatments have helped keep this window open. But these benefits have come at some cost. A generation of NIMH funding has been devoted to research that has helped sharpen the scientific questions. Yet this has diverted funding from clinical studies that might have led to an earlier establishment of the efficacy of ECT for psychotic depression, NMS, Parkinson's disease, or resistant mania. A clinical trial program interested in therapeutic outcomes would surely by now have produced some progress in delineating the schizophrenic syndromes that might be ECT-responsive.

ECT poses a vibrant challenge in areas besides psychopathology. It has been central to the genesis of informed consent in medicine. The patients likely to receive this treatment now are very often deluded, and as such they pose acute questions to our understanding of what informed consent means. But informed consent has changed in recent years from a formulation that emphasizes the disclosure of information into something closer to a risk assessment. Good clinical practice involves patients and their caregivers working with nursing staff and physicians to examine how the risks stack up in ECT and other procedures. A gut feeling or common sense may suggest that a weak or inappropriate course of drugs carries greater risk to the patient than modified ECT ever would. It can be difficult to know the answer; the bottom line will often be whether patients or their relatives are convinced that psychiatric staff would have ECT themselves if in the same position. On this point, lots of mental health professionals working with severely ill patients make informal living wills alerting their colleagues to the fact that they would wish to have ECT if they ever became this ill, whereas they would be far less likely to have DBS or VNS.

The complexity is layered. Was giving one's consent a good idea? It depends on when and how the question is asked. In chapter 9, we saw that physicians' and patients' assessments of benefit and harm can differ dramatically. This difference is something to celebrate in that nowhere else in psychiatry is there such systematic research available from multiple different viewpoints. One of the features of research undertaken by patient groups on ECT and other physical therapies is that assessments are made months after treatment has ended. This is in contrast to clinician-led research or drug trials, which typically are undertaken much closer to the treatment.

But the differences in results are not simply a matter of time frames: self-assessment is a problematic tool in psychiatry. It is not uncommon for patients, who are clearly improving in the course of ECT treatment to report that "everyone tells me this is helping, but I can't see it." Marked differences like this between points of view are phenomena that should challenge anyone with a real interest in the mysteries of psychiatry and consent. What does it mean if a treatment produces benefits readily apparent to disinterested observers but not apparent to the patient, and what are the implications of this for informed consent?

A history like this does not seek to answer questions about science, symptoms, or consent. It seeks instead to show how certain aspects of the mysteries involved in a domain like that of mental health come into and slip out of view at different points in time. What has happened in the case of ECT does not seem to sit comfortably beside either the dominant philosophies of science, which appeal to a steady accumulation of knowledge, nor with the business philosophies of modern clinical practice, which assume an ever more rational marketplace, in which it is almost inconceivable that a therapy of such importance could have been kicked aside for such trivial reasons as its image in a film. It is hard in fact to think of anywhere where the mismatch between rhetoric and reality is as great as it has been in the history of ECT. Medicine is clearly not vacuum-sealed against irrationality.

Notes

Abbreviations and Archives

AJP	*American Journal of Psychiatry*
Bini Papers	Menninger Archives, Kansas State Historical Society, Topeka
Cerletti Papers	Menninger Archives, Kansas State Historical Society, Topeka
GAP Papers (Diethelm)	Oskar Diethelm Library, Joan and Sanford I. Weill Medical College of Cornell University, New York City
GAP Papers (Menninger)	Menninger Archives, Kansas State Historical Society, Topeka
Hillside Hospital Archives	Hillside Hospital, Queens, New York
Impastato Papers	Oskar Diethelm Library, Joan and Sanford I. Weill Medical College of Cornell University, New York City
JAMA	*Journal of the American Medical Association*
JECT	*Journal of ECT*
Meduna Papers	Ladislas J. Meduna Papers, 1942–1959, University of Illinois at Urbana-Champaign Archives
Menninger Collection	Menninger Archives, Kansas State Historical Society, Topeka
Waggoner Collection	Bentley Historical Library, University of Michigan, Ann Arbor
Wortis Collection	Oskar Diethelm Library, Joan and Sanford I. Weill Medical College of Cornell University, New York City

Note: Throughout, all translations of quotations are by Edward Shorter.

CHAPTER ONE. The Penicillin of Psychiatry?

1. This, and all subsequent quotations relating to the patient, are from the Hillside Hospital Archives, reel 25, no. 2715.

2. Max Fink, "A Clinician-Researcher and ECDEU: 1959–1980," in Thomas Ban et al., eds., *The Triumph of Psychopharmacology and the Story of CINP* (Budapest: Animula, 2000), 82–92, quote on 92.

3. Cathy Sherbourne et al., "Characteristics, Treatment Patterns, and Outcomes of Persistent Depression despite Treatment in Primary Care," *General Hospital Psychiatry* 26 (2004): 106–114.

4. William Karliner, "Shock Treatments in Psychiatry," *American Practitioner and Digest of Treatment* 2 (1951): 511–516, quote on 511.

5. Richard Abrams, interview by David Healy, Chicago, May 20, 2003.

6. Hirsch L. Gordon, "Fifty Shock Therapy Theories," *Military Surgeon* 103 (1948): 397–401, quote on 398.

CHAPTER TWO. "Some Experiments on the Biological Influencing of the Course of Schizophrenia"

1. On Pascal's life, see Felicia Gordon, "French Psychiatry and the New Woman: The Case of Dr. Constance Pascal, 1877–1937," *History of Psychiatry* 17 (2006): 159–182. Gordon gives only passing and unsympathetic mention to Pascal's work on shock: "horrifying, the nakedly experimental nature of the treatments" (173).

2. C[onstance] Pascal and Jean Davesne, *Traitement des maladies mentales par les chocs* (Paris: Masson, 1926), vii. On her life, see Pierre Morel, *Dictionnaire biographique de la psychiatrie* (Paris: Les Empécheurs de Penser en Rond, 1996), 191.

3. Pascal and Davesne, *Traitement*, xv.

4. On these new approaches, see Edward Shorter, *A History of Psychiatry from the Age of the Asylum to the Era of Prozac* (New York: Wiley, 1997), 190–207.

5. In the extensive medical literature see, for example, Kenneth E. Appel et al., "Insulin in Undernutrition in the Psychoses," *AMA Archives of Neurology and Psychiatry* 21 (1929): 149–164. An overview of the subject (that does not mention Sakel) is Charlotte Munn, "Insulin in Catatonic Stupor," *AMA Archives of Neurology and Psychiatry* 34 (1935): 262–269.

6. Edith Klemperer, "Versuch einer Behandlung des Delirium tremens mit Insulin," *Psychiatrisch-Neurologische Wochenschrift* 29 (December 11, 1926): 549–551.

7. Julius Schuster, "Die Beinflussung psychischer Erkrankungen durch das Hervorrufen schweren anaphylaktischen Shocks," *Archiv für Psychiatrie und Nervenkrankheiten* 77 (1926): 314–316; Dezsö Miskolczy, "Insulinmastkur bei Nerven- und Geisteskranken," *Psychiatrisch-Neurologische Wochenschrift* 29 (January 8, 1927): 34–36; Julius Schuster, "Zur kombinierten Therapie der Psychosen durch Shock und Desensibilisierung, mit Anaphylaktogenen und Organextrakten," *Archiv für Psychiatrie und Nervenkrankheiten* 85 (1928): 779–794. In a later self-published monograph, c. 1938, *Zur Entdeckung der Insulinschocktherapie bei akuten Geisteskrankheiten, insbesondere bei der Schizophrenie,* Schuster claimed that since 1922 he had been treating schizophrenic patients with insulin coma and that he had reported on this in April 1926 in an oral communication to the

Psychiatric-Neurological Section of the Royal Hungarian Medical Society in Budapest. Yet Schuster's published work in the 1920s makes no mention of this. Indeed, to the contrary, in the above-cited 1926 article he speaks of treating "severe psychiatric illness" through emaciation. In his monograph he claimed for himself the priority for insulin therapy. The claim is not credible because, in discussing cases supposedly treated with insulin, he dates some as early as the summer of 1922. When asked about the possibility of this chronology, historian Michael Bliss, an authority on the history of insulin, replied: "I am certain the Hungarians would not have had any access to supplies of insulin [at that point]. No one in Europe that I know of was able to produce it before 1923" (personal communication, Michael Bliss to Edward Shorter, April 23, 2005). Interestingly, Schuster believed that insulin was discovered in 1920 (58). On the title page, Schuster identifies himself as "former I. Assistant at the Psychiatrisch-Neurologische Universitätsklinik of the Pazmany Peter University in Budapest." The undated work bears a handwritten acquisition date of 1938. We are grateful to Max Fink for calling our attention to the existence of the monograph.

8. Hans Steck, "Die Behandlung des Delirium tremens mit Insulin," *Schweizer Archiv für Neurologie und Psychiatrie* 29 (1932): 173. Steck, "Le traitement des agitations psychosiques aiguës (délire et agitation catatonique, delirium tremens) par l'insuline," in René Charpentier, ed., *Congrès des médecins aliénistes et neurologistes de France et des pays de langue française, 37e session, Rabat (7–13 avril 1933): Comptes rendus* (Paris: Masson, [1934]), 452–455: "Nous voudrions ... encore mettre en garde contre les états de chocs hypoglycémiques, qui sont d'autant plus à redouter si les malades sont déjà émaciés et faibles" (455). International attention was drawn to this work by Anton von Braunmühl, a staff psychiatrist at the Eglfing-Haar asylum near Munich—later a notorious center for Nazi euthanasia. See Braunmühl, *Die Insulinshockbehandlung der Schizophrenie* (Berlin: Springer, 1938), 14–15. See also Hjalmar Torp, who in July 1932 described a schizophrenic patient who had improved following a hypoglycemic coma. "Psykiske og nevrologiske forandringer efter hypoglykemisk koma hos en schizofren" ("Mental and Neurologic Changes after Hypoglycaemic Coma, in Case of Schizophrenia"), *Norsk Magazin for Laegevidenskaben* 93 (1932): 760–765.

9. Max Müller, *Erinnerungen: Erlebte Psychiatriegeschichte, 1920–1960* (Berlin: Springer, 1982), 71.

10. This, and all subsequent quotations relating to the patient, are from Manfred Sakel, "Schizophreniebehandlung mittels Insulin-Hypoglykämie sowie hypoglykämischer Shocks," *Wiener Medizinische Wochenschrift* 84 (December 1, 1934): 1326–1327; part 4 of a thirteen-part series.

11. In Sakel's parlance, wet shock meant comas; dry shock meant convulsions. Yet heavily sweating patients in a coma could easily convulse, and the distinction was not widely taken up. See Braunmühl, *Insulinshockbehandlung,* 37.

12. Obituary, "Manfred Sakel," *Lancet* 2 (December 14, 1957): 1235.

13. Braunmühl, in 1938 the first major German propagator of Sakel's treatment, considered that the convulsions had a therapeutic role, thus that the ostensible coma therapy was in fact a convulsive therapy. *Insulinshockbehandlung,* 41, 53. Joseph Wortis noted, however, that only 16 percent of insulin-coma patients actually had seizures: "Experiences with the Hypoglycemic Shock Treatment of

Schizophrenia," *AJP* 94 (1937): 159–169, see esp. 162. Phillip Polatin and coworkers at the New York State Psychiatric Institute reported that 36 percent of their insulin patients had convulsions, mostly in the context of long four- to five-hour comas: "Vertebral Fractures as a Complication of Convulsions in Hypoglycemic Shock and Metrazol Therapy in Psychiatric Disorders," *JAMA* 115 (August 10, 1940): 433–436, see esp. 436.

14. Sakel obituary, *New York Times*, December 3, 1957, 35. On Sakel's arrogance, see, among other sources, Otfried K. Linde, ed., *Pharmakopsychiatrie im Wandel der Zeit* (Klingenmünster: Tilia, 1988), 100–101.

15. See Manfred Sakel, "Schizophrenia: Most Disastrous Disease of Man; It Destroys His Mind Though Sparing His Body," in Henri Ey, ed., *Premier congrès mondial de psychiatrie, Paris, 1950*, vol. 4, *Thérapeutique biologique* (Paris: Hermann, 1952), 30–45; Manfred Sakel, "Über die Einführung der sog: Schocktherapie und Pötzl's Verdienst um ihre Einführung," in Hubert J. Urban, ed., *Festschrift zum 70. Geburtstag von Prof. Dr. Otto Pötzl* ([Vienna]: privately published, 1947), 403–407.

16. Heinz Lehmann, "Psychopharmacotherapy," in David Healy, ed., *The Psychopharmacologists*, vol. 1 (London: Chapman and Hall, 1996), 159–186, quote on 166.

17. William Karliner, interview by Edward Shorter, New York, April 6, 2004.

18. Sakel alluded to Bonhoeffer's initial benevolence in "Schizophrenia: Most Disastrous Disease of Man," 32.

19. Manfred Sakel, "Neue Behandlung der Morphinsucht," *Deutsche Medizinische Wochenschrift* 56 (October 17, 1930): 1777–1778.

20. Manfred Sakel, "Neue Behandlung der Morphinsucht," *Zeitschrift für die gesamte Neurologie und Psychiatrie* 143 (1933): 506–534.

21. Hans Hoff, "History of the Organic Treatment of Schizophrenia," in Max Rinkel and Harold E. Himwich, eds., *Insulin Treatment in Psychiatry* (New York: Philosophical Library, 1959), 10–11. Sakel does not mention Dussik and Palisa in his 1947 account but instead acknowledges the help of Otto Kauders and Hans Hoff. The book is the proceedings of a conference held in 1958. Herbert Pullar-Strecker dates the beginning of Sakel's work in Poetzl's clinic as October 1933. See Pullar-Strecker's letter "Insulin in Schizophrenia," *Lancet* 230 (June 27, 1936): 1498–1499. The diagnosis of schizophrenia was used casually in those days, tantamount to psychosis. More likely, the young woman in question had a psychotic depression, triggered by a disappointing life event. Insulin coma, however, would be quite effective for the psychotic part of her illness, and the depressive part she would get over naturally.

22. James Shields and Irving I. Gottesman, eds., introduction to *Man, Mind and Heredity: Selected Papers of Eliot Slater on Psychiatry and Genetics* (Baltimore: Johns Hopkins University Press, 1971), 21.

23. Manfred Sakel, "Neue Behandlungsart Schizophreniker und verwirrter Erregter," *Wiener Klinische Wochenschrift* 46 (November 10, 1933): 1372. The second phase of the procedure, Sakel said, consisted of "[die] Erzeugung von schweren hypoglykaemischen Schocks, eventuell mit Koma und epileptischen Anfällen." There was also a brief report of Sakel's November 3 lecture in the *Wiener Medizinische Wochenschrift* 83 (November 18, 1933): 1327.

24. Peter Berner, personal communication to Edward Shorter. It could also have been at a second Sakel lecture, to the Verein für Neurologie und Psychiatrie on November 14, that Wagner-Jauregg marched out. When English psychiatrist Isabel G. H. Wilson visited Vienna in 1936 to assess insulin coma, Wagner-Jauregg expressed to her his reservations about it. Wilson, *A Study of Hypoglycaemic Shock Treatment in Schizophrenia* (London: HMSO, 1936), 7.

25. Otto Poetzl, "Aussprache" [following Sakel's talk], *Wiener Klinische Wochenschrift* 46 (November 10, 1933): 1372–1373.

26. Joseph Wortis to Max Fink, June 24, 1983, Wortis Collection, box 7. Wortis asserted in the letter that Sakel had begun with camphor as a convulsive agent, which is almost certainly wrong.

27. Sakel, "Schizophrenia: Most Disastrous Disease of Man," 32.

28. In the discussion following Eugene Glynn, "Clinical Symposium: Insulin Coma Therapy," *Journal of Hillside Hospital* 4 (1955): 161–171, Sakel quote on 178.

29. Emil Fuhrmann, *Ärztliches Jahrbuch für Österreich, 1935* (Vienna: Rafael, 1935), 21. Karl Feiler was the other chief physician.

30. Reg[inald] S. Ellery, "Schizophrenia and Its Treatment by Insulin and 'Cardiazol,'" *Medical Journal of Australia* 2 (October 2, 1937): 552–564, esp. 555.

31. Manfred Sakel, "Schizophreniebehandlung mittels Insulin-Hypoglykämischer Schocks," *Wiener Medizinische Wochenschrift* 84 (November 3, 1934), in thirteen parts to February 9, 1935.

32. Manfred Sakel, *Neue Behandlungsmethode der Schizophrenie* (Vienna: Perles, 1935).

33. K[arl] Th[eo] Dussik and Manfred Sakel, "Ergebnisse und Grenzen der Hypoglykaemieschockbehandlung der Schizophrenie," *Zeitschrift für die gesamte Neurologie und Psychiatrie* 155 (1936): 351–415. The repeated "46's" are correct as written.

34. Sakel, *Neue Behandlungsmethode*, 8–13. For details of Poetzl's clinic and Sakel's, and Dussik's actual administration of insulin therapy, see Dussik and Sakel, "Ergebnisse und Grenzen der Hypoglykämieshockbehandlung der Schizophrenie"; see also Wilson, *Study of Hypoglycaemic Shock Treatment*, 9f.

35. Joseph Wortis, "On the Response of Schizophrenic Subjects to Hypoglycemic Insulin Shock," *Journal of Nervous and Mental Disease* 85 (1936): 497–506, quote on 498.

36. Deborah Blythe Doroshow, "The Injection of Insulin into American Psychiatry" (Senior thesis, Harvard University, 2004), 31–32. Max Fink was Doroshow's mentor for this project.

37. Linde, *Pharmakopsychiatrie*, 100. The wording is Linde's, not Müller's.

38. Sakel to Wortis, August 21, 1937, a handwritten postscript attached to a typewritten note. Wortis Collection, box 10. Nobody associated with insulin, Metrazol, or ECT ever received a Nobel Prize.

39. Sakel to Wortis, undated, sometime late in 1935, Wortis Collection, box 10. Excusing himself for not corresponding or going to work, Sakel said: "Ich war aus gewissen privaten Gründen in einer kleinen Tief."

40. Sakel to Wortis, April 11, 1935, Wortis Collection, box 10. The junior clinic member was Dussik.

41. "Aubrey Lewis's Report on His Visits to Psychiatric Centres in Europe in 1937," in Katherine Angel et al., eds., *European Psychiatry on the Eve of War: Aubrey Lewis, the Maudsley Hospital, and the Rockefeller Foundation in the 1930s* (London: Wellcome Trust Centre for the History of Medicine at UCL, 2003), 109. Lewis's report was written in 1938.

42. Josef Berze, "Die Insulin-Chok-Behandlung der Schizophrenie," *Wiener Medizinische Wochenschrift* 83 (December 2, 1933): 1365–1369.

43. In emulation of Sakel's work, other coma-inducing agents were tried, but none achieved the success of ICT. See, for example, Gabor Gazdag et al., "Atropine Coma: A Historical Note," *JECT* 21 (2005): 203–206.

44. Wilson, *Study of Hypoglycaemic Shock Treatment*, 21–22.

45. Lothar Kalinowsky, "The Various Forms of Shock Therapy in Mental Disorders and Their Practical Importance," *New York State Journal of Medicine* 41 (November 15, 1941): 2210–2215, quote on 2210.

46. See Max Fink, "Induced Seizures as Psychiatric Therapy: Ladislaus Meduna's Contributions in Modern Neuroscience," *JECT* 20 (2004): 133–136.

47. The following details are taken extensively from two manuscript versions of Meduna's autobiography in the Meduna Papers at the University of Illinois Archives. Version 1 is undated; on internal evidence, version 2 was written in 1954. A much-condensed rendition of version 2 was edited by Max Fink as "Autobiography of L. J. Meduna," in *Convulsive Therapy* 1 (1985): 43–57, and 121–135.

48. Laszlo J. Meduna, "The Convulsive Treatment: A Reappraisal," *Journal of Clinical and Experimental Psychopathology* 15 (1954): 219–233, quote on 219.

49. "Autobiography of L. J. Meduna," version 1, 12.

50. Ibid., 28.

51. Meduna, "The Convulsive Treatment: A Reappraisal," 220.

52. Béla Hechst, "Zur Histopathologie der Schizophrenie mit besonderer Berücksichtigung der Ausbreitung des Prozesses," *Zeitschrift für die gesamte Neurologie und Psychiatrie* 134 (1931): 163–267. "Im allgemeinen zeigt die Glia gegen die schizophrenen Veränderungen eine relative Insuffizienz: sie ist nicht imstande, die durch den Prozess verursachten Zellausfälle mit ihrer Wucherung zu ersetzen. Zur Erklärung dieser Insuffizienz müssen wir annehmen, dass infolge des schizophrenen Prozesses nicht nur die Nervenzellen untergehen, sondern dass der Prozess zum mindesten lähmend auf die Aktivität der Gliazellen einwirkt. . . . Wir glauben, dass wir hier mit einer Eigenerkrankung der Glia (im Sinne Schaffers) zu tun haben" (232).

53. Ladislaus v. Meduna, "Beiträge zur Histopathologie der Mikroglia," *Archiv für Psychiatrie und Nervenkrankheiten* 82 (1927): 123–193, quote on 184. On current thinking about the glia in ECT, see Dost Ongur and Stephan Heckers, "A Role for Glia in the Action of Electroconvulsive Therapy," *Harvard Review of Psychiatry* 12 (2004): 253–262.

54. "Autobiography of L. J. Meduna," version 1, 41. The publication was Meduna, "Klinische und anatomische Beiträge zur Frage der genuinen Epilepsie," *Deutsche Zeitschrift für Nervenheilkunde* 129 (1932): 17–42; yet this paper discussed only cell changes in epilepsy, not in schizophrenia. Meduna apparently never published his observations about glia cells in schizophrenia.

55. Robert Gaupp, "Die Frage der kombinierten Psychosen," *Archiv für Psychiatrie und Nervenkrankheiten* 76 (1926): 73–80, quote on 76.

56. Julius Nyirö and Albin Jablonszky, "Einige Daten zur Prognose der Epilepsie, mit besonderer Rücksicht auf die Konstitution," *Psychiatrisch-Neurologische Wochenschrift* 31 (November 2, 1929): 547–549, quote on 549.

57. On dubiety about the supposed antagonism, see, for example, P. H. Esser, "Die epileptiformen Anfälle der Schizophrenen und die differentialdiagnostischen Schwierigkeiten im Grenzgebiet von Epilepsie und Schizophrenie," *Zeitschrift für die gesamte Neurologie und Psychiatrie* 162 (1938): 1–24; and A. Yde, Edel Lohse, and A. Faurbye, "On the Relation between Schizophrenia, Epilepsy, and Induced Convulsions," *Acta Psychiatrica et Neurologica Scandinavica* 16 (1941): 325–388.

58. Quoted in Georges Heuyer et al., "Electro-choc chez des adolescents," *Annales Médico-Psychologiques* 100 (1942): 75–84, quote on 80. Heuyer felt that the success of ECT in adolescents with schizophrenia and manic-depression confirmed the accuracy of his earlier comment.

59. G. Steiner and A. Strauss, "Die körperlichen Erscheinungen," in Karl Wilmanns, ed., *Die Schizophrenie* (Berlin: Springer, 1932); vol. 9, part 5, of Oswald Bumke, ed., *Handbuch der Geisteskrankheiten,* see esp. 278–282.

60. Georg Müller, "Anfälle bei schizophrenen Erkrankungen," *Allgemeine Zeitschrift für Psychiatrie* 93 (1930): 235–240.

61. A[lfred] Glaus, "Über Kombinationen von Schizophrenie und Epilepsie," *Zeitschrift für die gesamte Neurologie und Psychiatrie* 135 (1931): 450–500, quote on 500.

62. See Meduna to Harry Brick, July 7, 1952, Meduna Papers, box 1. "I believe he should be considered the modern father of convulsive treatments."

63. "Autobiography of L. J. Meduna," version 1, 44.

64. See, for example, William Oliver, "Account of the Effects of Camphor in a Case of Insanity," *London Medical Journal* 6 (1785): 120–130. By Meduna's day, Oliver's interesting discovery had been completely lost sight of. A story circulated among Budapest insiders that Meduna conceived of camphor in schizophrenia because (according to the account in Nyirö's textbook of psychiatry) Meduna had "tried to break through catatonic inhibition with the administration of camphor injections. When, after the administration of a larger dose of camphor injections, his patient developed an epileptic fit, he stopped his experimentation. Nevertheless, since there was a marked improvement in his patient's condition, relying on Nyirö and Jablonszky's treatise, which established on the basis of a large sample that there was an antagonism between schizophrenia and epilepsy, Meduna continued with his therapeutic experiments." Gy Nyirö, *Psychiatria* [Hungarian], 11th unchanged printing (Budapest: Medicina, 1962), 319. We are grateful to Dr. Thomas Ban for an English translation of the Hungarian original.

65. Meduna, "Über experimentelle Campherepilepsie," *Archiv für Psychiatrie* 102 (1934): 333–339.

66. "Autobiography of L. J. Meduna," version 1, 50.

67. This anecdote about "Oh, Dr. Meduna" was included in version 2 of Meduna's autobiography (39), not in version 1.

68. "Autobiography of L. J. Meduna," version 1, 50–52.

69. Ibid., 53–54.

70. Meduna, "Versuche über die biologische Beeinflussung des Ablaufes der Schizophrenie: Campher und Cardiazol," *Zeitschrift für die gesamte Neurologie und Psychiatrie* 152 (1935): 235–262.

71. "Autobiography of L. J. Meduna," version 1, 68.

72. F. Hildebrandt, "Pentamethylentetrazol (Cardiazol)," *Naunyn-Schmiedebergs Archiv für Experimentelle Pathologie und Pharmakologie* 116 (1926): 100–116.

73. Whether all of these patients had "schizophrenia" is another question. When Aubrey Lewis visited Meduna in Budapest in 1937, he said: "[Meduna] has the common weakness of calling every anergic patient catatonic, so that some retarded depressions are likely to be diagnosed schizophrenic" (in Angel et al., *European Psychiatry on the Eve of War*, 107). Convulsive therapy, of course, later turned out to be more suitable for affective disorders than for schizophrenia, but it is not ineffective in the latter.

74. Meduna, *Die Konvulsionstherapie der Schizophrenie* (Halle, Germany: Marhold, 1937), 121.

75. Ellery, "Schizophrenia and Its Treatment by Insulin and 'Cardiazol,'" 562.

76. Lothar Kalinowsky, "Electric-Convulsion Therapy in Schizophrenia," *Lancet* 2 (December 9, 1939): 1232–1233, quote on 1233.

77. See Meduna, "The Significance of the Convulsive Reaction during the Insulin and the Cardiazol Therapy of Schizophrenia," *Journal of Nervous and Mental Disease* 87 (1938): 133–138.

78. Meduna, "Vierjährigen Erfahrungen mit der Cardiazol-Konvulsionstherapie," *Psychiatrisch-Neurologisch Blätter* (Amsterdam), nos. 5–6 (1938): 1–52; see also Meduna in discussion, 59–60.

79. See Esser, "Die epileptiformen Anfälle der Schizophrenen," and Yde, Lohse, and Faurbye, "On the Relation between Schizophrenia, Epilepsy, and Induced Convulsions," cited above, n. 57.

80. See P. Wolf and M. R. Trimble, "Biological Antagonism and Epileptic Psychosis," *British Journal of Psychiatry* 146 (1985): 272–276.

81. "Autobiography of L. J. Meduna," version 1, 64. While head of psychiatry at Debreczen, Ladislaus Benedek was greatly involved with insulin coma research. See his *Insulin-Schock-Wirkung auf die Wahrnehmung* (Berlin: Karger, 1935).

82. "Autobiography of L. J. Meduna," version 1, 7–68.

CHAPTER THREE. "Madness Cured with Electricity"

1. Cerletti, untitled lecture manuscript, c. 1956, quotes from the patient's chart, p. 7, Cerletti Papers, box 118-433.

2. See Max Fink, "Delirious Mania," *Bipolar Disorders* 1 (1999): 54–60.

3. Cerletti, untitled MS of a lecture he gave in Stockholm in the mid-1950s, p. 1, Cerletti Papers, box 118-433, file 10.

4. Cerletti manuscript on Perusini, given as a talk in 1957, Cerletti Papers, box 118-433, file 9.

5. Gaetano Perusini, "I corsi di perfezionamento nella clinica del Kraepelin," *Rivista Sperimentale di Freniatria* 33 (1907): 1009–1013.

6. Details of Cerletti's life are from [Cerletti], *Curriculum vitae e contributi scientifici del Prof. Ugo Cerletti* (Bari: Laterza, 1928); and MS, "Curriculum" in the Cerletti Papers, box 118-433. On the "Rome school" of neuropsychiatry, see Roberta Passione, "Italian Psychiatry in an International Context: Ugo Cerletti and the Case of Electroshock," *History of Psychiatry* 15 (2004): 83–104.

7. Viale was of course aware of a tradition in electrophysiology of inducing epileptic fits experimentally in animals with electric currents. See, for example, Stéphane Leduc, "Production du sommeil et de l'anesthésie générale et locale par les courants électriques," *Académie des Sciences—Comptes Rendus* 135 (1902): 199–200; M. F. Battelli, "Production d'accès épileptiformes par les courants électriques industriels," *Société de Biologie: Comptes Rendus* 55 (1903): 903–904. Erich Schilf, "Über experimentelle Erzeugung epileptischer Anfälle durch dosierte Starkstromenergie," *Zeitschrift für die gesamte experimentelle Medizin* 28 (1922): 127–143, found that potassium bromide raised the seizure threshold. Although medicine had a history of experimentally inducing fits in humans with electricity going back to Cincinnati physician Robert Bartholow in 1874, no previous worker, to our knowledge, had speculated about the potential therapeutic use of this procedure in humans. On Bartholow and subsequent experiments on the human cortex with electricity, see James P. Morgan, "The First Reported Case of Electrical Stimulation of the Human Brain," *Journal of the History of Medicine* 37 (1982): 51–64. For a general history of electricity in medicine, see Margaret Rowbottom and Charles Susskind, *Electricity and Medicine: History of Their Interaction* (San Francisco: San Francisco Press, 1984), that contains as well a brief account of electroconvulsive therapy (193–194).

8. A[ngelo?] Chiauzzi, "Richerche sperimentali sull'epilessia col metodo di Viale," *Pathologica* 26 (1934): 18–23.

9. These facts are basically from Cerletti's introductory essay in the special issue on "L'elettroshock," *Rivista Sperimentale di Freniatria* 64, nos. 2–4 (1940): 4–11.

10. This was the reasoning that Cerletti explained in 1950, at the time of the Paris World Psychiatry Congress, to French psychiatrist Jean Thuillier. See Thuillier, "Rencontre avec Ugo Cerletti, l'inventeur de l'électrochoc," *Revue du Practicien* 42 (1992): 80–82, esp. 81.

11. Lothar Kalinowsky, "Lothar B. Kalinowsky," in Ludwig J. Pongratz, ed., *Psychiatrie in Selbstdarstellungen* (Berne: Huber, 1977), 147–164, see esp. 154. Bini may have undertaken several visits to Vienna, because Charlotte Frisch-Walker, a former assistant of Poetzl, wrote to Bini in 1940 saying she recalled his visit with Accornero when they came to see ICT. Frisch-Walker to Bini, March 8, 1940. Bini Papers, box 1.

12. See Bini and Accornero, "La insulina-shock-terapia nella Clinica Neuropsichiatrica di Roma," in Max Müller, ed., "Bericht über die wissenschaftlichen Verhandlungen auf der Versammlung der Schweizerischen Gesellschaft für Psychiatrie in Münsingen bei Bern am 29.–31. Mai 1937: Die Therapie der Schizophrenie—Insulinshock, Cardiazol, Dauerschlaf," *Schweizer Archiv für Neurologie und Psychiatrie* 39, supplement (1937).

13. "Autobiography of L. J. Meduna," Meduna Papers, version 2 [1954], 52.

14. These events are reported in Accornero, undated manuscript, Cerletti Papers, box 118-433, file 8, pp. 3–8. Accornero gave a considerably abridged account in "Testimonianza oculare sulla scoperta dell'elettroshock," *Pagine di Storia della Medicina* 14 (1970): 38–52. On a lethal dose (450 volts for 50 seconds), see, for example, Bini, "La tecnica e le manifestazioni dell'elettroshock," *Rivista Sperimentale di Freniatria* 64 (1940): 361–458, esp. 382.

15. Accornero MS cited note 14, 9.

16. Quoted in Giorgio Sogliani, "Elettroshockterapia e cardiazolterapia," *Rassegna di Studi Psichiatrici* 28 (1939): 652–661, quote on 652.

17. There is even a list of those who claimed to have conducted ECT on humans before Cerletti's trial in April 1938. Erwin Stransky, a Viennese psychiatrist, said in his unpublished manuscript autobiography that he and electropathologist Stephan Jellinek had done so in Vienna, yet he provided no details nor record of publication. See his "Autobiographie," 508, in the archives of the Vienna Institut für Geschichte der Medizin. On June 4, 1940, psychiatrist Vittore Negri at the psychiatric hospital in Sondrio, Italy, told Bini that he and colleague Giorgio Sogliani were doing research on provoking epileptic fits experimentally, as though this were independent of the Cerletti-Bini publication in the *Rivista Sperimentale di Freniatria* in 1940. Although Sogliani did later publish on ECT, it is intriguing that joint work with Negri might have preceded that of Cerletti (see Bini Papers, box 2). On the long history of the use of electricity in psychiatry, see our discussion of the origins of magnetic stimulation treatments in chapter 11. Cerletti was the discoverer not of electrical therapy but of electroconvulsive therapy. The many researchers who applied electricity therapeutically, such as Giovanni Aldini, professor of physics in Bologna (who described in 1804 the application of electricity to the heads of psychiatry patients), did not induce convulsions. Yet Aldini might be deemed the pioneer of petit mal treatments (shock without a full seizure): Tom Bolwig has shared with us the text of Aldini's *Essai théorique et expérimental sur le galvanisme, avec une série d'expériences* (Paris: Fournier, 1804 [An XII]), 219–224, in which it is apparent that Aldini successfully treated a melancholic twenty-seven-year-old farmer with electrotherapy, but did not induce convulsions. On Aldini, see André Bourguignon, "La découverte par Aldini (1804) des effets thérapeutiques de l'électrochoc sur la mélancholie," *Annales Médico-Psychologiques* 122 (1964): 29–36. Bourguignon claims implausibly (29) that "one must attribute the merit of this therapeutic discovery" to Italy. Finally, the amnesia often following applications of electricity to the head has been known since the days of Benjamin Franklin. See Stanley Finger and Franklin Zaromb, "Benjamin Franklin and Shock-Induced Amnesia," *American Psychologist* 61 (2006): 240–248.

18. G. Alberti, untitled news story, *Sapere*, May 1941, 290. His anecdotes of the trial ring true but are doubtless secondhand.

19. See Cerletti to Balduzzi, August 7, 1957, and Accornero to Izikowitz, October 16, 1958, Cerletti Papers, box 118-433, file 9; Cerletti MS, "Storia dell'elettroshock," version of mid-1950s, Cerletti Papers, box 118-433, file 8, p. 8; and David J. Impastato, "The Story of the First Electroshock Treatment," *AJP* 116

(1960): 1113–1114, an interview in which Cerletti mentioned "Fleischer." Giovanni Flescher's contribution on "L'amnesia retrograda dopo l'elettroshock," *Schweizer Archiv für Neurologie und Psychiatrie* 48 (1941): 1–28, represents the first study of memory loss in ECT. It was possibly not published in the special issue of the *Rivista Sperimentale di Freniatria* in 1940 because Flescher had some rather dispiriting things to say about patients' fears and "permanent" memory loss (13).

20. The account in Bini's notebook no. 1 is preserved in Bini Papers, box 1. E. Bruno Magliocco translated the note of the trial of April 11, 1938, into English, and Max Fink published it as "an historical note" in *Convulsive Therapy* 11 (1995): 260–261. The rest of the notebook remains untranslated and unpublished. In Bini's manuscript notebook the patient is not named, but Cerletti's 1956 manuscript paper, the first page of which is titled simply "Prefazione," Cerletti Papers, box 118-433, identifies the first patient as Enrico X (7).

21. Accounts vary about exactly what phrase Enrico X called out. The most accessible published version is Accornero's, cited above.

22. Enrico X is mentioned by family name in the notebook only for the treatment series beginning on April 20 (92 volts, one-half second).

23. Ugo Cerletti and Lucio Bini, "Un nuovo metodo di shockterapia: 'L'elettroshock' (Riassunto)," *Communicazione alla Seduta del 28 maggio 1938–XVI della Reale Accademia Medica di Roma,*" 5 pp. Kalinowsky, in Pongratz, *Psychiatrie in Selbstdarstellungen,* 154, says that this patient was in fact the first patient, namely, Enrico X.

24. "'L'elettroshock': Nuovo brillante metodo di cura delle psicosi," *Il Messaggero,* May 29, 1938. Clipping in Bini Papers, box 1.

25. For these events, see Cerletti, "Prefazione," 9.

26. See, for example, Cerletti, "Electroshock Therapy," *Journal of Clinical and Experimental Psychopathology* 15 (1954): 191–217; see the narrative on 193–194.

27. Cerletti Papers, box 118-433, file 10.

28. Eugenio Giovannetti, "La pazzia curata con la scossa elettrica," *Il Giornale d'Italia,* August 26, 1938.

29. Accornero, untitled and undated MS, Cerletti Papers, box 118-433, file 8, pp. 14–15; Cerletti in a news interview, "Anzitutto i malati non sono affatto riluttanti per la cura con l'elettroshock," *Annali Ravasini,* November 10, 1938.

30. Bini notebook no. 2. The patients are numbered from "nr. 2" to "nr. 21." These figures do not include several patients whose series were broken off early, a line drawn through their pages in the notebook.

31. Lucie Jessner and V. Gerard Ryan's *Shock Treatment in Psychiatry: A Manual* (New York: Grune and Stratton, 1941) was mainly about insulin coma and Metrazol and had only twenty-one pages on ECT.

32. Cerletti MS, "Storia dell'elettroshock," version written in mid-1950s, 7.

33. See Bini notebook no. 2, entry for patient 17 for October 15, 1938.

34. Director to Bini, January 5, 1940, Bini Papers, box 1.

35. See letters to Bini of March 12 and June 27, 1940, Bini Papers, box 1.

36. See the director of the Consiglio Superiore di Sanità to Cerletti, June 10, 1940, asking him for a report on the question, Cerletti Papers, box 118-433.

37. As Cerletti wrote in his article in the *Rivista Sperimentale di Freniatria* in 1940: "Risultati ancor più brillanti che nella schizofrenia si sono ottenuti nella frenosi maniaco-depressiva, particolarmente negli episodi depressivi" (225).

38. See Cerletti, "Prefazione," 12.

39. Cerletti pointed out Bini's contribution here in the MS, "Annotazione sull'elettroshock" [c. 1940], 4–5, Cerletti Papers, box 118-433.

40. Bini had first suggested the "annichilimento" approach in 1940. He mentioned it to an English-speaking audience in his paper "Electroplexy in the Treatment of Depression," in E. Beresford Davies, ed., *Depression: Proceedings of the Symposium Held at Cambridge 22 to 26 September 1959* (Cambridge: Cambridge University Press, 1964), 263–273, esp. 266–267.

41. See Ugo Cerletti, "Résumés des rapports publiés avant le congrès," in Henri Ey, ed., *Premier congrès mondial de psychiatrie, Paris, 1950*, vol. 4, *Thérapeutique biologique* (Paris: Hermann, 1952), 10–15, esp. 11–12.

42. Etta Cerletti to Menninger Foundation, March 11, 1965, Bini Papers, box 1.

43. Kalinowsky, in Pongratz, *Psychiatrie in Selbstdarstellungen*, 153. These biographical details are taken almost entirely from this autobiography.

44. Ey, *Premier congrès mondial de psychiatrie, Paris, 1950*, 4:144.

45. Max Müller mentions the loss of the designs. *Erinnerungen: Erlebte Psychiatriegeschichte, 1920–1960* (Berlin: Springer, 1982), 247. But in Kalinowsky's papers it is clear that he gave the designs to the Duflot Company, evidently in Paris, in the hopes of a licensing fee, which however he never obtained. See Kalinowsky to Duflot, May 11, 1940, Bini Papers, box 1.

46. Kalinowsky to Bini, December 7, 1939, Bini Papers, box 1.

47. See Kalinowsky's rueful note to Bini, August 13, 1940, Bini Papers, box 1.

CHAPTER FOUR. From the University Clinic to the Psychiatric Institute: Shock Therapy Goes Global

1. This, and all subsequent quotations relating to the patient, are from Hillside Hospital Archives, reel 11, no. 1182. The records of the first insulin patient at Hillside are on reel 9, no. 1069.

2. Details on Nijinsky are taken from Richard Buckle, *Nijinsky* (1971; rpt. Harmondsworth: Penguin, 1975), 512–521; "Aid Offered Nijinski [*sic*] for Cure in America," *New York Times*, December 10, 1939, 43; "Consulate Blocks Nijinsky Trip Here," *New York Times*, May 10, 1940, 10.

3. For background, see Max Müller, *Erinnerungen: Erlebte Psychiatriegeschichte, 1920–1960* (Berlin: Springer, 1982), 167–170.

4. Otfried K. Linde, *Pharmakopsychiatrie im Wandel der Zeit* (Klingenmünster: Tilia, 1988), 101.

5. "Die Therapie der Schizophrenie," *Schweizer Archiv für Neurologie und Psychiatrie* (*Ergänzungsheft* [suppl.]) 39 (1937); the conference also considered Metrazol, but the bulk of the discussion was about insulin treatment. See Wortis to Fink, February 16, 1983, Wortis Collection, box 7.

6. On sterilization, see the 1938 report to the Rockefeller Foundation by English psychiatrist Aubrey Lewis, in Katherine Angel et al., eds., *European Psychiatry*

on the Eve of War: Aubrey Lewis, the Maudsley Hospital and the Rockefeller Foundation in the 1930s (London: Wellcome Trust Centre for the History of Medicine at UCL, 2003), 90.

7. Sakel to Wortis, May 3, 1936, Wortis Collection, box 10.

8. See Isabel G. H. Wilson, *A Study of Hypoglycaemic Shock Treatment in Schizophrenia* (London: HMSO, 1936), 56; Pullar-Strecker alludes to this in a letter, "Insulin in Schizophrenia," *Lancet* 230 (June 27, 1936): 1498–1499.

9. See Wilson, *Study of Hypoglycaemic Shock Treatment,* passim.

10. Angel, *European Psychiatry on the Eve of War,* mentions the date November 1938 (14); see also William Sargant, "Insulin Treatment in England," in Max Rinkel and Harold E. Himwich, eds., *Insulin Treatment in Psychiatry* (New York: Philosophical Library, 1959), 146.

11. Sargant, "Insulin Treatment in England," 146.

12. W[illi] Mayer-Gross, "Insulin Coma Therapy of Schizophrenia: Some Critical Remarks on Dr. Sakel's Report," *Journal of Mental Science* 97 (1951): 132–135.

13. Denbighshire Record Office, file HD/I/II, Denbigh Mental Hospital, *Annual Report of the Medical Superintendent,* 1940, 21.

14. On the four, see Samuel Atkin's discussion comments in Eugene Glynn, "Clinical Symposium: Insulin Coma Therapy," *Journal of Hillside Hospital* 4 (1955): 161–189, esp. 182.

15. See Marvin Stein, "The Establishment of the Department of Psychiatry in the Mount Sinai Hospital: A Conflict between Neurology and Psychiatry," *Journal of the History of the Behavioral Sciences* 40 (2004): 285–309, esp. 289 and passim.

16. See Hillside Hospital Archives, reel 9, no. 1069.

17. See Hilary Richardson, "The Fate of Kingsley Porter," *Donegal Annual,* no. 45 (1993): 83–87.

18. Most of this information comes from an information sheet on Wortis at the Diethelm Library as part of a calendar of his papers.

19. On these details, see Wortis to Porter, April 20, 1937, Wortis Collection, box 10. Wortis's chief early publications on insulin coma were "On the Response of Schizophrenic Subjects to Hypoglycemic Insulin Shock," *Journal of Nervous and Mental Disease* 84 (November 1936): 497–506; "Cases Illustrating the Treatment of Schizophrenia by Insulin Shock," *Journal of Nervous and Mental Disease* 85 (April 1937): 446–456, a paper he first gave at the meeting of the New York Society of Clinical Psychiatry, November 12, 1936; "Early Experiences with Sakel's Hypoglycemic Insulin Treatment of Psychoses in America," *Schweizer Archiv für Neurologie und Psychiatrie (Ergänzungsheft* [suppl.]) 39 (1937): 208; and Wortis et al., "Further Experiences at Bellevue Hospital with the Hypoglycemic Insulin Treatment of Schizophrenia," *AJP* 94 (July 1937): 153–158.

20. Wortis to Jelliffe, June 1, 1937, Wortis Collection, box 8.

21. Alexander Thomas, *History of Bellevue Psychiatric Hospital, 1736–1994* (New York: privately published, 1999), 116. Wortis left Bellevue in 1942 to work for the U.S. Public Health Service during the war.

22. Sakel to Wortis, telegram, July 13, 1936, Wortis Collection, box 10, in which Sakel asks Wortis to negotiate an honorarium on his behalf in that range.

23. William Karliner, interview by Edward Shorter, New York, April 6, 2004.

24. Kalinowsky to Bini, May 18, 1940, Bini Papers, box 1. (Hereafter in this chapter, unless noted otherwise, all correspondence involving Bini comes from this collection.)

25. Meduna to Pullar-Strecker, January 31, 1949, Meduna Papers, box 1. (Hereafter in this chapter, unless noted otherwise, all correspondence involving Meduna comes from this collection.)

26. "Dinner on Friday to Advance Plan of Medical Fund," *New York Times,* October 19, 1958, 102.

27. "Sakel Will Probated," *New York Times,* December 24, 1957, 21.

28. See Harold Himwich to Wortis, October 4, 1937. Wortis Collection, box 8.

29. See D. Ewen Cameron and R. G. Hoskins, "Some Observations on Sakel's Insulin-Hypoglycemia Treatment of Schizophrenia," *Schweizer Archiv für Neurologie und Psychiatrie (Ergänzungsheft* [suppl.]) 39 (1937): 180–182; Cameron and Hoskins, "Experiences in the Insulin-Hypoglycemia Treatment of Schizophrenia," *Journal of the American Medical Association* 109 (October 16, 1937): 1246–1249.

30. Glueck's was one of the earliest American reports on insulin coma: "The Hypoglycemic State in the Treatment of Schizophrenia," *JAMA* 107 (September 26, 1936): 1029–1031.

31. Sakel said in 1935 that Meyer was applying insulin coma treatment "indiscriminately [*wahllos*]." Sakel to Wortis, June 27, 1935. Wortis Collection, box 10. Late in 1938, Wortis traveled down to Baltimore to teach the proper application of the technique.

32. "Dementia Praecox Curbed by Insulin," *New York Times,* January 13, 1937, 11; editorial, "Insulin and the Mind," January 14, 1937, 20.

33. See the following articles by John R. Ross and coauthors at Harlem Valley: John R. Ross, "Report of the Hypoglycemic Treatment in New York State Hospitals," *AJP* 94 (1937): 131–134; Ross and Benjamin Malzberg, "A Review of the Results of the Pharmacological Shock Therapy and the Metrazol Convulsive Therapy in New York State," *AJP* 96 (1939): 297–316; Ross, "The Pharmacological Shock Treatment of Schizophrenia," *AJP* 95 (1939): 769–779; and Ross et al., "The Pharmacological Shock Treatment of Schizophrenia: A Two-Year Follow-up Study from the New York State Hospitals," *AJP* 97 (1941): 1007–1023.

34. Wortis told the story to Georgetown University psychiatry professor Zigmond M. Lebensohn. See Lebensohn, "The History of Electroconvulsive Therapy in the United States and Its Place in American Psychiatry: A Personal Memoir," *Comprehensive Psychiatry* 40 (1999): 173–181, see 174. According to a letter Lebensohn wrote at the time, the presentation at St. Elizabeths took place on January 14, 1938, not in February, as Wortis later told Lebensohn. See Lebensohn to Wortis, January 2, 1938, Wortis Collection, box 9.

35. William Laurence, "Insulin Therapy," *New York Times,* August 8, 1943, E9. Laurence, the science reporter, tended to idolize Sakel.

36. Paul H. Hoch, "Insulin Therapy as Compared to Drug Treatment in Psychiatry," in Rinkel and Himwich, *Insulin Treatment,* 181–221, quote on 185.

37. Benjamin Malzberg, "Outcome of Insulin Treatment of One Thousand Patients with Dementia Praecox," *Psychiatric Quarterly* 12 (1938): 528–553, quotes on 548, 552.

38. T. D. Rivers and Earl D. Bond, "Follow-up Results in Insulin Shock Therapy after One to Three Years," *AJP* 98 (1941): 382–384, quote on 384.

39. See Manfred Sakel, "The Methodical Use of Hypoglycemia in the Treatment of Psychoses," *AJP* 94 (July 1937): 111–130.

40. Lawrence Kolb and Victor H. Vogel, "The Use of Shock Therapy in 305 Mental Hospitals," *AJP* 99 (1942): 90–100.

41. Deborah Blythe Doroshow, "The Injection of Insulin into American Psychiatry" (Senior thesis, Harvard University, 2004), 38–39. She cataloged its spread on the basis of mentions in state and regional medical journals.

42. Kalinowsky to Bini, April 24, 1941.

43. State of New York, *Seventeenth Annual Report of the Director of the Psychiatric Institute to the Department of Mental Hygiene for the Fiscal Year Ended March 31, 1946* (Utica: State Hospitals Press, 1946), 17. "The nursing shortage also has been a handicap, not only here but in other hospitals where the treatments have been completely discontinued."

44. "Creedmoor Patients Facing a Time of Uncertainty," *New York Times,* November 20, 1968, 34. See also H. Peter Laqueur to Raymond W. Waggoner, March 18, 1960, Waggoner Collection, box 3.

45. The correspondence of Raymond G. Waggoner, professor of psychiatry at the University of Michigan, gives a more nuanced picture of the decline in the United States. In 1959, he quizzed the directors of the state hospitals of Michigan about the current status of insulin coma therapy. The responses converged on a temporary abandonment of the treatment during the war owing to a shortage of nurses, then a brief postwar revival, followed by the definitive abandonment of insulin coma and insulin subcoma during the 1950s. See Waggoner Collection, box 3.

46. Harold Bourne, "The Insulin Myth," *Lancet* 2 (November 7, 1953): 964–968.

47. See letters in the *Lancet* 2 (November 14, 1953): 1047–1048; (November 28, 1953): 1151–1153.

48. Brian Ackner, Arthur Harris, and A. J. Oldham, "Insulin Treatment of Schizophrenia: A Controlled Study," *Lancet* 1 (March 23, 1957): 607–611.

49. Max Fink et al., "Comparative Study of Chlorpromazine and Insulin Coma in Therapy of Psychosis," *JAMA* 166 (April 12, 1958): 1846–1850. In fact, the first presentation of these findings occurred six months previously, in September 1957, at the Second International Congress of Psychiatry in Zurich. See Fink, "Alteration of Brain Function in Therapy," in Nathan S. Kline, ed., *Psychopharmacology Frontiers* (Boston: Little Brown, [1957]), 325–338, esp. 326–327. Yet the later article in *JAMA* enjoyed far more currency than this conference paper.

50. Max Fink, interview by Edward Shorter, Nissequogue, N.Y., July 13, 2004.

51. Max Fink, "A Clinician-Researcher and ECDEU: 1959–1980," in Thomas Ban et al., eds., *The Triumph of Psychopharmacology and the Story of CINP* (Budapest: Animula, 2000), 82–92, quote on 84.

52. Rinkel and Himwich, *Insulin Treatment,* passim.

53. Sylvia Nasar, *A Beautiful Mind: The Life of Nobel Laureate and Mathematical Genius John Nash* (New York: Simon and Schuster, 1998), 288–294.

54. Ladislaus v. Meduna, "Versuche über die biologische Beeinflussung des Ablaufes der Schizophrenie," *Zeitschrift für die Gesamte Neurologie und Psychiatrie* 152 (1935): 235–262.

55. S[alvatore] Gullotta, "Narcosi, catatonia ed epilessia provocate sperimentalmente mediante la corrente elettrica," *Rivista Sperimentale di Freniatria* 58 (1934): 417–424.

56. See Michael Burleigh, *Death and Deliverance: "Euthanasia" in Germany, 1900–1945* (Cambridge: Cambridge University Press, 1994), 252, 272, 275–276.

57. Meduna to A. E. Bennett, December 20, 1945.

58. [Adolf] Wahlmann, "Vorläufige Mitteilung über Konvulsionstherapie der Psychosen," *Psychiatrisch-Neurologische Wochenschrift* 38 (February 15, 1936): 78–79.

59. E. Küppers, "Die Insulin- und Cardiazolbehandlung der Schizophrenie," *Allgemeine Zeitschrift für Psychiatrie* 107 (1938): 76–96, esp. 76, 79–80.

60. A[nton] von Braunmühl, "Das 'Azoman' bei der Krampfbehandlung der Schizophrenie," *Psychiatrisch-Neurologische Wochenschrift* 40 (November 5, 1938): 515–519, quote on 515.

61. Meduna, "Allgemeine Betrachtungen über die Cardiazoltherapie," *Schweizer Archiv für Neurologie und Psychiatrie (Ergänzungsheft* [suppl.]) 39 (1937): 32–37; Müller, *Erinnerungen,* 168–170.

62. See L. C. Cook, "Cardiazol Convulsion Therapy in Schizophrenia," *Proceedings of the Royal Society of Medicine* 31 (1938): 567–577. Cook, then the deputy superintendent of Bexley Hospital for Nervous and Mental Disorders, had visited Meduna in Budapest. On Cardiazol in psychotic depression and mania, see Cook and W. Ogden, "Cardiazol Convulsion Therapy in Non-schizophrenic Reaction States," *Lancet* 2 (October 15, 1938): 885–887.

63. Meduna, "Il trattamento della schizofrenia negli ospedali di stato," *Rassegna di Studi Psichiatrici* 27 (1938): 883–896, see table 1, 889.

64. Ervin Varga, "Horus: Meduna," *Orvosi Hetilap,* no. 21 (1965): 1999–2000. On Gonda's role, see "Autobiography of L. J. Meduna," Meduna Papers, version 1, 72–76.

65. Meduna to R. W. Medlicott, August 27, 1947.

66. State of New York, *Psychiatric Institute and Hospital, Eighth Annual Report for the Fiscal Year Ending June 30, 1937* (Utica: State Hospitals Press, 1938), 6.

67. Hans H. Reese and August Sauthoff, "Insulin and Metrazol Treatment in Schizophrenia," *Wisconsin Medical Journal* 37 (1938): 816–820.

68. This is mentioned in Meduna to H. L. Gordon, September 30, 1947.

69. Cook and Ogden, "Cardiazol Convulsion Therapy in Non-schizophrenic Reaction States," *Lancet* 2 (October 15, 1938): 885–887.

70. A. E. Bennett, "Convulsive (Pentamethylenetetrazol) Shock Therapy in Depressive Psychoses," *American Journal of the Medical Sciences* 196 (1938): 420–428; Bennett, "Metrazol Convulsive Shock Therapy in Affective Psychoses: A Follow-up Report of Results Obtained in Sixty-one Depressive and Nine Manic Cases," *American Journal of the Medical Sciences* 198 (1939): 695–701, quote on 701.

71. Kolb and Vogel, "The Use of Shock Therapy in 305 Mental Hospitals," 94.

72. Irving J. Sands gives this background on the case conference in "The First

Twenty-five Years of Hillside Hospital," *Journal of Hillside Hospital* 2 (1953): 199–206, see esp. 203. The case of Jack X itself, and all related quotations given here, is in Hillside Hospital Archives, reel 11, no. 1168.

73. Louis Wender and M[orris] D[avid] Epstein, "Disturbances in the Reticulo-Endothelial System during the Course of Metrazol Treatment," *Psychiatric Quarterly* 13 (1939): 534–538. Epstein became known as a pioneer of insulin therapy as well as electroconvulsive therapy. See the interview with his son, Dr. Fred J. Epstein, *New York Times*, April 11, 1993, A1, under the category "Connecticut Q&A."

74. Hillside Hospital Archives, reel 11, no. 1193.

75. Ibid., reel 13, no. 1385.

76. Karl Theo Dussik to Wortis, August 26, 1937, Wortis Collection, box 6.

77. Phillip Polatin et al., "Vertebral Fractures Produced by Metrazol-Induced Convulsions," *JAMA* 112 (April 29, 1939): 1684–1687.

78. Harold A. Palmer, "Vertebral Fractures Complicating Convulsion Therapy," *Lancet* 2 (July 22, 1939): 181–183.

79. Bennett, "Metrazol Convulsive Shock Therapy in Affective Psychoses," 698.

80. Hillside Hospital Archives, reel 11, no. 1195.

81. Arcioni, list of ECT apparatus sales, October 1, 1939, updated in Bini's hand to January 1940, Bini Papers, box 1.

82. Müller to G. Corberi, November 25, 1939. Corberi fowarded the letter to Cerletti, where it was found in the Cerletti Papers, box 118-434. The account of Müller's experience with ECT is from Müller, *Erinnerungen*, 245–247.

83. Max Müller, "Die Elektroschocktherapie in der Psychiatrie," *Schweizerische Medizinische Wochenschrift* 70 (April 13, 1940): 323–326, quote on 326.

84. Christian Müller, *Vom Tollhaus zum Psychozentrum: Vignetten und Bausteine zur Psychiatriegeschichte in zeitlicher Abfolge* (Hürtgenwald: Pressler, 1993), 201.

85. Schweizerische Gesellschaft für Psychiatrie, "Einladung zur 96. Versammlung," November 15–16, 1941, Basel, in Cerletti Papers, box 118-434.

86. Arcioni to Bini, July 25, 1939.

87. G. Alberti, news story, *Sapere*, May 1941, 290.

88. Kalinowsky to Bini, May 26, 1940.

89. A. Bingel and F. Meggendorfer, "Über die ersten deutschen Versuche einer Elektrokrampfbehandlung der Geisteskranken," *Psychiatrisch-Neurologische Wochenschrift* 42 (February 3, 1940): 41–43.

90. Müller, *Erinnerungen*, 248.

91. A[nton] von Braunmühl, "Die kombinierte Shock-Krampfbehandlung der Schizophrenie am Beispiel der 'Blockmethode,'" *Zeitschrift für die gesamte Neurologie und Psychiatrie* 164 (1938): 69–92.

92. A[nton] von Braunmühl, "Der Elektrokrampf in der Psychiatrie," *Münchner Medizinische Wochenschrift* 87 (May 10, 1940): 511–514. Braunmühl recommended a stimulus duration of 0.5 seconds at 110 volts giving 400–600 mA of electricity. He elaborated the "block method"—a combination of ECT and insulin—in the second edition of his textbook, published after the war: Anton v. Braunmühl, *Insulinshock und Heilkrampf in der Psychiatrie: Ein Leitfaden für die Praxis*, 2nd ed. (Stuttgart: Wissenschaftliche Verlagsgesellschaft, 1947), 191–194. At this point Braunmühl had become director of Eglfing-Haar. For a rather antipsychiatric

discussion of insulin coma at Eglfing-Haar, see Burleigh, *Death and Deliverance,* 84–89.

93. Zigmond Lebensohn MS, "Rough Notes at ECT Hearings, American Psychiatric Association, Tuesday, May 11, 1976," 1, in Max Fink's personal archive, Nissequogue, N.Y. Henri Claude and P. Rubenovitch, in *Thérapeutiques biologiques des affections mentales* (Paris: Masson, 1940), describe animal research but say they are only contemplating the introduction of ECT (330–331). Yet the text must have been drafted earlier.

94. Claude apparently told Kalinowsky that, after the invasion, he wished to undertake ECT somewhere in the provinces. See Kalinowsky to Bini, May 26, 1940. Duflot was supposed to make a machine for Claude before the invasion, and in fact did so afterward. Further details are not known. See Kalinowsky to Bini, August 13, 1940. In the discussion of the Lapipe-Rondepierre paper at the French Medical-Psychological Society on April 28, 1941 (see n. 95, below), Claude said that his group had renounced applying ECT to humans because they were unable to obtain convulsions in animal experiments (94).

95. M[arcel] Lapipe and J[ean-Jacques] Rondepierre, "Essais d'un appareil français pour l'électro-choc," *Annales Médico–Psychologiques* 99 (1941): 87–94. The first publication in France on ECT was André Plichet, "L'électro-choc: Le traitement des affections mentales par les crisis convulsives électriques," *Presse Médicale* 48 (November 20–23, 1940): 937–939; it was, however, a review of the German and Italian literature rather than a presentation of findings. The first book was Lapipe and Rondepierre, *Contribution à l'étude physique, physiologique et clinique de l'électro-choc* (Paris: Maloine, 1942).

96. Perret said that it was impossible to obtain an ECT machine in France at that time; Perret to Cerletti, February 19, 1942, Cerletti Papers, box 118-433, file 10. But Lapipe and Rondepierre, in an article a month later, said their machine was available in "fifteen or so" (*une quinzaine*) psychiatric hospitals and private clinics. "L'électro-choc en psychiatrie," *Presse Médicale* 50 (March 10, 1942): 269–272. On October 26, 1942, they presented their new "Sismothère" apparatus to the Société Médico-Psychologique; see Lapipe and Rondepierre, "Présentation d'un nouvel appareil portatif à reglage automatique," *Annales Médico-Psychologiques* 100 (1942): 346–350.

97. Oscar Forel, *La mémoire du chêne* (Montreux: Favre, 1980), 106.

98. In discussion following Jean Laboucarié, "Un cas de mort après électrochoc," *Annales Médico-Psychologiques* 103 (1945): 430–431; comments on 434.

99. Stephen Barber, *Antonin Artaud: Blows and Bombs* (London: Faber, 1993), 105–107, 113.

100. Arianna Stassinopoulos Huffington, *Picasso: Creator and Destroyer* (New York: Avon Books, 1989), 300, 324.

101. Jean Delay, *L'électro-choc et la psycho-physiologie* (Paris: Masson, 1946), 20–43, 97–98, 105–130.

102. Henri Baruk, *Traité de psychiatrie* (Paris: Masson, 1959), 2:794.

103. Jean Thuillier interview in David Healy, ed., *The Psychopharmacologists,* vol. 3 (London: Arnold, 2000), 543–559, quote on 548.

104. P[aul] Delmas-Marsalet, discussion, in Henri Ey, ed., *Premier congrès mon-*

dial de psychiatrie, Paris, 1950, vol. 4, *Thérapeutique biologique* (Paris: Hermann, 1952), 98–99.

105. "Thomas Percy Rees," *Lives of the Fellows of the Royal College of Physicians* (Munk's *Roll*) (London: Royal College of the Physicians of London, 1968), 5:344–345.

106. Arcioni to Bini, August 8, 1939.

107. Lothar Kalinowsky, "Electric Convulsion Therapy in Schizophrenia," *Lancet* 2 (December 9, 1939): 1232–1233.

108. G[erald] W.T.H. Fleming, F[rederick] L. Golla, and W. Grey Walter, "Electric-Convulsion Therapy of Schizophrenia," *Lancet* 2 (December 30, 1939): 1353–1355.

109. Kalinowsky to Bini, December 7, 1939: " . . . Devono usare correnti più alti (140 volt e di più) perchè la resistenza con quali efferatore è 'alta.'"

110. William H. Shepley and J. S. McGregor, "Electrically Induced Convulsions in Treatment of Mental Disorders," *British Medical Journal* 3 (December 30, 1939): 1269–1271, quote on 1271.

111. "Reports of Societies: Electrically Induced Convulsions" [meeting of the Section of Psychiatry of the Royal Society of Medicine], *British Medical Journal* 1 (January 20, 1940): 104–106.

112. "Eric Strauss," *Munk's Roll,* 5:404. See E. B. Strauss and Angus MacPhail, "The Treatment of Out-patients by Electrical Convulsant Therapy with a Portable Apparatus," *British Medical Journal* 2 (December 7, 1940): 779–782, esp. 780. They also administered ECT once a week in the department of psychological medicine at "Bart's." Strauss is arguably more remembered for having furthered, together with Joshua Bierer, the "therapeutic social clubs" that were the basis of social psychiatry in Britain. See E[ric] B. Strauss, R. Ström-Olsen, and J[oshua] Bierer, "Memorandum on Therapeutic Social Clubs in Psychiatry," *British Medical Journal* 2 (December 30, 1944): 861.

113. Jonathan Andrews et al., *The History of Bethlem* (London: Routledge, 1997), 693.

114. A. Spencer Paterson, discussion, in E. Beresford Davies, ed., *Depression: Proceedings of the Symposium Held at Cambridge, 22 to 26 September 1959* (Cambridge: Cambridge University Press, 1964), 354.

115. L[eslie] C[olin] Cook, "The Place of Physical Treatments in Psychiatry," *Journal of Mental Science* 104 (1958): 933–942, quote on 934.

116. M[ichael] Shepherd, "Evaluation of Psychotropic Drugs (2), Depression, Part I—1959," reprinted in E. L. Harris et al., eds., *The Principles and Practice of Clinical Trials* (Edinburgh: Livingstone, 1970), 199–207, quote on 202.

117. Kalinowsky to Meduna, November 18, 1947.

118. C[yril] R[obert] Birnie comment, "Reports of Societies: Electrically Induced Convulsions," *British Medical Journal* 1 (January 20, 1940): 106.

119. Cerletti MS, "Storia dell'elettroshock," draft from the mid-1950s, 7–8, Cerletti Papers, box 118-433, file 8.

120. Müller, *Erinnerungen,* 247.

121. Tom Bolwig, telephone interview by David Healy, July 17, 2004.

122. Snorre Wohlfahrt, discussion, in Ey, *Premier congrès mondial de psychiatrie,* 4:141.

123. Castelluci to Bini, January 31, 1940.

124. He lamented to Bini that he had sold only eight machines (Castelluci to Bini, February 25, 1943).

125. The machine was supposed to arrive in early November, but whether it actually did so and when it was used are unknown (Hirsch to Bini, September 9, 1939; October 23, 1939). Hirsch addressed Bini as *tu,* and it is likely that Hirsch had been a resident under Cerletti as well. Hirsch had a brother-in-law, Max Friedmann, in Milan.

126. Kalinowsky memoir, in Ludwig J. Pongratz, ed., *Psychiatrie in Selbstdarstellungen* (Berne: Huber, 1977), 156.

127. Walter E. Barton, *The History and Influence of the American Psychiatric Association* (Washington, D.C.: American Psychiatric Press, 1987), 164.

128. Kalinowsky to Bini, May 26, 1940, said that Goldman demonstrated ECT at the meeting. The program of the session of May 23, 1940, mentions that Kalinowsky, Meduna, Sakel, and Gonda took part in the discussion but says nothing about a demonstration, which presumably was arranged informally; "Proceedings of Societies," *AJP* 97 (1940): 436.

129. Obituary of Douglas Goldman, *Cincinnati Enquirer,* February 8, 1986, C3.

130. Lebensohn, "Rough Notes at ECT Hearings," 1.

131. This dating is dependent on the manuscript account of David J. Impastato's son, David Impastato Jr., "Notes on the First Use of ECT in the U.S.," version C, deposited in 1992 in the Impastato Papers at the Oscar Diethelm Library. In a letter to Zigmond Lebensohn of January 26, 1998, David Impastato Jr. noted that the possible office treatment of Miss X on January 7, 1940, could well have occurred in 1941 (Impastato Papers).

132. Renato Almansi and David J. Impastato, "Electrically Induced Convulsions in the Treatment of Mental Disease," *New York State Journal of Medicine* 40 (1940): 1315–1316.

133. Viktor [*sic*] Gonda, "Rasche Heilung der Symptome der im Kriege enstandenen 'traumatische Neurose,'" *Wiener Klinische Wochenschrift* 29 (1916): 950–951.

134. The son, unidentified by name but probably psychiatrist William Gonda, gave this account to Sydney E. Pulver, "The First Electroconvulsive Treatment Given in the United States," *AJP* 117 (1961): 845–846.

135. Kalinowsky to Bini, May 26, 1940: "in una maniera proprio adatta da discreditare il metodo."

136. Victor E. Gonda, "Treatment of Mental Disorders with Electrically Induced Convulsions," *Diseases of the Nervous System* 2 (1941): 84–92; quote on 89.

137. Lauren H. Smith, Joseph Hughes, and Donald W. Hastings, "First Impressions of Electroshock Treatment," *Pennsylvania Medical Journal* 44 (1941): 452–455. On the May 1 date, see Pulver, "The First Electroconvulsive Treatment Given in the United States," 845.

138. For these details, see David J. Impastato, "Beginnings of EST in Boston Area," in Impastato Papers. The main scientific paper to emerge from this work was Louis Feldman and Frederick T. Davis, "An Improved Apparatus for Convulsive Therapy," *Archives of Physical Therapy* 22 (1941): 89–91.

139. On October 21, 1940, Joseph Wortis told Harold Himwich that they were just about to start ECT at Bellevue: "S. B. Wortis is already doing work on rats after ES convulsions." Wortis Papers, box 8.

140. Thomas, *History of Bellevue Psychiatric Hospital,* 129n33.

141. Impastato MS, "Beginnings of EST in New York Area," Impastato Papers. See Kalinowsky to Bini, June 17, 1940, for the date of the first ECT.

142. See Kalinowsky to Bini, May 18, 1940.

143. State of New York, *Eleventh Annual Report of the Director of the Psychiatric Institute and Hospital to the Department of Mental Hygiene for the Fiscal Year Ending June 30, 1940* (Utica: State Hospitals Press, 1941), 8.

144. "Insanity Treated by Electroshock," *New York Times,* July 6, 1940, 16.

145. Undated letter, Almansi to Bini, c. May 1941, on basis of internal evidence.

146. Kalinowsky to Bini, May 18, 1940.

147. Cerletti MS, "L'elettroshock: L'epilessia curativa," c. 1945, 2, Cerletti Papers, box 118-436.

148. Lothar Kalinowsky and S[evero] Eugene Barrera, "Electric Convulsion Therapy in Mental Disorders," *Psychiatric Quarterly* 14 (1940): 719–730, quote on 727.

149. Kalinowsky to Bini, July 6, 1940.

150. State of New York, *Fourteenth Annual Report of the Director of the Psychiatric Institute and Hospital to the Department of Mental Hygiene for the Fiscal Period Ending March 31, 1943* (Utica: State Hospitals Press, 1943), 14.

151. State of New York, *Sixteenth Annual Report of the Director of the Psychiatric Institute to the Department of Mental Hygiene for the Fiscal Year Ended March 31, 1945* (Utica: State Hospitals Press, 1945), 19.

152. Kalinowsky, in Pongratz, *Psychiatrie in Selbstdarstellungen,* 161.

153. For these details, see ibid., 156–157.

154. Ibid., 160.

155. An obituary of Taylor claimed that at some unspecified time he had worked with Sakel as well. "Dr. J. H. Taylor Jr., Trenton Therapist," *New York Times,* May 4, 1948, 26.

156. Louis Linn, "Dr. Linn Reminisces," *American Psychiatric Association, Area II Council, Bulletin* (March–April 1991): 5–6, quote on 5.

157. Kolb and Vogel, "The Use of Shock Therapy in 305 Mental Hospitals," 94, fig. 3.

158. Lucy Freeman, "Shock Treatment Held Not Enough," *New York Times,* April 14, 1947, 27. Jones deplored the widespread use of shock therapy and preferred psychotherapy.

159. Theodore Robie, "Is Shock Therapy on Trial?" *AJP* 106 (1950): 902–909. The APA had invited members across the country to write in with their opinions.

160. Benjamin Wiesel, oral history interview, p. 7, T. Stewart Hamilton Archives, Hartford Hospital, Hartford, Conn.

161. Kenneth J. Tillotson and Wolfgang Sulzbach, "A Comparative Study and Evaluation of Electric Shock Therapy in Depressive States," *AJP* 101 (1945): 455–459.

162. See Max Fink, *Convulsive Therapy: Theory and Practice* (New York: Raven Press, 1979), 22–23.

163. Lothar Kalinowsky, "The Various Forms of Shock Therapy in Mental Disorders and Their Practical Importance," *New York State Journal of Medicine* 41 (1941): 2210–2215, quotes on 2213, 2214.

164. *Dow v. State of New York*, 183 Misc. 674, 50 N.Y.S. 2d 342 (1944), LexisNexis Academic, LEXIS 2323, 2–3.

165. Pennsylvania Department of Justice, 64 Pa. D. & C. 14 (1948), LexisNexis Academic, LEXIS 182.

CHAPTER FIVE.   The Couch or the Treatment Table?

1. Joseph J. Schildkraut, "The Catecholamine Hypothesis," in David Healy, ed., *The Psychopharmacologists,* vol. 3 (London: Arnold, 2000), 111–134, quote on 115–116.

2. Fred H. Frankel, "Reasoned Discourse or a Holy War? Postscript to a Report on ECT," *AJP* 132 (1975): 77–79, quote on 77.

3. Ernest Jones in discussion, "Royal Medico-Psychological Association of July 13, 1950," *Journal of Mental Science* 97 (1951): 147.

4. Tom Bolwig, telephone interview by David Healy, July 17, 2004.

5. William Karliner, interview by Edward Shorter, New York, April 6, 2004.

6. D[onald] W[oods] Winnicott, "Physical Therapy of Mental Disorder," *British Medical Journal* 1 (May 17, 1947): 688–689, quote on 688.

7. Aubrey Lewis, in discussion, in E. Beresford Davies, ed., *Depression: Proceedings of the Symposium Held at Cambridge, 22 to 26 September 1959* (Cambridge: Cambridge University Press, 1964), 74–75.

8. Edith Vowinckel Weigert, "Psychoanalytic Notes on Sleep and Convulsion Treatment in Functional Psychoses," *Psychiatry* 3 (1940): 189–209, quote on 209.

9. Otto Fenichel, *The Psychoanalytic Theory of Neurosis* (New York: Norton, 1945), 568.

10. Lauretta Bender, "The Life Course of Children with Schizophrenia," *AJP* 130 (1973): 783–786. The treatment facilitated a number of remissions.

11. In addition to Kaufman, the eight analyst members of GAP's Committee on Therapy were Daniel Blain, Moses M. Frohlich, Maxwell Gitelson, Robert P. Knight, Maurice Levine, Betram Lewin, Alfred O. Ludwig, and Sydney G. Margolin. The two nonanalyst members were Travis E. Dancey (an asylum psychiatrist in Montreal), and George M. Raines (a former navy psychiatrist, at Georgetown University).

12. Group for the Advancement of Psychiatry (GAP), Circular Letter no. 16, "Report of Committee on Therapy," January 22, 1947. GAP Papers (Menninger).

13. GAP, *Report No. 1: Shock Therapy* (September 15, 1947), 1. GAP Papers (Menninger).

14. See undated MS, "Suggestions for the Third Day," GAP Papers (Diethelm), box 4.

15. GAP, Circular Letter no. 51, October 6, 1947, 2.

16. MS, "Proceedings: Meeting of the Group for the Advancement of Psychiatry," November 14, 1948, 107, GAP Papers (Menninger), box 118-256.

17. GAP, Circular Letter no. 132, February 16, 1949.

18. Quoted in Lucy Freeman, "New Roles Urged for Psychiatrists," *New York Times,* May 28, 1949, 16. Freeman, not exactly a model of journalistic principle, had wanted permission to cover GAP meetings and told Menninger she would be willing to let him censor her copy. See Freeman to Menninger, October 19, 1948, GAP Papers (Diethelm), box 4: "I should be glad to submit my articles to you or a person appointed by you before I telegraphed them to The Times."

19. See the Circular Letter no. 141, May 4, 1949, issued by the Committee on Therapy, to the effect that in the forthcoming revised report both sides in the "issue of ambulatory electroshock therapy" would have a chance to state their case.

20. Knight to Menninger, September 14, 1949, Menninger Collection, box 118-252.

21. Gitelson to Menninger, October 16, 1950, Menninger Collection, box 118-252. It was Gitelson's letter of resignation from the Therapy Committee and from GAP.

22. Menninger to Gitelson, February 15, 1950, Menninger Collection, box 118-252.

23. Menninger to Gitelson, April 24, 1950, ibid.

24. William Menninger to Henry Brosin, July 21, 1950, GAP Papers (Diethelm), box 4.

25. GAP, Committee on Therapy, "Revised Electro-Shock Therapy Report," *Report No. 15* (August 1950), 3.

26. Meeting of GAP, April 1, 1951, "Proceedings," p. 38, GAP Papers (Diethelm), box 48.

27. Margolin to Menninger, March 27, 1951, Menninger Collection, box 118-251.

28. Irving Burt Harrison, letter to the editor, *New York Times,* November 1, 1953, SM4.

29. Stanley F. Hansen to Ladislaus Meduna, August 16, 1951. Meduna Papers, box 1.

30. Robert Cancro, "The Uncompleted Task of Psychiatry," in Thomas Ban et al., eds., *From Psychopharmacology to Neuropsychopharmacology in the 1980s* (Budapest: Animula, 2002), 237–241, quote on 238.

31. Fred Frankel, interview by David Healy, Boston, October 3, 2004.

32. Arthur Gabriel, interview by Edward Shorter, New York, April 8, 2004.

33. Louis Linn, interview by Edward Shorter, New York, July 12, 2004.

34. Maximilian Fink, "Clinical Conference: Homosexuality with Panic and Paranoid States," *Journal of Hillside Hospital* 2 (1953): 164–173, quote on 172.

35. Hillside Hospital Archives, reel 14, no. 1546.

36. Quoted in Lucy Freeman, "State's Research Aids Mentally Ill," *New York Times,* February 4, 1949, 16.

37. State of New York, *Twenty-third Annual Report of the Director of the New York State Psychiatric Institute to the Department of Mental Hygiene for the Fiscal Year Ended March 31, 1952* (Utica: State Hospitals Press, 1952), 11–13.

38. Lothar B. Kalinowsky and Paul H. Hoch, *Shock Treatments and Other Somatic Procedures in Psychiatry* (New York: Grune and Stratton, 1946).

39. *Warner Williams v. United States of America,* 133 F. Supp. 319 (U.S. Dist. 1955), LexisNexis Academic, LEXIS 2884.

40. George Simpson interview, "Clinical Psychopharmacology," in David Healy, ed., *The Psychopharmacologists*, vol. 2 (London: Arnold, 1998), 285–305, quote on 297.

41. Peter G. Cranford, *But for the Grace of God: The Inside Story of the World's Largest Insane Asylum* (Augusta, Ga.: Great Pyramid Press, 1981), 86–87, 138. As noted in the text, Milledgeville was not, in fact, the world's largest mental hospital.

42. Sociologist Ivan Belknap offered a hostile view of ECT at "Southern State Hospital," apparently Milledgeville, in *Human Problems of a State Mental Hospital* (New York: McGraw-Hill, 1956), 162, 191–195.

43. Michael Taylor, interview by Max Fink, Ann Arbor, Mich., March 19, 2004.

44. On the 80 percent rule, see John D. Little et al., "Right Unilateral Electroconvulsive Therapy at Six Times the Seizure Threshold," *Australian and New Zealand Journal of Psychiatry* 37 (2003): 715–719: "As to patient selection, there is a body of evidence to suggest that a response rate above 80% . . . should now be routine. If the technique is unable to achieve this result, then either that technique or the patients selected, need to change" (719).

45. Giorgio Sogliani, "Elettroshockterapia e Cardiazolterapia," *Rassegna di Studi Psichiatrici* 28 (1939): 652–661. Several researchers had previously called attention to the effectiveness of Metrazol in depression. See A. A. Low et al., "Metrazol Shock Treatment of the 'Functional' Psychoses," *AMA Archives of Neurology and Psychiatry* 39 (1938): 717–736; table 2, 721, shows that 82 percent of the sixteen patients with "affective psychoses" recovered after Metrazol treatment.

46. Giorgio Sogliani, "Eine neue Methode der Krampftherapie: Die Elektroshocktherapie," *Deutsche Zeitschrift für Nervenheilkunde* 149 (1939): 159–168, quote on 166.

47. Ugo Cerletti, "L'elettroshock," *Rivista Sperimentale di Freniatria* 64 (1940): 209–310, see esp. 225.

48. A[bram] E. Bennett, "Metrazol Convulsive Shock Therapy in Affective Psychoses," *American Journal of the Medical Sciences* 198 (1939): 695–701. He filed a preliminary report on ten cases in 1938: "Convulsive (Pentamethylenetetrazol) Shock Therapy in Depressive Psychoses," *American Journal of the Medical Sciences* 196 (1938): 420–428.

49. Abraham Myerson, "Experience with Electric-Shock Therapy in Mental Disease," *New England Journal of Medicine* 224 (June 26, 1941): 1081–1085. Victor Gonda had published some statistics previously but had only eight depressives in his series (seven of whom recovered following ECT). See his "Treatment of Mental Disorders with Electrically Induced Convulsions," *Diseases of the Nervous System* 2 (March 1941): 84–92.

50. L. H. Smith et al., "Electroshock Treatment in the Psychoses," *AJP* 98 (1942): 558–561.

51. Lothar Kalinowsky, "Experience with Electric Convulsive Therapy in Various Types of Psychiatric Patients," *Bulletin of the New York Academy of Medicine* 20 (1944): 485–494.

52. Kenneth J. Tillotson and Wolfgang Sulzbach, "A Comparative Study and Evaluation of Electric Shock Therapy in Depressive States," *AJP* 101 (1945): 455–459.

53. U.S. Bureau of the Census, *Historical Statistics of the United States, Colonial Times to 1970, Bicentennial Edition, Part 1* (Washington, D.C.: Superintendent of Documents, 1975), 414, table H, 971–986.

54. Ugo Cerletti, "Résumé des rapports publiés avant le congrès," in Henri Ey, ed., *Premier congrès mondial de psychiatrie, Paris 1950*, vol. 4, *Thérapeutique biologique* (Paris: Hermann, 1952), 10–15, quote on 12.

55. Cerletti, untitled MS (1956), first page of which begins "Prefazione," 54, 57.

56. Nathan Savitsky and William Karliner, "Electroshock Therapy for Depression: Report of 200 Cases," *Medical Clinics of North America* 33 (1949): 515–526, quote on 516.

57. Theodore R. Robie, "Is Shock Therapy on Trial?" *AJP* 106 (1950): 902–910, quote on 903.

58. Eugene Ziskind, Esther Somerfeld-Ziskind, and Louis Ziskind, "Metrazol and Electric Convulsive Therapy of the Affective Psychoses: A Controlled Series of Observations Covering a Period of Five Years," *AMA Archives of Neurology and Psychiatry* 53 (1945): 212–217.

59. Paul E. Huston and Lillian M. Locher, "Manic-Depressive Psychosis: Course When Treated and Untreated with Electric Shock," *AMA Archives of Neurology and Psychiatry* 60 (1948): 37–48.

60. Charles H. Kellner et al., "Relief of Expressed Suicidal Intent by ECT: A Consortium for Research in ECT Study," *AJP* 162 (2005): 977–982. See also David Avery and George Winokur, "Suicide, Attempted Suicide, and Relapse Rates in Depression," *Archives of General Psychiatry* 35 (1978): 749–753.

61. Lothar B. Kalinowsky, S. Eugene Barrera, and William A. Horwitz, "Electric Convulsive Therapy of the Psychoneuroses," *AMA Archives of Neurology and Psychiatry* 52 (1944): 498–504, quotes on 499, 504.

62. Lothar B. Kalinowsky, "Experience with Electric Convulsive Therapy in Various Types of Psychiatric Patients," *Bulletin of the New York Academy of Medicine* 20 (1944): 485–494, quote on 488.

63. "12-Day Sneezer Leaves Hospital," *New York Times*, April 21, 1944, 34. On the stammerer, see "Notes on Science—Stammering," *New York Times*, February 29, 1948, E11.

64. Eugene Ziskind and Esther Somerfeld-Ziskind, "Metrazol Therapy in Chronic Encephalitis with Parkinsonism," *Bulletin of the Los Angeles Neurological Society* 3 (1938): 186–188.

65. Osvaldo Meco, "De l'origine psychique du syndrome neurologique parkinsonien révélée par les effets de l'électrochoc," in Ey, *Premier congrès mondial de psychiatrie, Paris 1950*, 4:278–281, quote on 280.

66. On Richard Abrams's efforts to rehabilitate ECT in the treatment of Parkonsonism, see his editorial, "ECT for Parkinson's Disease," *AJP* 146 (1989): 1391–1393.

67. "Dr. Linn Reminisces," *American Psychiatric Association, Area II Council, Bulletin* 33 (March–April 1991): 5, 12; quote on 5.

68. William Karliner, interview by Edward Shorter, New York, April 6, 2004.

69. Arcioni [company], Milan, "Apparecchio per l'elettroshock," Cerletti Papers, box 118-433, file 10.

70. Unidentified discussant, "McGill University Conference on Depression and Allied States, March 19–21, 1959," *Canadian Psychiatric Association Journal* 4, special suppl. (1959): S67.

71. Robie, "Is Shock Therapy on Trial?" 903. "Proceedings of Societies," Friday morning, May 9, 1941, session on "Electric Shock Treatment," mentions Abraham Myerson, "The Out-Patient Electric Shock Treatment of Manic-Depressive Psychoses," *AJP* 98 (1941): 280.

72. Kalinowsky to Bini, April 24, 1941, Bini Papers, box1.

73. Kalinowsky, "Experience with Electric Convulsive Therapy in Various Types of Psychiatric Patients," 492.

74. William Karliner, interview by Max Fink, Palm Beach, Fla., January 27, 2003.

75. See Savitsky and Karliner, "Electroshock Therapy for Depression"; Karliner, "Shock Treatments in Psychiatry," *American Practitioner and Digest of Treatment* 2 (1951): 511–516; Karliner, "Office Electroshock Therapy," *Journal of Hillside Hospital* 1 (1952): 131–144; Karliner, "Office Electroshock Therapy," *New York State Journal of Medicine* 54 (1954): 1338–1340.

76. American Psychiatric Association, "Standards of Electroshock Treatment: Practice Guideline, Approved by the Council," May 1953, retired, 1959. APA Archives.

CHAPTER SIX. "ECT Does Not Create Zombies"

1. A Practising Psychiatrist [pseud.], "The Experience of Electro-Convulsive Therapy," *British Journal of Psychiatry* 111 (1965): 365–367.

2. Max Fink, personal communication to Edward Shorter, 2005.

3. Lothar Kalinowsky, "Shock Treatment with Electric Current as the Exciting Agent," *Medical Times* 70 (July 1942): 238–240, quote on 238.

4. Arthur Cherkin, "Possible Brain Damage by Electroconvulsive Therapy: Memory Impairment and Cultural Resistance," *Behavioral and Brain Sciences* 7 (1984): 25–26, quote on 25; italics in original.

5. See the UK ECT Review Group, "Efficacy and Safety of Electroconvulsive Therapy in Depressive Disorders: A Systematic Review and Meta-analysis," *Lancet* 361 (March 8, 2003): 799–808, esp. 804

6. This and all subsequent quotes about the patient are from Tom Bolwig, telephone interview by David Healy, July 17, 2004.

7. Lothar B. Kalinowsky and S. Eugene Barrera, "Electric Convulsion Therapy in Mental Disorders," *Psychiatric Quarterly* 14 (1940): 719–730, quote on 726.

8. Victor E. Gonda, "Treatment of Mental Disorders with Electrically Induced Convulsions," *Diseases of the Nervous System* 2 (1941): 84–92, quote on 88.

9. Max Müller, *Erinnerungen: Erlebte Psychiatriegeschichte, 1920–1960* (Berlin: Springer, 1982), 245.

10. O[scar] L. Forel, "L'électrochoc en psychiatrie," *Annales Médico-Psychologiques* 99 (1941): 32–40, quote on 40.

11. Louis Wender, "Hillside Reminiscences," *Journal of Hillside Hospital* 5 (1956): 145–155, see esp. 154.

12. Hillside Hospital Archives, reel 14, no. 1546.

13. Ibid., reel 14, no. 1549.

14. Ibid., reel 14, no. 1561.

15. Ibid., reel 14, no. 1515.

16. Ibid., reel 14, no. 1541.

17. Ibid., reel 14, no. 1547

18. Ibid., reel 14, no. 1484.

19. We searched the records for the first twenty-five, but were unable to locate, among the extensive microfilm files, the charts for patients with ECT numbers 7, 19, 20, and 21.

20. Hillside Hospital Archives, reel 14, no. 1567.

21. Abraham Myerson, "Experience with Electric-Shock Therapy in Mental Disease," *New England Journal of Medicine* 224 (June 26, 1941): 1081–1085, quote on 1083.

22. G[iovanni] Flescher, "L'amnesia retrograda dopo l'elettroshock," *Schweizer Archiv für Neurologie und Psychiatrie* 48 (1941): 1–28, quote on 11.

23. Louis Wender, Benjamin H. Balser, and David Beres, "Extra-mural Shock Therapy," *AJP* 99 (1943): 712–718, quote on 713.

24. Alfred Gallinek, "Fear and Anxiety in the Course of Electroshock Therapy," *AJP* 113 (1956): 428–434, quote on 433. See also Herbert A. Fox, "Patients' Fear of and Objection to Electroconvulsive Therapy," *Hospital and Community Psychiatry* 44 (1993): 357–360.

25. Meduna to H. L. Gordon, September 30, 1947, Meduna Papers, box 1. The paper in question was Hirsch Loeb Gordon, "Objectors to Electric Shock Treatment Are Refractory to Its Therapy," *New York State Journal of Medicine* 46 (1946): 407–410.

26. Ugo Cerletti, untitled MS (1956), first page of which begins "Prefazione," 54, Cerletti Papers, box 118-433. "Paura postuma": "Che il paziente non sa assolutamente motivare ma che lo turba talora a tal punto che egli si rifiuta di continuare la cura."

27. Veterans Administration Center, Neuropsychiatric Hospital, Los Angeles, California, "Procedure for Electro Convulsive Treatment," March 1956, 5.

28. Sidney Malitz, interview by David Healy, Edward Shorter, and Max Fink, New York, October 5, 2004.

29. Mme. M—— to Cerletti, March 4, 1948, Cerletti Papers, box 118-433.

30. Fred Frankel, interview by David Healy, Boston, October 3, 2004.

31. C.P.L. Freeman and R. E. Kendell, "ECT: I. Patients' Experiences and Attitudes," *British Journal of Psychiatry* 137 (1980): 8–16, quote on 12. Most of the patients received bilateral ECT. Further technical details of the treatments are not known, although the authors said that an anesthetist was involved. A majority of the interviews were in 1976 but not all. A similar survey of ECT patients in South Carolina in 1998 asked the "dentist question," and a majority of ECT-treated patients said they feared the dentist more. Hilary J. Bernstein et al. "Patient Attitudes about ECT after Treatment," *Psychiatric Annals* 28 (1998): 524–527.

32. *Supreme Court of New Jersey, in the Matter of H. Albert Hyett,* 61 N.J. 518, 296 A.2d 306 (1972), LexisNexis Academic, LEXIS 202, 9.

33. Ladislaus von Meduna, *Die Konvulsionstherapie der Schizophrenie* (Halle, Germany: Marhold, 1937), 119–120.

34. Meduna to Gerty, March 14, 1947, Meduna Papers.

35. Hugo [*sic*] Cerletti, "Bemerkungen über den Elektroschock," *Wiener Medizinische Wochenschrift* 90 (December 28, 1940): 1000–1002, quote on 1002. In "Prefazione" (see note 26 in this chapter) Cerletti said that ECT-induced memory loss and disorientation were "tutti transitori." Cerletti Papers, box 118-433.

36. Jean Delay, "Les amnésies expérimentales après électro-choc," *Revue Neurologique* 75 (1943): 20–22, quote on 22.

37. Eugene Ziskind, Robert Loken, and J. A. Gengerelli, "Effect of Metrazol on Recent Learning," *Proceedings of the Society for Experimental Biology and Medicine* 43 (1940): 64–65, quote on 65.

38. Eugene Ziskind, "Memory Defects during Metrazol Therapy," *AMA Archives of Neurology and Psychiatry* 45 (1941): 223–234, quotes on 224, 234.

39. G[iovanni] Flescher, "L'amnesia retrograda dopo l'elettroshock," *Schweizer Archiv für Neurologie und Psychiatrie* 48 (1941): 1–28, quote on 13.

40. Bernard L. Pacella, "Sequelae and Complications of Convulsive Shock Therapy," *Bulletin of the New York Academy of Medicine* 20 (1944): 575–587, quote on 584.

41. P[aul] Delmas-Marsalet, *Électro-choc et thérapeutiques nouvelles en neuropsychiatrie* (Paris: Baillière, 1946), 34.

42. A[dolf?] Bingel, "Über die psychischen und chirurgischen Komplikationen des Elektrokrampfes," *Allgemeine Zeitschrift für Psychiatrie* 115 (1940): 325–343, quotes on 330, 331.

43. Lothar B. Kalinowsky, "Organic Psychotic Syndromes Occurring during Electric Convulsive Therapy," *AMA Archives of Neurology and Psychiatry* 53 (1945): 269–273, quotes on 269.

44. The essential point of Michael Taylor and Max Fink, *Melancholia: The Diagnosis, Pathophysiology, and Treatment of Depressive Illness* (New York: Cambridge University Press, 2006), is to separate within the syndromes of "major depression" those that are melancholic from those that are not, the former being responsive to tricyclic antidepressants and ECT.

45. Erwin Stengel, in discussion, Henri Ey, ed., *Premier congrès mondial de psychiatrie, Paris 1950,* vol. 4, *Thérapeutique biologique* (Paris: Hermann, 1952), 55.

46. Lothar B. Kalinowsky, "Present Status of Electric Shock Therapy," *Bulletin of the New York Academy of Medicine* 25 (1949): 541–553, quote on 552.

47. Lothar B. Kalinowsky, "Problems in Research on Electroconvulsive Therapy," *Behavioral and Brain Sciences* 7 (1984): 28–29, quote on 28.

48. Robert Levine, interview by Edward Shorter, New York, April 8, 2004.

49. For an overview, see Leo Alexander, *Treatment of Mental Disorder* (Philadelphia: Saunders, 1953), 83–94.

50. Max Fink, *Convulsive Therapy: Theory and Practice* (New York: Raven Press, 1979), 108.

51. Lothar Kalinowsky, S. Eugene Barrera, and William A. Horwitz, "The 'Petit Mal' Response in Electric Shock Therapy," *AJP* 98 (1942): 708–711, quote on 711. The paper was first given at a meeting of the American Psychiatric Association in 1941.

52. Lucio Bini, "La tecnica e le manifestazioni dell'elettroshock," *Rivista Sperimentale di Freniatria* 64 (1940): 361–458. Bini, in table 1 (374), gives somewhat higher milliamperes.

53. Emerick Friedman and Paul H. Wilcox, "Electrostimulated Convulsive Doses in Intact Humans by Means of Unidirectional Currents," *Journal of Nervous and Mental Disease* 96 (1942): 56–63.

54. Ibid., 57.

55. Emerick Friedman, "Unidirectional Electrostimulated Convulsive Therapy," *AJP* 99 (1942): 218–223, quote on 223.

56. Paul Delmas-Marsalet, "L'électro-choc par courant continu," *Annales Médico-Psychologiques* 100 (1942): 70–74.

57. Kalinowsky, "Present Status of Electric Shock Therapy," information on 542–543, quote on 544.

58. David J. Impastato, "The Use of Barbiturates in Electroshock Therapy," *Confinia Neurologica* 4 (1954): 269–275, quote on 271.

59. Joseph Epstein and Louis Wender, "Alternating Current vs. Unidirectional Current for Electroconvulsive Therapy—Comparative Studies," *Confinia Neurologica* 16 (1956): 137–146, quotes on 142, 144.

60. W[ladimir] T. Liberson, "New Possibilities in Electric Convulsive Therapy: 'Brief Stimuli' Technique," *Institute of Living, Abstracts and Translations* 12 (1944): 368–369. Liberson's lengthier report, from which the above technical details are drawn, was "Time Factors in Electric Convulsive Therapy," *Yale Journal of Biology and Medicine* 17 (1945): 571–578. The quotation, however, is from the 1944 article (368).

61. See Franklin Offner, "Stimulation with Minimum Power," *Journal of Neurophysiology* 9 (1946): 387–390.

62. W[ladimir] T. Liberson, "Brief Stimulus Therapy," *AJP* 105 (1948): 28–39. The paper had been delivered to the American Psychiatric Association a year previously. For a wrap-up on different wave forms, see Liberson, "Current Evaluation of Electric Convulsive Therapy: Correlation of the Parameters of Electric Current with Physiologic and Psychologic Changes," in Association for Research in Nervous and Mental Disease, *Psychiatric Treatment: Proceedings, December 14–15, 1951* (Baltimore: Williams and Wilkins, 1953), 199–231.

63. Douglas Goldman, "Brief Stimulus Electric Shock Therapy," *Journal of Nervous and Mental Disease* 110 (1949): 36–45, quote on 39.

64. Ibid.

65. See, for example, Jean Delay et al., "Appareillage pour l'électrochoc par stimuli brefs rectangulaires," in Ey, *Premier congrès mondial, Paris 1950*, 4:157–159.

66. Jan-Otto Ottosson, *Experimental Studies of the Mode of Action of Electroconvulsive Therapy* (Copenhagen: Munksgaard, 1960; *Acta Psychiatrica et Neurologica Scandinavica,* supplement 1945), 136.

67. See Arthur Gabriel, "The Renaissance of ECT," *American Psychiatric Association, Area II Council, Bulletin* 33 (5) (March–April 1991): 3–5.

68. Bernard L. Pacella and David J. Impastato, "Focal Stimulation Therapy," *American Journal of Psychiatry* 110 (1954): 576–578.

69. Neville Peel Lancaster, Reuben Ralph Steinert, and Isaac Frost, "Unilateral Electro-Convulsive Therapy," *Journal of Mental Science* 104 (1958): 221–227.

70. S[tanley] M. Cannicott, "Unilateral Electro-Convulsive Therapy," *Postgraduate Medical Journal* 38 (1962): 451–459.

71. David J. Impastato and William Karliner, "Control of Memory Impairment in EST by Unilateral Stimulation of the Non-dominant Hemisphere," *Diseases of the Nervous System* 27 (1966): 183–188, quotes on 187–188.

72. Kalinowsky, "Problems in Research on Electroconvulsive Therapy," 29.

73. William Karliner, "Present Status of Unilateral Shock Treatments," *Behavioral Neuropsychiatry* 4 (1972–73): 2–5, 12, quote on 3.

74. William Karliner, interview by Edward Shorter, New York, April 6, 2004.

75. John C. Krantz Jr. et al., "A New Pharmaco-convulsive Agent," *Science* 126 (August 23, 1957): 353–354, quote on 354.

76. John C. Krantz Jr. et al., "Hexafluordiethyl Ether (Indoklon)—an Inhalant Convulsant: Its Use in Psychiatric Treatment," *JAMA* 166 (March 29, 1958): 1555–1562.

77. State of New York. *Twenty-ninth Annual Report of the Director of the New York State Psychiatric Institute to the Department of Mental Hygiene for the Fiscal Year Ended March 31, 1958* (Utica: State Hospitals Press, [1958]), 10. *Annual Report, 1959,* 5.

78. William Karliner and Louis J. Padula, "The Use of Hexafluorodiethyl Ether in Psychiatric Treatment," *Journal of Neuropsychiatry* 38 (1960): 67–70.

79. William Karliner, interview by Edward Shorter, New York, April 6, 2004.

80. William Karliner, "Clinical Experiences with Intravenous Indoklon: A New Convulsant Drug," *Journal of Neuropsychiatry* 4 (1963): 184–189, quote on 186.

81. Ibid., 186. It was Karliner's concern for his outpatients that led him to propose maintenance ECT as a means of keeping them well. See Karliner and H. K. Wehrheim, "Maintenance Convulsive Treatments," *AJP* 121 (1965): 1113–1115. Yet Karliner was not the first to suggest maintenance ECT. See Norman P. Moore, "The Maintenance Treatment of Chronic Psychotics by Electrically Induced Convulsions," *Journal of Mental Science* 89 (1943): 257–269; Stephen Weisz and Jane N. Creel, "Maintenance Treatment in Schizophrenia," *Diseases of the Nervous System* 9 (1948): 10–14; J[ohn] J. Geoghegan and G[eorge] H. Stevenson, "Prophylactic Electroshock," *AJP* 105 (1949): 494–495.

82. "Drug Is Approved for Inhalation Use as Anti-depressant," *New York Times,* January 9, 1964, 15.

83. Max Fink et al., "Inhalant-Induced Convulsions," *Archives of General Psychiatry* 4 (1961): 259–266.

84. Joyce G. Small and Iver F. Small, "Clinical Results: Indoklon versus ECT," *Seminars in Psychiatry* 4 (1972): 13–25, quote on 23.

85. Max Fink, "Induced Seizures as Psychiatric Therapy: Ladislaus Meduna's Contributions in Modern Neuroscience," *JECT* 20 (2004): 133–136.

86. Phillip Polatin et al., "Vertebral Fractures Produced by Metrazol-Induced Convulsions," *JAMA* 112 (April 29, 1939): 1684–1687.

87. Cerletti, "Bemerkungen über den Elektroschock," 1002.

88. Renato Almansi and David J. Impastato, "Electrically Induced Convulsions

in the Treatment of Mental Diseases," *New York State Journal of Medicine* 40 (1940): 1315–1316, quote on 1316.

89. Donald Blair, in discussion, "Reports of Societies: Electrically Induced Convulsions," *British Medical Journal* 1 (January 20, 1940): 104–105, quote on 105.

90. Bingel, "Über die psychischen und chirurgischen Komplikationen des Elektrokrampfes," 342.

91. L[auren] H. Smith, J[oseph] Hughes, and D[onald] W. Hastings, "Electroshock Treatment in the Psychoses," *AJP* 98 (1942): 558–561.

92. Eric Samuel, "Some Complications Arising during Electrical Convulsive Therapy," *Journal of Mental Science* 89 (1943): 81–84.

93. Kalinowsky to Bini, August 13, 1940, Bini Papers, box 1.

94. Lothar B. Kalinowsky, "The Various Forms of Shock Therapy in Mental Disorders and Their Practical Importance," *New York State Journal of Medicine* 41 (1941): 2210–2215, quote on 2211.

95. State of New York, *Nineteenth Annual Report of the Director of the New York State Psychiatric Institute to the Department of Mental Hygiene for the Fiscal Year Ended March 31, 1948* (Utica: State Hospitals Press, [1948]), 13.

96. Victor E. Gonda, "Treatment of Mental Disorders with Electrically Induced Convulsions," *Diseases of the Nervous System* 2 (1941): 84–92, quote on 86.

97. Harry J. Worthing and Lothar B. Kalinowsky, "The Question of Vertebral Fractures in Convulsive Therapy and in Epilepsy," *AJP* 98 (1942): 533–537, quote on 534.

98. The Committee on Therapy of the American Psychiatric Association expressed dubiety in 1953 about hyperextension in its "Standards for Electroshock Treatment: Practice Guideline," a document retired in 1959 (American Psychiatric Association Archives). It did not mention Kalinowsky's evidence, and it is unclear what other data the members had at their disposal.

99. Frank Ayd interview, in David Healy, ed., *The Psychopharmacologists,* vol. 1 (London: Chapman and Hall, 1996), 81–110, quote on 95.

100. Nathan Savitsky and William Karliner, "Electroshock Therapy for Depression: Report of 200 Cases," *Medical Clinics of North America* 33 (1949): 515–526; see esp. 523.

101. Harold A. Palmer, "Vertebral Fractures Complicating Convulsion Therapy," *Lancet* 2 (July 22, 1939): 181–182.

102. W. R. Hamsa, and A[bram] E. Bennett, "Traumatic Complications of Convulsive Shock Therapy: A Method of Preventing Fractures of the Spine and Lower Extremities," *JAMA* 112 (June 3, 1939): 2244–2246.

103. Louis S. Goodman and Alfred Gilman, *The Pharmacological Basis of Therapeutics,* 2nd ed. (New York: Macmillan, 1955), 607.

104. A[bram] E. Bennett, "Preventing Traumatic Complications in Convulsive Shock Therapy by Curare," *JAMA* 114 (January 27, 1940): 322–324, quote on 323. For Bennett's further report, see "Curare: A Preventive of Traumatic Complications in Convulsive Shock Therapy," *AJP* 97 (1941): 1040–1060. Both papers concerned Metrazol.

105. Byron Stewart, "Electro-Shock Therapy," *Bulletin of the Los Angeles Neurological Society* 7 (2) (June 1942): 88–94, quote on 89.

106. Snorre Wohlfahrt et al., "The Prevention of Skeletal Complications in Electroshock Therapy," in Ey, *Premier congrès mondial de psychiatrie, Paris 1950*, 4:235–239.

107. David J. Impastato and Renato J. Almansi, "A Study of over Two Thousand Cases of Electrofit-Treated Patients," *New York State Journal of Medicine* 43 (1943): 2057–2064, see esp. 2060.

108. Lothar B. Kalinowsky, "Present Status of Electric Shock Therapy," *Bulletin of the New York Academy of Medicine* 25 (1949): 541–553, quote on 545.

109. New York State Psychiatric Institute, *Annual Report, 1948*, 13.

110. Gabriel, "The Renaissance of ECT," 4.

111. D[aniel] Bovet et al., "Proprietà farmacodinamiche di alcuni derivati della succinilcolina dotati di azione curarica," *Rendiconti: Istituto Superiore di Sanità* 12 (1949): 106–137.

112. G[unnar] Holmberg and S[tephen] Thesleff, "Succinyl-Choline-Iodide as a Muscular Relaxant in Electroshock Therapy," *AJP* 108 (1952): 842–846, quotes on 843. Among the earliest investigators to propose the use of oxygen in ECT was Anne Holovachka (at St. Luke's Hospital in Chicago), "Oxygen in Electro-Shock Therapy," *Journal of Nervous and Mental Disease* 98 (1943): 485–487.

113. See D. J. Addersley and Max Hamilton, "Use of Succinylcholine in E.C.T.," *British Medical Journal* 1 (1953): 195–197.

114. It is claimed that Jean Delay was first to introduce anesthesia into ECT, evidently during World War II, and that as early as 1943 it was used in Barcelona, Spain, and in Portugal. See Ey, *Congrès mondial psychiatrie, Paris 1950*, 4:49. We have not seen this documented and welcome communications that help establish it.

115. Max Fink, interview by Edward Shorter and David Healy, Nissequogue, N.Y., October 25, 2002.

116. B[enjamin] F. Moss, C[orbett] H. Thigpen, and W[illiam] P. Robison, "Report on the Use of Succinyl Choline Dichloride (a Curare-like Drug) in Electroconvulsive Therapy," *AJP* 109 (1953): 895–898, quote on 898.

117. Max Hamilton, in discussion, in Donald M. Gallant and George M. Simpson, eds., *Depression: Behavioral, Biochemical, Diagnostic and Treatment Concepts* (New York: Spectrum Publications, 1976), 149.

118. Zigmond M. Lebensohn, "The History of Electroconvulsive Therapy in the United States and Its Place in American Psychiatry: A Personal Memoir," *Comprehensive Psychiatry* 40 (1999): 173–181, quote on 177. He was quoting an unnamed "authority," yet he obviously shared the sentiment.

119. Ugo Cerletti and Lucio Bini, "Le alterazioni istopatologiche del sistema nervoso in seguito all'E. S.," *Rivista Sperimentale di Freniatria* 64 (1940): 311–359, see esp. summary of findings, 353.

120. Phillip Polatin, Hans Strauss, and Leon L. Altman, "Transient Organic Mental Reactions during Shock Therapy of the Psychoses: A Clinical Study with Electroencephalographic and Psychological Performance Correlates," *Psychiatric Quarterly* 14 (1940): 457–465, quote on 464.

121. Ziskind, "Memory Defects during Metrazol Therapy," 232.

122. William L. Laurence, "Report Sakel Cure Aids Mentally Ill," *New York*

Times, May 20, 1942, 16. Laurence idolized Sakel, often referring to him as "the new Pasteur."

123. Ey, *Premier congrès mondial de psychiatrie, Paris, 1950,* 4:37.

124. B[ernard] L. Pacella, S. E[ugene] Barrera, and L[othar] Kalinowsky, "Variations in Electroencephalogram Associated with Electric Shock Therapy of Patients with Mental Disorders," *AMA Archives of Neurology and Psychiatry* 47 (1942): 367–384, quote on 384. For similar findings in another EEG study, see Norman A. Levy, H. M. Serota, and Roy R. Grinker, "Disturbances in Brain Function Following Convulsive Shock Therapy," *AMA Archives of Neurology and Psychiatry* 47 (1942): 1009–1029: "Recovery from these disturbances of cerebral function occurred in most patients in a few weeks. In the more severely affected patients evidences of impaired cerebral function sometimes lasted as long as six months" (1027). In other words, none of the twenty-three patients studied experienced cerebral changes of a duration greater than six months. Nevertheless, psychoanalyst Roy R. Grinker of Chicago, one of the coauthors, delivered in the discussion a blast against shock therapy: "This mechanistic approach to psychiatry is being used extensively at present; I think it can be stated unequivocally that it is fraught with extreme danger. . . . Those who have seen fighters that have been in many battles know the 'punch-drunk' or 'slap-happy' conditions and may recognize a similar state in some patients after shock therapy" (1028).

125. S. Eugene Barrera et al., "Brain Changes Associated with Electrically Induced Seizures: A Study in the Macacus Rhesus," *American Neurological Association Transactions* 68 (1942): 31–45.

126. N. W[illiam] Winkelman and Matthew T. Moore, "Neurohistologic Findings in Experimental Electric Shock Treatment," *Journal of Neuropathology and Experimental Neurology* 3 (1944): 199–209.

127. Eugene Ziskind, Esther Somerfeld-Ziskind, and Louis Ziskind, "Metrazol and Electric Convulsive Therapy of the Affective Psychoses," *AMA Archives of Neurology and Psychiatry* 53 (1945): 212–217, quote on 216.

128. Richard D. Weiner, "Does Electroconvulsive Therapy Cause Brain Damage?" *Behavioral and Brain Sciences* 7 (1984): 1–22.

129. Joyce G. Small and Iver F. Small, "Current Issues in ECT Practice and Research," *Behavioral and Brain Sciences* 7 (1984): 33–34, quote on 34.

130. Steven F. Zornetzer, "Out of the Shadows and into the Light," *Behavioral and Brain Sciences* 7 (1984): 41. Italics in original in this and following quotes.

131. Larry Squire and Pamela C. Slater, "Electroconvulsive Therapy and Complaints of Memory Dysfunction: A Prospective Three-Year Follow-up Study," *British Journal of Psychiatry* 142 (1983): 1–8.

132. Max Fink, "ECT—Verdict: Not Guilty," *Behavioral and Brain Sciences* 7 (1984): 26–27, quote on 26.

133. Weiner, "Does Electroconvulsive Therapy Cause Brain Damage?" 42.

134. C. Edward Coffey et al., "Brain Anatomic Effects of Electroconvulsive Therapy: A Prospective Magnetic Resonance Imaging Study," *Archives of General Psychiatry* 48 (1991): 1013–1021.

135. Andrew J. Dwork et al., "Absence of Histological Lesions in Primate Models of ECT and Magnetic Seizure Therapy," *AJP* 161 (2004): 576–578, quotes on 578.

136. *Gary C. Aden et al. v. Evelle J. Younger,* 57 Cal. App. 3d 662, 129 Cal. Rptr. 535 (1976), LexisNexis Academic, LEXIS 1482, footnote 5.

137. Oscar Forel, *La mémoire du chêne* (Paris: Favre, 1980), 111–112.

138. Hans Löwenbach and Edward J. Stainbrook, "Observations of Mental Patients after Electro-Shock," *AJP* 98 (1942): 828–833, quote on 833.

139. Edward A. Tyler and Hans Löwenbach, "Polydiurnal Electric Shock Treatment in Mental Disorders," *North Carolina Medical Journal* 8 (1947): 577–582.

140. Giorgio Sogliani, "Elettroshockterapia e Cardiazolterapia," *Rassegna di Studi Psichiatrici* 28 (1939): 652–661, quote on 657.

141. Giorgio Sogliani, "Eine neue Methode der Krampftherapie: Die Elektroshocktherapie," *Deutsche Zeitschrift für Nervenheilkunde* 149 (1939): 159–168, see esp. 163–164. For this German audience he stated that he administered treatments "every second day."

142. L[ucio] Bini and T. Bazzi, "L'elettroshockterapia col metodo dell'annichilimento nelle forme gravi di psiconevrosi," *Rassegna di Neuropsichiatria e Scienze Affini* 1 (1947): 59–70. The table on 63–65 shows they were administering about one treatment a day.

143. Lauretta Bender, "One Hundred Cases of Childhood Schizophrenia Treated with Electric Shock," *American Neurological Association, Transactions* 72 (1947): 165–169.

144. W. Liddell Milligan, "Psychoneuroses Treated with Electrical Convulsions: The Intensive Method," *Lancet* 2 (October 12, 1946): 516–520, quote on 516.

145. In 1943, Abraham Myerson provided a rationale for it, though he did not in fact treat his patients intensively. In describing the remedy for "anhedonic unreality syndrome," a "borderline mental state," he said: "The mechanism of improvement and recovery seems to be to knock out the brain and reduce the higher activities, to impair the memory, and thus the newer acquisition of the mind, namely, the pathological state, is forgotten." Myerson, "Borderline Cases Treated by Shock," *AJP* 100 (1943): 355–357, quote on 357.

146. New York State Psychiatric Institute, *Annual Report,* 1947, said it had tried twenty treatments in two weeks on one schizophrenic patient, with disappointing results (18); the *Annual Report* for 1949 reported failure in two female patients diagnosed with "tension" (12).

147. New York State Psychiatric Institute, *Annual Report,* 1949, 12.

148. New York State Psychiatric Institute, *Annual Report,* 1955, 34.

149. Cyril J. C. Kennedy and David Anchel, "Regressive Electric-Shock in Schizophrenics Refractory to Other Shock Therapies," *Psychiatric Quarterly* 22 (1948): 317–320, quote on 317.

150. Ephraim S. Garrett and Charles W. Mockbee, "New Hope for Far Advanced Schizophrenia: Intensive Regressive Electroconvulsive Therapy in Treatment of Severely Regressed Schizophrenics," *Ohio State Medical Journal* 48 (1952): 505–509, quotes on 508.

151. John E. Exner and Luis G. Murillo, "A Long-Term Follow-up of Schizophrenics Treated with Regressive ECT," *Diseases of the Nervous System* 38 (1977): 162–168, quote on 167. Their original report, Murillo and Exner, "The Effects of Regressive ECT with Process Schizophrenics," appeared in *AJP* 130 (1973): 269–273.

152. D. Ewen Cameron, J. G. Lohrenz, and K. A. Handcock, "The Depatterning Treatment of Schizophrenia," *Comprehensive Psychiatry* 3 (1962): 65–76. Much has been made of Cameron's involvement, along with Harold A. Abramson, Robert W. Hyde, Carl Pfeiffer, and Louis Jolyon West (all of whom studied LSD), in the CIA's "Project Bluebird" (later called "Project Artichoke"). See "Private Institutions Used in C.I.A. Effort to Control Behavior," *New York Times*, August 2, 1977, 61. Yet Cameron would doubtless have done the same research without CIA contact of any kind.

153. Gerald Garmany and Donald F. Early, "Electronarcosis" (letter), *Lancet* 1 (1948): 614.

154. Paul H. Blachly and David Gowing, "Multiple Monitored Electroconvulsive Treatment," *Comprehensive Psychiatry* 7 (1966): 100–109.

155. Richard Abrams and Max Fink, "Clinical Experiences with Multiple Electroconvulsive Treatments," *Comprehensive Psychiatry* 13 (1972): 115–121.

156. Max Fink, interview by Edward Shorter and David Healy, Nissequogue, N.Y., October 25, 2002.

157. Max Fink, personal communication to Edward Shorter, 2005.

158. Almansi and Impastato, "Electrically Induced Convulsions in the Treatment of Mental Diseases."

159. Hans Strauss and Walter E. Rahm Jr., "The Effect of Metrazol Injections on the Electroencephalogram," *Psychiatric Quarterly* (January 1940): 43–48. Rahm was a technician at the New York State Psychiatric Institute who built an ECT device and founded his own company.

160. W[olfgang] Holzer and K[urt] Polzer, "Elektroschock und Elektrokardiogramm," *Archiv für Kreislaufforschung* 8 (1941): 382–396 (Holzer was a psychiatrist, Polzer a cardiologist; the authors are better known for their work on rheography in cardiology); Jean Delay et al., "Électro-encéphalogramme et électro-choc," paper at the Société de Biologie, May 13, 1944, reported in Paul Delmas-Marsalet, *Électro-choc et thérapeutiques nouvelles en neuro-psychiatrie* (Paris: Baillière, 1946), 146–147, 358.

CHAPTER SEVEN. "They're Going to Fry Your Brains!"

1. Michele Greenwald, unpublished account, "A Winter of Despair." All subsequent details about this case are from this source, unless otherwise indicated. We are grateful to Dr. Greenwald, a senior medical student at Albert Einstein College of Medicine at the time she wrote it, for sharing this report with us. We have suppressed the name of the patient in question and have suppressed some personal details to protect his privacy.

2. Tom Bolwig, personal communication to Edward Shorter, January 11, 2006.

3. "Two Health Plans Augment Benefits," *New York Times*, November 19, 1959, 1.

4. Victor Bockris, *Transformer: The Lou Reed Story* (New York: Da Capo, 1995).

5. Haroutun M. Babigian and Laurence B. Guttmacher, "Epidemiologic Considerations in Electroconvulsive Therapy," *Archives of General Psychiatry* 41 (1984): 246–253; see table 3, 248. The rate is for first receipt of ECT.

6. James L. Hedlund et al., "Electroconvulsive Therapy in Missouri State Facilities: 1971–75," *Journal of Operational Psychiatry* 9 (1978): 40–56, table 1, 43.

7. Max Fink, interview by Edward Shorter and David Healy, Nissequogue, N.Y., October 25, 2002.

8. James W. Thompson and Jack D. Blaine, "Use of ECT in the United States in 1975 and 1980," *AJP* 144 (1987): 557–562, see table 1, 558; quote on 561.

9. *International Psychiatric Association for the Advancement of Electrotherapy, Summer Newsletter,* 1985, 3.

10. *International Psychiatric Association for the Advancement of Electrotherapy, Spring–Summer Newsletter,* 1986, 6.

11. Samuel H. Bailine and John H. Rau, "The Decision to Use ECT: A Retrospective Study," *Comprehensive Psychiatry* 22 (1981): 274–281, esp. 274.

12. In a personal communication to Edward Shorter, December 18, 2004, Thomas Ban describes his own experiences at the World Health Organization in the early 1980s getting third-world psychiatrists to substitute antipsychotics for ECT: "During the two years I spent with WHO I learned that ECT was far more extensively used on the poor than on the rich (I'm not talking about the USA). I had many conversations on site with WHO regional representatives in countries like India, Thailand, etc. who complained that they use ECT extensively because they don't have enough money for drugs. In 1982 I was trying to solve this issue in India by having long acting (generic) fluphenazine manufactured locally. By using long acting generic preparations they could reduce the cost to the level that pharmacotherapy became affordable."

13. Joseph P. Morrissey et al., "Developing an Empirical Base for Psycho-Legal Policy Analyses of ECT: A New York State Survey," *International Journal of Law and Psychiatry* 2 (1979): 99–111, quote on 103.

14. S. V. Eranti and D. M. McLoughlin, "Author's Reply," *British Journal of Psychiatry* 183 (2003): 172–173.

15. Jonathan Andrews et al., *The History of Bethlem* (London: Routledge, 1997), 694.

16. Max Fink, personal communication to Edward Shorter, May 14, 2004.

17. Michael Taylor, interview by Max Fink, Ann Arbor, Mich., March 19, 2004.

18. Elissa Ely, "Shock Therapy Deserves Better . . . Treatment: Its Stark Image Belies Its Helpful Impact," *Boston Globe,* March 21, 1999, 2 (ProQuest printout).

19. Martha Manning, *Undercurrents: A Therapist's Reckoning with Her Own Depression* (San Francisco: Harper San Francisco, 1994), 165.

20. William Styron, *Darkness Visible: A Memoir of Madness* (New York: Random House, 1990), 43, 46, 50, 70. The text first appeared as an article in *Vanity Fair* in 1989. Abbott Laboratories helped distribute a reprint as a small book.

21. *Donato Delicata v. Ann Bourlesses,* 9 (Mass. Ct. App. 1980) 713, 404 N.E. 2d 667, LexisNexis Academic, LEXIS 1154.

22. "Psychiatric Care Close to Home," *New York Times,* March 31, 1985, LI18. The colleague was Michael W. Slome at nearby Stony Brook.

23. Thompson and Blaine, "Use of ECT in the United States in 1975 and 1980," 558, table 1.

24. William R. Breakey and Gary J. Dunn, "Racial Disparity in the Use of ECT for Affective Disorders," *AJP* 161 (2004): 1635–1641.

25. Mark Moran, "Culture, History Can Keep Blacks from Getting Depression Treatment," *Psychiatric News,* June 4, 2004, 12.

26. Michael Taylor, interview by Max Fink, Ann Arbor, Mich., March 19, 2004.

27. Conrad Swartz, interview by Edward Shorter, Springfield, Ill., May 11, 2004.

28. "Opposition to Shock Therapy Diverse," *Houston Chronicle,* January 26, 1997, 4 (ProQuest printout).

29. U.S. Census Bureau, "State and County QuickFacts," http://quickfacts .census.gov/qfd/states/48000.html, accessed December 15, 2004.

30. On the basis of no evidence, Roland Littlewood and Maurice Lipsedge argue that in the United Kingdom blacks are more likely to receive ECT; whites, psychotherapy. *Aliens and Alienists: Ethnic Minorities and Psychiatry* (1982), 3rd ed. (London: Routledge, 1997), 302.

31. Louis Linn, interview by Edward Shorter, New York, July 12, 2004.

32. Mary Jane Ward, *The Snake Pit* (New York: Random House, 1946); "Dr. Gerard Chrzanowski, Innovative Psychoanalyst, Dies at 87," *New York Times,* November 12, 2000, 46.

33. See the list of films in Andrew McDonald and Garry Walter, "The Portrayal of ECT in American Movies," *JECT* 17 (2001): 264–274; a partial list of films depicting ECT between 1948 and 2000 is found on 265. For several additional films, see David Griner, "Electroshock Therapy Emerges from Disrepute," *Journal Gazette* (Ft. Wayne, Ind.), April 7, 2002, 5–6 (ProQuest printout).

34. "Manic Attack," *Sunday Times* (London), October 19, 2003, 2 (ProQuest printout).

35. Elissa Ely, "Doctor Files: Despite Social Stigmas, ECT Can Play a Vital Role," *Los Angeles Times,* November 17, 2003, 1–2 (ProQuest printout).

36. Josephine Marcotty, *Star Tribune* (Minneapolis), November 17, 1999, 3 (ProQuest printout).

37. Michael Taylor, interview by Max Fink, Ann Arbor, Mich., March 19, 2004.

38. Richard Weiner, interview by Heather Dichter, Durham, N.C., January 6, 2005.

39. See A. E. Hotchner, *Papa Hemingway: A Personal Memoir* (New York: Random House, 1966), 284; for other details, see Jeffrey Meyers, *Hemingway: A Biography* (New York: Harper and Row, 1985), 538–554. Michael Reynolds lists some of Hemingway's medications before his first admission to the Mayo Clinic in *Hemingway: The Final Years* (New York: Norton, 1999), 301. Reynolds suggests that one of them, reserpine (Serpasil), might have caused his depression (350), yet the view that reserpine caused depression is probably a canard. It was more likely an antidepressant.

40. "The Hero of the Code," *Time,* July 14, 1961, 69–71. All of Hemingway's biographers, beginning with Aaron E. Hotchner, presented ECT as having destroyed Hemingway's memory. For example, in *Papa Hemingway,* Hotchner has Hemingway saying: "What is the sense of ruining my head and erasing my memory, which is my capital, and putting me out of business. It was a brilliant cure but we lost the patient" (280).

41. Meyers, *Hemingway,* 550.

42. David Healy, *Let Them Eat Prozac: The Unhealthy Relationship between the Pharmaceutical Industry and Depression* (New York: New York University Press, 2004), 80.

43. Sylvia Plath, *The Bell Jar* (1971), 25th anniversary ed. (New York: Harper-Collins, 1996), 161.

44. Edward de Grazia, review of Thomas Szasz's *Law, Liberty, and Psychiatry*, *New York Times*, January 26, 1964, BR6.

45. Millen Brand, *Savage Sleep* (New York: Crown, 1968); quote from Bantam ed., 5.

46. Thomas Lask, review of Millen Brand's *Savage Sleep*, *New York Times*, November 5, 1968, BR45.

47. Joan Didion, review of Doris Lessing's *Briefing for a Descent into Hell* (London: Cape, 1971), *New York Times*, March 14, 1971, BR1.

48. Adrienne Rich, review of Phyllis Chesler's *Women and Madness*, *New York Times*, December 31, 1972, BR1.

49. Seymour Peck, review of Gene Tierney's *Self-Portrait*, *New York Times*, April 8, 1979, BR3.

50. See, for example, William Laurence, "Psychiatrist Hits Misuse of Shocks," *New York Times*, August 21, 1953, 9.

51. Mark E. Rosenzweig, "Biologists Try to Learn Exactly How We Learn," *New York Times*, January 12, 1970, 85.

52. Elizabeth Wertz, "The Fury of Shock Treatment—A Patient's View," *Washington Post*, December 10, 1972, PO36.

53. Zigmond M. Lebensohn, letter to the editor, *Washington Post*, March 4, 1973, PO8.

54. Berton Roueché, "As Empty as Eve," *New Yorker*, September 9, 1974, 84–100. Max Fink later wrote to Roueché: "I am disappointed that the *New Yorker* . . . saw fit to publish a single case report, with many errors of fact in discussion—thereby doing a disservice to the many patients who will undoubtedly read or be given this article, and who will be scared out of their wits if a physician recommends this therapy. The harm that has been done will never be known by you, but the many therapists who will find it more difficult to use this therapy when it is useful will have reason to remember you, as will the families that will have lost a member by suicide." Fink to Roueché, September 24, 1974, Fink's personal archive.

55. See, for example, "Eagleton Tells of Shock Therapy on Two Occasions," *New York Times*, July 26, 1972, 1.

56. "Eagleton Is Firm despite Pressure by 2 Party Chiefs," *New York Times*, July 31, 1972, 1.

57. "States' Rights vs. Victims' Rights," *New York Times*, May 8, 1977, 146.

58. Material on the lawsuit and a partial transcript of the show are on file in the archives of the Jimmy Carter Library and Museum in Atlanta, Peter Bourne Papers, box 13, O/A 6042.

59. Dwayne DeLong affidavit of October 18, 1977, Bourne Papers (see n. 58).

60. Robert H. Hicks Jr. affidavit of October 13, 1977.

61. Leonard Cammer to "William" Lewis, November 18, 1976, Bourne Papers (see n. 58).

62. Richard D. Weiner, "ECT: Facts, Affects, and Ambiguities," *Behavioral and Brain Sciences* 7 (1984): 42–47, quote on 46.

63. All quotes relating to this case are from Anthony D'Agostino, "Depression: Schism in Contemporary Psychiatry," *AJP* 132 (1975): 629–632.

64. Spencer Paterson, discussion, in E. Beresford Davies, ed., *Depression: Proceedings of the Symposium Held at Cambridge 22 to 26 September 1959* (Cambridge: Cambridge University Press, 1964), 354.

65. Max Fink, "Die Geschichte der EKT in den Vereinigten Staaten in den letzten Jahrzehnten," *Nervenarzt* 64 (1993): 689–695, see esp. 690.

66. Quoted in Jack E. Rosenblatt, "Interview with Max Fink, M.D.," *Currents in Affective Illness* 13 (1994): 5–14, quote on 10 (interview in December 1993). See also Fink and Richard Abrams, "Qualification for ECT," *Convulsive Therapy* 8 (1992): 1–4.

67. Zigmond M. Lebensohn, "The History of Electroconvulsive Therapy in the United States and Its Place in American Psychiatry: A Personal Memoir," *Comprehensive Psychiatry* 40 (1999): quote on 174.

68. Robert O. Friedel, "The Combined Use of Neuroleptics and ECT in Drug Resistant Schizophrenic Patients," *Psychopharmacology Bulletin* 22 (1986): 928–930.

69. Max Fink, interview by Edward Shorter and David Healy, Nissequogue, N.Y., October 25, 2002.

70. Steven M. Paul et al., "Use of ECT with Treatment-Resistant Depressed Patients at the National Institute of Mental Health," *AJP* 138 (1981): 486–489, quote on 488.

71. Matthew Rudorfer, interview by Max Fink, Boca Raton, Fla., February 9, 2004.

72. Alexander Thomas, *History of Bellevue Psychiatric Hospital, 1736–1994* (New York: privately published, 1999), 120.

73. S. B. Sutton, *Crossroads in Psychiatry: A History of the McLean Hospital* (Washington, D.C.: American Psychiatric Press, 1986), 274.

74. David Healy, interview with Mandel Cohen, "Mandel Cohen and the Origins of the *Diagnostic and Statistical Manual of Mental Disorders, Third Edition: DSM–III*," *History of Psychiatry* 13 (2002): 209–230, quote on 217.

75. American Psychiatric Association, *Report of the Task Force on Electroconvulsive Therapy* (Task Force Report No. 14) (Washington, D.C.: APA, 1978), 1–6.

CHAPTER EIGHT. The End of "Bedlam" and the Age of Psychopharmacology

1. Elliot S. Valenstein, *Great and Desperate Cures: The Rise and Decline of Psychosurgery and Other Radical Treatments for Mental Illness* (New York: Basic Books, 1986), 272.

2. Nathan S. Kline, "Use of *Rauwolfia serpentina* Benth in Neuropsychiatric Conditions," *Annals of the New York Academy of Sciences* 59 (1954): 107–132.

3. Wilfred Overholser, "Foreword," in Nathan S. Kline, ed., *Psychopharmacology: A Symposium . . . December 30, 1954* (Washington, D.C.: American Association for the Advancement of Science, 1956), iii–iv, quote on iii.

4. Jean Delay, Pierre Deniker, and J. M. Harl, "Utilisation en thérapeutique psychiatrique d'une phénothiazine d'action centrale élective (4560 RP)," *Annales Médico-Psychologiques* 110 (1952): 112–117; Delay, Deniker, and Harl, "Traitement des états d'excitation et d'agitation par une méthode médicamenteuse dérivée de l'hibernothérapie," *Annales Médico-Psychologiques* 110 (1952): 267–273.

5. Jean Delay and Pierre Deniker, "Neuroleptic Effects of Chlorpromazine in Therapeutics of Neuropsychiatry," *International Record of Medicine* 168 (1955): 318–326, quote on 320.

6. Jean Thuillier, "Ten Years That Changed Psychiatry," in David Healy, ed., *The Psychopharmacologists,* vol. 3 (London: Arnold, 2000), 543–559, quotes on 551, 553.

7. Collective: Comité Lyonnais de Recherches Thérapeutiques en Psychiatrie, "The Birth of Psychopharmacotherapy," in Healy, *Psychopharmacologists,* 3:1–52, quotes on 10–11.

8. Jean Delay, Pierre Deniker, and R. Ropert, "Étude de 300 dossiers de malades psychotiques traités par la chlorpromazine en service fermé depuis 1952," in Jean Delay, ed., *Colloque international sur la chlorpromazine, Paris, 20, 21, 22 octobre 1955* (Paris: Doin, 1956; special ed. of papers appearing in *L'Encéphale*), 228–235, see esp. 229.

9. J. D. Aulnay and R. Malineau, "Depuis l'avénement de la chlorpromazine la cure de Sakel est-elle condamnée?" in Delay, *Colloque international,* 356–360.

10. Delay, "Introduction au colloque international," in *Colloque international,* 3–12, quote on 4.

11. Raymond Battegay, "Forty-four Years of Psychiatry and Psychopharmacology," in Healy, *Psychopharmacologists,* 3:371–394, quote on 372.

12. J[oel] Elkes and Charmian Elkes, "Effect of Chlorpromazine on the Behaviour of Chronically Overactive Psychotic Patients," *British Medical Journal* 2 (September 4, 1954): 560–565.

13. W[illy] Mayer-Gross, "A Survey of the Pharmacological Possibilities in Psychiatry," in Delay, *Colloque international,* 7–12.

14. Max Fink, "Neglected Disciplines in Human Psychopharmacology," in Healy, *Psychopharmacologists,* 3:431–457, quote on 434.

15. N[athaniel] William Winkelman, "Chlorpromazine in the Treatment of Neuropsychiatric Disorders," *JAMA* 155 (May 1, 1954): 18–21, quote on 21.

16. H[einz] E. Lehmann and G[orman] E. Hanrahan, "Chlorpromazine: A New Inhibiting Agent for Psychomotor Excitement and Manic States," *A.M.A. Archives of Neurology and Psychiatry* 71 (1954): 227–237; quotes on 235. See also Willis H. Bower, "Chlorpromazine in Psychiatric Illness," *New England Journal of Medicine* 251 (October 21, 1954): 689–692, who started trials at McLean Hospital in September 1953, and who published after Lehmann and Hanrahan.

17. Donald Klein, "Reaction Patterns to Psychotropic Drugs and the Discovery of Panic Disorder," in David Healy, *The Psychopharmacologists,* vol. 1 (London: Chapman and Hall, 1996), 329–352, quote on 345–346.

18. Charles D. Yohe, discussion comment, in Smith Kline and French Laboratories, ed., *Chlorpromazine and Mental Health: Proceedings of the Symposium* (Philadelphia: Lea and Febiger, 1955), 96.

19. Leo Hollister, "From Hypertension to Psychopharmacology: A Serendipitous Career," in Healy, *Psychopharmacologists,* 2:215-236, quote on 221.

20. Max Fink et al., "Comparative Study of Chlorpromazine and Insulin Coma in Therapy of Psychosis," *JAMA* 166 (April 12, 1958): 1846–1850.

21. Fritz Freyhan, "The Immediate and Long Range Effects of Chlorpromazine on the Mental Hospital," in Smith Kline and French, *Chlorpromazine and Mental Health,* 71–84, see esp. 83. The reference was to "maintenance ECT."

22. Frank Ayd, testimony, U.S. Congress, Senate, Select Committee on Small Business, Subcommittee on Monopoly, December 11, 17, 18, 19, 1968, and January 23, 1969, *Hearings . . . on Present Status of Competition in the Pharmaceutical Industry* (Washington, D.C.: GPO, 1969), part 10, 4163. He did specify that insulin and electroshock were unhelpful to those "continuously ill for more than 2 years," but he did not point out insulin's track record of success in treating recently ill schizophrenics.

23. Philip R. A. May, "Anti-psychotic Drugs and Other Forms of Therapy," in Daniel H. Efron, ed., *Psychopharmacology: A Review of Progress, 1957–1967,* Public Health Service pub. no. 1836 (Washington, D.C.: GPO, 1968), 1155–1176, quotes on 1156–1157.

24. See Thomas Ban, *Psychopharmacology* (Baltimore: Williams and Wilkins, 1969), 439, table 1.

25. Max Fink, personal communication to Edward Shorter, December 10, 2004.

26. Max Fink interview, "Neglected Disciplines in Human Psychopharmacology: Pharmaco-EEG and Electroshock," in Healy, *Psychopharmacologists,* 3:431–457, quote on 453.

27. Max Fink and Jan-Otto Ottosson, "A Theory of Convulsive Therapy in Endogenous Depression: Significance of Hypothalamic Functions," *Psychiatric Research* 2 (1980): 49–61.

28. Félix Martí-Ibáñez et al., "The Challenge of Bio- and Chemotherapy in Psychiatry," *Journal of Clinical and Experimental Psychopathology* 17 (1956): 15–18, quote on 15. (The quote from Paracelsus also appears in Martí-Ibáñez's article.)

29. Alex A. Cardoni, "Fifty Years of Psychopharmacology: Interview with Benjamin Wiesel, M.D.," *Connecticut Medicine* 55 (1991): 409–411, quote on 410.

30. P[er] Bech, "A Review of the Antidepressant Properties of Serotonin Reuptake Inhibitors," *Advances in Biological Psychiatry* 17 (1988): 58–60, see fig. 1:60.

31. Kurt Schneider, "Die Schichtung des emotionalen Lebens und der Aufbau der Depressionszustände," *Zeitschrift für die gesamte Neurologie und Psychiatrie* 59 (1920): 281–286.

32. Quoted in Thomas A. Ban et al., eds., *From Psychopharmacology to Neuropsychopharmacology in the 1980s* (Budapest: Animula, 2002), 334–335. Kuhn's first report was "Über die Behandlung depressiver Zustände mit einem Iminodibenzylderivat (G 22355)," *Schweizer Medizinische Wochenschrift* 87 (August 31, 1957): 1135–1140.

33. Tofranil advertisement, *Journal of Neuropsychiatry* 1 (April 1960): n.p.

34. Nathan S. Kline, "Clinical Experience with Iproniazid (Marsilid)," *Journal of Clinical and Experimental Psychopathology* 19, suppl. 1 (1958): 72–79.

35. Benjamin Pollack, "Clinical Findings in the Use of Tofranil in Depressive and Other Psychiatric States," *AJP* 116 (1959): 312–317, quote on 312.

36. Bernard B. Brodie, "Some Ideas on the Mode of Action of Imipramine-Type Antidepressants," in John Marks and C.M.B. Pare, eds., *The Scientific Basis of Drug Therapy in Psychiatry: A Symposium at St. Bartholomew's Hospital, London, 7th and 8th September, 1964* (Oxford: Pergamon, 1965), 127–146, quote on 128–129.

37. D. H. Clark, in discussion, in E. Beresford Davies, ed., *Depression: Proceedings of the Symposium Held at Cambridge 22 to 26 September 1959* (Cambridge: Cambridge University Press, 1964), quote on 80.

38. "New Mood Drug Appraised Here," *New York Times*, June 19, 1959, 11.

39. Fritz A. Freyhan, "Zur modernen psychiatrischen Behandlung der Depressionen," *Nervenarzt* 31 (1960): 112–118.

40. J. R[ichard] Wittenborn et al., "A Comparison of Imipramine, Electroconvulsive Therapy and Placebo in the Treatment of Depressions," *Journal of Nervous and Mental Disease* 135 (1962): 131–137.

41. Linford Rees and S. Benaim, "An Evaluation of Iproniazid (Marsilid) in the Treatment of Depression," *Journal of Mental Science* 106 (1960): 193–202, quote on 200.

42. A. Leitch and C. P. Seager, "A Trial of Four Anti-depressant Drugs," *Psychopharmacologica* 4 (1963): 72–77, quote on 76.

43. Henry Wechsler, George H. Grosser, and Milton Greenblatt, "Research Evaluating Antidepressant Medications on Hospitalized Mental Patients: A Survey of Published Reports during a Five-Year Period," *Journal of Nervous and Mental Disease* 141 (1965): 231–239, quote on 236.

44. Thomas Ban, *Depression and the Tricyclic Antidepressants* (Montreal: Ronalds, 1974), quote on 30.

45. Jonathan O. Cole, "The Future of Psychopharmacology," in Ronald R. Fieve, ed., *Depression in the 1970's: Modern Theory and Research* (Amsterdam: Excerpta Medica, 1971), 81–86, quotes on 82–83. On the subject of antidepressants possibly increasing suicidcal behavior, at a conference in Cambridge in 1959, E. S. Kristiansen, a psychiatrist in Lyngby, Denmark, offered that "during the [imipramine] treatment I have seen now and then delirious periods of three to four days' duration, where patients complain of dreams of aggressive content. . . . This state is accompanied by great anxiety, and sometimes also by suicidal impulses. The symptoms disappear when imipramine is withdrawn or dosage reduced. . . ." See discussion in Davies, ed., *Depression: Proceedings,* 82. Sir Martin Roth noted at a conference in 1973: "Among the disadvantages of the widespread use of antidepressive substances has been the increasing prevalence of suicidal attempts with these compounds." See discussion in Jules Angst, ed., *Classification and Prediction of Outcome in Depression* (New York: Schattauer, 1974), 199. In 1980, investigators found lower-than-expected suicidal behavior among patients on imipramine, higher than expected on dothiepin. See R. G. Priest et al., "Suicide, Attempted Suicide and Antidepressant Drugs," *Journal of International Medical Research* 8, suppl. 3 (1980): 8–13: "The results of this investigation sugggest that there are observable differences between antidepressants in the extent to which they are associated with suicidal behavior" (12).

46. F[elix] Labhardt, "Technik, Nebenerscheinungen und Komplikationen der Largactiltherapie," *Schweizer Archiv für Neurologie und Psychiatrie* 73 (1954): 338–345, quote on 341.

47. R[ichard] Avenarius, discussion, ibid., 353–354.

48. H[ans] Steck, "Le syndrome extrapyramidal et diencéphalique au cours des traitements au largactil et au serpasil," *Annales Médico-Psychologiques* 112 (1954): 737–744; H[ans]-J[oachim] Haase, "Über Vorkommen und Deutung des psychomotorischen Parkinsonsnydroms bei Megaphen-bzw: Largactil-Dauerbehandlung," *Nervenarzt* 25 (1954): 486–492.

49. George W. Brooks, in discussion, in Smith Kline and French, *Chlorpromazine and Mental Health*, 51.

50. Vernon Kinross-Wright, "Clinical Application of Chlorpromazine," in Nathan S. Kline, ed., *Psychopharmacology: A Symposium Organized by the Section on Medical Sciences of the A.A.A.S. . . . Presented at the Berkeley Meeting December 30, 1954* (Washington, D.C.: American Association for the Advancement of Science, 1956), 31–38, quote on 33.

51. [Herman C. B.] Denber, in discussion, in Kline, *Psychopharmacology*, 75. Denber had been born in Europe, trained in Switzerland and the United States, and was at the time on staff at Manhattan State Hospital in New York.

52. J[ean] Sigwald, D. Bouttier, and P. Nicolas-Charles, "'Ambulatory' Treatment with Chlorpromazine," *Journal of Clinical and Experimental Psychopathology* 17 (1956): 57–69, see esp. 62.

53. "Psychiatrist Hails Drug Therapy," interview with Frank Ayd Jr., *JAMA* 210 (October 6, 1969): 24.

54. Mark Olfson et al., "Predicting Medication Noncompliance after Hospital Discharge among Patients with Schizophrenia," *Psychiatric Services* 51 (2000): 216–222.

55. J. S. McCombs et al., "Use Patterns for Antipsychotic Medications in Medicaid Patients with Schizophrenia," *Journal of Clinical Psychiatry* 60, suppl. 19 (1999): 5–11.

56. Paul Janssen interview, "From Haloperidol to Risperidone," in Healy, *Psychopharmacologists*, 2:49.

57. Ibid., 61.

58. Thorazine advertisement, *Diseases of the Nervous System* 16 (1955): 227.

59. Maurice R. Nance, director of clinical investigation at Smith Kline and French, opening remarks, in Smith Kline and French, *Chlorpromazine and Mental Health*, 11–16, quote on 14.

60. Elavil advertisement, *Mental Hospitals* 16 (1965): n.p.

61. Marplan advertisement, *Diseases of the Nervous System* 27 (1966): n.p.

62. Tofranil advertisement, *Diseases of the Nervous System* 27 (1966): n.p. It was quoting an academic study, but still, drug companies are not obliged to print in their advertisements findings that reflect well on the competition.

63. Estes Kefauver, quoted in U.S. Congress, Senate, Committee on the Judiciary, Subcommittee on Antitrust and Monopoly, 87th Cong., 1st sess., 1961, *Study of Administered Prices in the Drug Industry* (Washington, D.C.: GPO, 1961), 143.

64. See David Schwartzman, *Innovation in the Pharmaceutical Industry* (Baltimore: Johns Hopkins University Press, 1976), 124, table 6.1.

65. For more on this topic, see David Healy, *Let Them Eat Prozac: The Unhealthy Relationship between the Pharmaceutical Industry and Depression* (New York: New York University Press, 2004), passim.

66. We have not seen all the transcripts of PDAC meetings in the 1980s and after, but we have seen a good number of them. Although the subject of ECT almost never comes up for discussion, there was one significant exception, in 1990, at a meeting of the PDAC to consider sertraline (Zoloft): Paul Leber, head of the Neuropsychopharmaceutical Drugs Division of FDA, allowed that for inpatients, ECT, as opposed to drugs, would "give you your biggest bang over the shortest period of time." FDA, Psychopharmacological Drugs Advisory Committee, November 19, 1990, 64; transcript of meeting obtained through the Freedom of Information Act.

67. P[aul] H. Blachly, "New Developments in Electroconvulsive Therapy," *Diseases of the Nervous System* 37 (1976): 356–358, quote on 357.

68. Arthur Zitrin, interview by Edward Shorter, New York, July 13, 2004.

CHAPTER NINE. The Swinging Pendulum: The Effects of Politics, Law, and Changes in Medical Culture on ECT

1. David Healy, *The Creation of Psychopharmacology* (Cambridge, Mass.: Harvard University Press, 2002); Norman Dain, "Critics and Dissenters: Reflections on 'Anti-psychiatry' in the United States," *Journal of the History of the Behavioral Sciences* 25 (1989): 3–25.

2. David Healy et al., "Psychiatric Bed Utilisation: 1896 and 1996 Compared," *Psychological Medicine* 31 (2001): 779–790.

3. David Rosenhan, "On Being Sane in Insane Places," *Science* 179 (1973): 250–258.

4. Healy, *Creation of Psychopharmacology,* 176.

5. David Healy, "Conflicting Interests: The Evolution of an Issue," *Monash Review of Bioethics* 23 (2004): 8–18.

6. Thomas Szasz, *The Myth of Mental Illness* (New York: Hoeber-Harper, 1961); T. Szasz, *The Manufacture of Madness* (New York: Dell, 1970).

7. Thomas S. Szasz, "What Psychiatry Can and Cannot Do," *Harper's Magazine,* February 1964, 50–53.

8. See Leonard R. Frank, in John Friedberg, *Shock Treatment Is Not Good for Your Brain* (San Francisco: Glide, 1976), 62–81.

9. Leonard Roy Frank, *The History of Shock Treatment* (San Francisco: LR Frank, 1978).

10. From the cover, ibid.

11. "Consumer/Survivor-Operated Self-Help Programs: A Technical Report," U.S. Department of Health and Human Services, Center for Mental Health Services, http://mentalhealth.samhsa.gov/publications/allpubs/SMA01-3510, accessed September 19, 2004; L. Van Tosh, R. O. Ralph, and J. Campbell, "The Rise of Consumerism," *Psychiatric Rehabilitation Skill* 4 (2000): 383–409.

12. Clifford Beers, *A Mind That Found Itself* (1908; repr., New York: Doubleday, 1953).

13. Judi Chamberlin, *On Our Own: Patient Controlled Alternatives to the Mental Health System* (New York: McGraw-Hill, 1978); Chamberlin, "The Ex-Patients' Movement: Where We've Been and Where We're Going," *Journal of Mind and Behaviour* 11 (1990): 323–336; Chamberlin, "Rehabilitating Ourselves: The Psychiatric Survivor Movement," *International Journal of Mental Health* 24 (1995): 39–46.

14. Ruby Rogers Advocacy and Drop-in Center, "Your Rights as a Mental Patient in Massachusetts," *Handbook for Patients (In-patients, Outpatients, and Pre-patients) by Ex-patients* (Somerville, Mass.: Ruby Rogers Advocacy and Drop-in Center, 1994).

15. National Association for Rights Protection and Advocacy, "Mental Health Advocacy, from Then to Now," http://www.narpa.org/webdoc6.htm, accessed September 16, 2004.

16. Mind,   http://www.mind.org.uk/NR/exeres/9AC202AF-6738-47F3-B136-ECC6E7E055AC.htm?NRMODE=Published&wbc_purpose=Basic&WBCMODE=PresentationUnpublished, accessed September 19, 2004.

17. Editorial, "Antipsychiatrists and ECT," *British Medical Journal* 2 (October 4, 1975): 1–2.

18. *Martin Salgo v. Leland Stanford Jr. University Board of Trustees,* 317 Cal. P.2d 170, 181 (1957).

19. R. R. Faden and T. L. Beauchamp, *History and Theory of Informed Consent* (New York: Oxford University Press, 1986), 125.

20. *Schloendorff v. Society of New York Hospitals,* 211 N.Y. 125, 126, 105 n.e. 92, 95.

21. Martin S. Pernick, "The Patient's Role in Medical Decision Making: A Social History of Informed Consent in Medical Therapy," in *President's Commission for the Study of Ethical Problems in Medicine and Biomedical and Behavioral Research, Making Health Care Decisions* (Washington, D.C.: GPO, 1982), 3:3.

22. Jay Katz, *The Silent World of Doctor and Patient* (New York: Free Press, 1984).

23. Benjamin Rush, *Sixteen Introductory Lectures* (Philadelphia: Bradford and Innskeep, 1811), 65, quoted in Faden and Beauchamp, *History and Theory of Informed Consent.*

24. N. J. Demy, "Informed Opinion on Informed Consent." *JAMA* 217 (1971): 696–697.

25. Carl H. Fellner and John R. Marshall, "The Myth of Informed Consent," *AJP* 126 (1970): 1245–1250.

26. Henry K. Beecher, "Ethics and Clinical Research," *New England Journal of Medicine* 74 (1966): 1354–1360.

27. David Rothman, *Strangers at the Bedside: A History of How Law and Bioethics Transformed Medical Decision Making* (New York: Basic Books, 1991).

28. Barron H. Lerner, *The Breast Cancer Wars* (New York: Oxford University Press, 2001).

29. *Irma Natanson v. John Kline,* 186 Kan. 393, 350 P.2d (1960).

30. Ellen Leopold, "Irma Natanson and the Legal Landmark, *Natanson v Kline*," *Breast Cancer Action Newsletter,* no. 83 (Fall 2004).

31. *William Mitchell v. G. Wilse Robinson Jr. et al.*, 334 Mo. SW 2d 11 (1960).

32. *John Bolam v. Friern Hospital Management Committee,* Queens Bench Division, Mcnair J (February 20–26, 1957). All subsequent quotations about the trial are from this source.

33. American Psychiatric Association, "Standards for Electroshock Treatment: Practice Guideline, Approved May 1953."

34. *Mitchell v. Robinson,* 17, 18, 19.

35. Fred Frankel, interview by David Healy, Boston, October 3, 2004.

36. Interview of Joseph J. Schildkraut, in David Healy, *The Psychopharmacologists,* vol. 3 (London: Arnold, 2000): 111–134.

37. The situation was dramatically presented in a *Washington Post* article by Elizabeth Wertz, "The Fury of Shock Treatment—A Patient's View," December 10, 1972, 36, 45, 58. Bournewood Hospital does teach Harvard psychiatry residents, but it is not a full-fledged teaching hospital as McLean Hospital is.

38. Fred H. Frankel, "Psychiatry Beleaguered: The Psychiatric Identity Crisis," *Psychiatric Quarterly* 43 (1969): 410–413; Fred H. Frankel, "Reasoned Discourse or a Holy War? Postscript to a Report on ECT," *AJP* 132 (1975): 77–79.

39. *Ricky Wyatt v. Stonewall B. Stickney,* 325 F. Supp. 781 (M.D. Ala. 1971); 334 F. Supp. 1341 (M.D. Ala. 1971).

40. Appeal docketed sub nom *Wyatt v. Aderholt,* no. 72-2634, 5th Cir., filed August 1, 1973.

41. Quoted in Jean Dietz, "Shock Therapy's Comeback," *Boston Globe,* January 14, 1985, 37.

42. The task force consisted of Robert Arnot, Donald Bowen, Gerald Caplan, Jonathan Cole, Donald Gair, David Langau, Phillip Quinn, Gershon Rosenblum, Carl Salzman, and Daniel Weiss.

43. Jean Deitz and Richard Knox, "Shock Therapy Ranks High for VP Problems," *Boston Globe,* July 27, 1972, 1 et seq. Also, Stuart Auerbach, "Shock Treatment Still Controversial," *Washington Post,* July 26, 1972, 1.

44. Fred H. Frankel, "Electro-Convulsive Therapy in Massachusetts: A Task Force Report," *Massachusetts Journal of Mental Health* 3 (1973): 3–29; Fred H. Frankel, "Current Perspectives on ECT: A Discussion." *AJP* 134 (1977): 1014–1019.

45. The issue remains controversial at this writing. There are possible exceptions, such as catatonia in adolescents.

46. Paul Appelbaum, "The Right to Refuse Treatment with Anti-psychotic Drugs: Retrospect and Prospect," *AJP* 145 (1988): 513–519.

47. California Welfare and Institutions Code 5326.85 (West 1980); C. Levine, "Voting 'Yes' to a Ban on Electroshock," *Hastings Center Report* 2 (1982): 19.

48. Ernest Rudin, "Psychiatric Treatment: General Implications and Lessons from Recent Court Decisions in California," *Western Journal of Medicine* 128 (1978): 459–466; G. N. Peterson, "Regulation of Electroconvulsive Therapy: The California Experience," in H. I. Schwartz, ed., *Psychiatric Practice under Fire: The Influence of Government, the Media, and Special Interests on Somatic Therapies* (Washington, D.C.: American Psychiatric Press, 1994), 29–62.

49. See *Gary Aden et al. v. Evelle J. Younger, Attorney General,* 57 Cal. App. 3d 662, 129 Cal. Rptr. 535 (1976) (Cal. App. LEXIS 1482).

50. Wade Hudson, "NAPA Battles Shock," in Frank, *History of Shock Treatment*, 146–152.

51. John Pippard, interview by David Healy, London, July 16, 2004. The following presentation of Pippard's experiences and impressions is also derived from this interview.

52. John Pippard and Les Ellam, *Electroconvulsive Treatment in Great Britain* (London: Gaskill, 1980); John Pippard and Les Ellam, "Electroconvulsive Treatment in Great Britain, 1981," *British Journal of Psychiatry* 139 (1981): 563–568.

53. American Psychiatric Association, *Electroconvulsive Therapy*, 2–5.

54. Sven O. Frederiksen and Gaetano D'Elia, "Electroconvulsive Therapy in Sweden," *British Journal of Psychiatry* 134 (1979): 283–287.

55. Charles J. Clark, *Report of the Electro-Convulsive Therapy Review Committee*, sent to Murray J. Elston, Minister for Health, Canada, 1985.

56. John Pippard, "Audit of Electroconvulsive Treatment in Two National Health Service Regions," *British Journal of Psychiatry* 160 (1992): 621–637.

57. Richard Duffett and Paul Lelliott, "Auditing Electroconvulsive Therapy: The Third Cycle," *British Journal of Psychiatry* 172 (1998): 401–405.

58. Fraser N. Watts et al., "Memory Deficit in Clinical Depression: Processing Resources and Structure of Material," *Psychological Medicine* 20 (1990): 345–349.

59. Diana Rose et al., "Patients' Perspectives on Electroconvulsive Therapy: Systematic Review," *British Medical Journal* 326 (2003): 1363–1364.

60. Anne B. Donahue, "Electroconvulsive Therapy and Memory Loss: A Personal Journey," *JECT* 16 (2000): 133–143.

61. Berton Roueché, "As Empty as Eve," *New Yorker*, September 9, 1974, 84–100.

62. Excerpts from Rice's deposition in *Rice v. Nardoni* (see note 63), quoted in Frank, *History of Shock Treatment*, 95–97.

63. Complaint in the Superior Court for the District of Columbia, Civil action 703-74, *Marilyn Rice v. Dr. John E. Nardini*.

64. Committee for Truth in Psychiatry (CTIP), "What You Should Know about ECT," http://www.harborside.com/~equinox/ect.htm, accessed September 17, 2004; L. Andre, "CTIP—The Committee for Truth in Psychiatry," 2004, http://www.ect.org/ctip_about.shtml, accessed July 7, 2004.

65. *Peggy Salters v. Palmetto Health Alliance, Inc.*, 20 P.N.L.R. 153 (2005), no. PN739.

66. Peter R. Breggin, *Electroshock: Its Brain-Disabling Effects* (New York: Springer, 1979).

67. D. W. Abse, "Theory of the Rationale of Convulsion Therapy," *British Journal of Medical Psychology* 19 (1944): 262–270; R. Good, "Some Observations on the Psychological Aspects of Cardiazol Therapy," *Journal of Mental Science* 86 (1940): 491–501.

68. E. Stainbrook, "Shock Therapy, Psychological Theory and Research," *Psychological Bulletin* 43 (1946): 21–60; T. D. Power, "Psychosomatic Regression in Therapeutic Epilepsy," *Psychosomatic Medicine* 7 (1945): 279–290; E. P. Mosse, "Electroshock and Personality Structure," *Journal of Nervous and Mental Disease* 104 (1946): 296–302.

69. Thelma G. Alper, "An Electric Shock Patient Tells His Story," *Journal of Abnormal and Social Psychology* 43 (1948): 201–210.

70. M. Gordon, "50 Shock Therapy Theories," *Military Surgery* 103 (1958): 397–401.

71. Joseph Brady, "The Evolution of Behavioural Pharmacology," in David Healy, *The Psychopharmacologists,* vol. 2 (London: Arnold, 1998), 71–92.

72. R. Good et al., "The Role of Fear in Electroconvulsive Treatment," *Journal of Nervous and Mental Disease* 136 (1963): 9–33.

73. Edgar Miller, "Psychological Theories of ECT: A Review," *British Journal of Psychiatry* 113 (1967): 301–311.

74. S. M. Corson, "The Successful Treatment of an Obsessive Compulsive Neurosis with Narcosynthesis Followed by Daily Electroshocks," *Journal of Nervous and Mental Disease* 109 (1949): 37–41.

75. C. P. Duncan, "The Retroactive Effect of Electroshock on Learning," *Journal of Comparative Physiological Psychology* 42 (1949): 32–44; M. C. Madsen and J. L. McGaugh, "The Effects of ECS on One Trial Avoidance Learning," *Journal of Comparative Physiology* 54 (1961): 522–523.

76. D. Ewen Cameron, "The Production of Differential Amnesia as a Factor in the Treatment of Schizophrenia," *Comprehensive Psychiatry* 1 (1960): 26–34.

77. I. L. Janis, "Psychological Effects of Electric Convulsive Therapies: Post Treatment Amnesias," *Journal of Nervous and Mental Disease* 111 (1950): 359–382.

78. Bernard C. Glueck Jr., Harry Reiss, and Louis E. Bernard, "Regressive Shock Therapy," *Psychiatric Quarterly* 31 (1957): 117–136.

79. R. Thompson and W. Dean, "A Further Study of the Retroactive Effect of ECS," *Journal of Comparative and Physiological Psychology* 48 (1955): 488–491.

80. H. E. Adams and D. J. Lewis, "Electroconvulsive Shock, Retrograde Amnesia and Competing Responses," *Journal of Comparative and Physiological Psychology* 55 (1962): 299–305.

81. F. Joseph et al., "The Effect of Electroconvulsive Shock on a Conditioned Emotional Response as a Function of the Temporal Distribution of the Treatment," *Journal of Comparative and Physiological Psychology* 47 (1954): 451–457. (Brady was actually the key author.)

82. Edward Weinstein and Robert L. Kahn, *Denial of Illness* (Springfield, Ill.: Charles C. Thomas, 1955).

83. Max Fink, "Neglected Disciplines in Psychopharmacology: Electroshock Therapy and Quantitative EEG," in Healy, *Psychopharmacologists,* 3:431–458.

84. L. Madow, "Brain Changes in Electroshock Therapy," *AJP* 113 (1956): 337–347.

85. See, for example, Breggin, *Electroshock.*

86. L. C. Epstein and Louis Lasagna, "Obtaining Informed Consent: Form or Substance?" *Archives of Internal Medicine* 123 (1969): 682–688.

87. See Leo Hollister, "From Hypertension to Psychopharmacology: A Serendipitous Career," in Healy, *Psychopharmacologists,* 2:215–236.

88. Letter from Ken Kesey to Thomas Szasz, February 28, 1963, at http://www.szasz.com/kesey.pdf.

89. Harold A. Sackeim, editorial, "Memory and ECT: From Polarization to Reconciliation," *JECT* 16 (2000): 87–96.

90. Timothy Garton-Ash, *The File: A Personal History* (New York: Vintage Books, 1998).

91. Elizabeth Loftus, "Planting Misinformation in the Human Mind: A 30-Year Investigation of the Malleability of Memory," *Learning & Memory* 12 (2005): 361–366.

92. Carl Elliott and Tod Chambers, *Prozac as a Way of Life* (Chapel Hill: University of North Carolina Press, 2004).

93. Bruce Stutz, "Pumphead," *Scientific American* 289 (2003): 68–73.

94. Mark F. Newman et al., "Longitudinal Assessment of Neurocognitive Function after Coronary Artery Bypass Surgery," *New England Journal of Medicine* 344 (2001): 395–402; Ola A. Selnes and Guy M. McKhann, "Coronary-Artery Bypass Surgery and the Brain," *New England Journal of Medicine* 344 (2001): 451–452; D. Van Dijk et al., "Cognitive Outcome after Off-pump and On-pump Coronary Artery Bypass Graft Surgery: A Randomized Trial," *JAMA* 287 (2002): 1405–1412.

95. Newman et al., "Longitudinal Assessment."

96. John Geddes, U.K. ECT Review Group, "Efficacy and Safety of Electroconvulsive Therapy in Depressive Disorders: A Systematic Review and Meta-analysis," *Lancet* 361 (2003): 799–808.

97. Mind, "Mind Comment on ECT Report in the *Lancet*," March 7, 2003, http://www.mind.org.uk/News+policy+and+campaigns/Press+archive/Mind+comment+on+ECT+report+in+the+Lancet.htm.

98. Rose et al., "Patients' Perspectives on Electroconvulsive Therapy: Systematic Review."

99. David Healy, *The Suspended Revolution: Psychiatry and Psychotherapy Reexamined* (London: Faber and Faber, 1990).

100. David Healy, "The Assessment of Outcome in Depression: Measures of Social Functioning," *Reviews in Contemporary Pharmacotherapy* 11 (2000): 295–301.

101. David Healy, *Let Them Eat Prozac* (New York: New York University Press, 2004).

102. Leon E. Rosenberg, "Brain Sick: A Physician's Journey to the Brink," *Cerebrum* 4 (2002): 43–60. (Rosenberg was formerly a dean at Yale University.)

103. Sherwin B. Nuland, *Lost in America* (New York: Knopf, 2003).

104. Norman S. Endler and E. Persad, *Electroconvulsive Therapy: The Myths and the Realities* (Toronto: Hans Huber, 1988).

CHAPTER TEN.   Electrogirl and the New ECT

1. *In the Matter of W.S., Jr., a Patient in the United States Veterans Administration Hospital, Lyons, New Jersey,* 152 N.J. Super. 298, 377 A.2d 969 (1977), LexisNexis Academic, LEXIS 1058. Informed consent in this case was mandated by the Veterans Omnibus Health Care Act of 1976, not by the State of New Jersey.

2. Margo L. Rosenbach et al., "Use of Electroconvulsive Therapy in the Medicare Population between 1987 and 1992," *Psychiatric Services* 48 (1997): 1537–1542.

3. Richard C. Hermann et al., "Variation in ECT Use in the United States," *AJP* 152 (1995): 869–875.

4. Srinivasa Reddy, telephone interview by Heather Dichter, January 20, 2005.

5. Don St. John, "Pharmacotherapeutic Approaches to Treatment-Resistant Depression," *Journal of the American Academy of Physician Assistants* 16 (2003): 32–48, quote on 47.

6. Although Leonhard had been playing with this distinction for a number of years, the first comprehensive presentation of his ideas was in Leonhard, *Aufteilung der endogenen Psychosen* (Berlin: Akademie-Verlag, 1957), see esp. 273–274. For an overview of Leonhard's ideas, see Frank Fish, "A Guide to the Leonhard Classification of Chronic Schizophrenia," *Psychiatric Quarterly* 38 (1964): 438–450.

7. Christian Astrup, "The Effects of Ataraxic Drugs on Schizophrenic Subgroups Related to Experimental Findings," *Acta Psychiatrica et Neurologica Scandinavica* 34, suppl. 136 (1959): 388–393, see table 1, 389.

8. Frank Fish, "The Influence of the Tranquillisers on the Leonhard Schizophrenic Syndromes," *L'Encéphale* 53 (1964): 245–249, see table 1, 248.

9. Kurt Witton, "Efficacy of ECT Following Prolonged Use of Psychotropic Drugs," *AJP* 119 (1962): 79.

10. Turan M. Itil, Ali Keskiner, and Max Fink, "Therapeutic Studies in 'Therapy Resistant' Schizophrenic Patients," *Comprehensive Psychiatry* 7 (1966): 488–493.

11. Max Fink, interview by David Healy, Toronto, May 1998.

12. Ole Bratfos and John Otto Haug, "Electroconvulsive Therapy and Antidepressant Drugs in Manic-Depressive Disease," *Acta Psychiatrica et Neurologica Scandinavica* 41 (1965): 588–596.

13. [Corbett Hilsman] Thigpen, discussion comment, in William Karliner, "Clinical Experiences with Intravenous Indoklon: A New Convulsant Drug," *Journal of Neuropsychiatry* 4 (1963): 184–187, see esp. 189.

14. Alexander H. Glassman et al., "Depression, Delusions, and Drug Response," *AJP* 132 (1975): 716–719.

15. Alexander Glassman, interview by Edward Shorter and David Healy, New York, October 5, 2004.

16. Conrad M. Swartz, "The Justification for Electroconvulsive Therapy," *Behavioral and Brain Sciences* 7 (1984): 37–38, quote on 37.

17. Trevor R. P. Price, "Modern ECT: Effective and Safe," *Behavioral and Brain Sciences* 7 (1984): 31–32, quote on 31.

18. Cathy Sherbourne et al., "Characteristics, Treatment Patterns, and Outcomes of Persistent Depression despite Treatment in Primary Care," *General Hospital Psychiatry* 26 (2004): 106–114.

19. "Suit Filed against Anti-ECT Statute," *Psychiatric Times,* August 1987, 20.

20. "Psychiatrists Explain Medical Facts in Depression Controversy," *New York Times,* July 29, 1972, 11.

21. Gary C. Aden, "The International Psychiatric Association for the Advancement of Electrotherapy: A Brief History," *American Journal of Social Psychiatry* 4 (1984): 9–10.

22. Fred Frankel, interview by David Healy, Boston, October 3, 2004.

23. See Frankel memo, "Report on the First Meeting of the APA Task Force on ECT . . . September 25–26, 1975," Max Fink's personal archive, Nissequogue, N.Y.

24. Max Fink's comments were made during an interview with Sidney Malitz by Edward Shorter, David Healy, and Max Fink, New York, October 5, 2004.

25. See Fred Frankel to task force, July 6, 1977, enclosing draft "Report on Electroconvulsive Therapy," 4, Max Fink's personal archive.

26. Leonard Cammer to Lester Grinspoon, December 12, 1977, Max Fink's personal archive.

27. On the December 9 meeting, see Frankel to Grinspoon, December 12, 1977, Max Fink's personal archive.

28. American Psychiatric Association, *Report of the Task Force on Electroconvulsive Therapy,* Task Force Report no. 14 (Washington, D.C.: APA, 1978), 161–162.

29. See Frankel to task force, November 23, 1977, 5, Max Fink's personal archive.

30. Fink, personal communication to Edward Shorter, December 21, 2004.

31. Lothar B. Kalinowsky and Paul H. Hoch, *Shock Treatments and Other Somatic Procedures in Psychiatry* (New York: Grune and Stratton, 1946). After Hoch's death, Kalinowsky and Hanns Hippius in Munich collaborated on a sequel, titled *Pharmacological, Convulsive, and Other Treatments in Psychiatry* (New York: Grune and Stratton, 1972).

32. Richard Abrams, interview by David Healy, Chicago, May 20, 2003.

33. American Psychiatric Association, *Report of the Task Force,* 166.

34. Iverson O. Brownell to Henry H. Work, November 14, 1977, Max Fink's personal archive.

35. Outpatient ECT services based in hospitals are alive and resurging. These incorporate many features of Karliner's practice. Yet office-practice ECT is dead.

36. Max Fink, "Toward a Rational Theory of Behavior," *Careers in Biological Research* 7 (1981): 2–12, quote on 3; this was first published in 1971 (Sandoz, *Career Directions*) and then updated.

37. Max Fink, Robert L. Kahn, and Edwin Weinstein, "Relation of Amobarbital Test to Clinical Improvement in Electroshock," *AMA Archives of Neurology and Psychiatry* 76 (1956): 23–29; he published two other ECT articles that year as well.

38. John P. Feighner et al., "Diagnostic Criteria for Use in Psychiatric Research," *Archives of General Psychiatry* 26 (1972): 57–63.

39. Robert L. Spitzer, Jean Endicott, and Eli Robins, "Research Diagnostic Criteria," *Archives of General Psychiatry* 35 (1978): 773–782.

40. American Psychiatric Association, *Diagnostic and Statistical Manual of Mental Disorders,* 3rd ed. (Washington, D.C.: APA, 1980).

41. Robert Levine, interview by Edward Shorter, New York, April 8, 2004.

42. Michael Taylor, interview by Max Fink, Ann Arbor, Mich., March 19, 2004.

43. Richard Abrams, *Electroconvulsive Therapy,* 4th ed. (Oxford: Oxford University Press, 2002).

44. Richard Abrams, "Daily Administration of Unilateral ECT," *AJP* 124 (1967): 384–386.

45. On these details, see Abrams to Fink, undated letter, Max Fink's personal archive.

46. Herbert Fox, interview by Edward Shorter, New York, April 8, 2004.

47. Richard Abrams and Michael A. Taylor, "Anterior Bifrontal ECT: A Clinical Trial," *British Journal of Psychiatry* 122 (1973): 587–590.

48. Max Fink and Richard Abrams, "Answers to Questions about ECT," *Seminars in Psychiatry* 4 (1972): 33–38; Fink, "The Therapeutic Process in Induced Convulsions (ECT)," *Seminars in Psychiatry* 4 (1972): 39–46.

49. Jan Volavka, "Neurophysiology of ECT," *Seminars in Psychiatry* 4 (1972): 55–66; Rhea Dornbush, "Memory and Induced ECT," ibid., 47–54. See also Jan Volavka et al., "EEG and Clinical Change after Bilateral and Unilateral Electroconvulsive Therapy," *Electroencephalography and Clinical Neurophysiology* 32 (1972): 631–639.

50. Max Fink, personal communication to Edward Shorter, January 7, 2005.

51. Richard Abrams and Michael Alan Taylor, "Catatonia: A Prospective Clinical Study," *Archives of General Psychiatry* 33 (1976): 579–581.

52. Max Fink and Michael Alan Taylor, *Catatonia: A Clinician's Guide to Diagnosis and Treatment* (Cambridge: Cambridge University Press, 2003).

53. Max Fink, personal communication to Edward Shorter, February 13, 2005.

54. [Thomas W. Williams] to chairman and members, conference planning committee, January 4, 1971, Max Fink's personal archive.

55. Max Fink et al., eds., *Psychobiology of Convulsive Therapy* (New York: Wiley, 1974).

56. ClinicalTrials.gov, http://www.clinicaltrials.gov, accessed December 30, 2004.

57. Martin M. Katz to members of Ad Hoc Planning Group for Electroconvulsive Therapy Conference, November 3, 1975, Max Fink's personal archive.

58. See Max Fink to Seymour Kety, February 28, 1976; also Fink to Jonathan Cole, February 28, 1976, Max Fink's personal archive.

59. Zigmond Lebensohn to Henry H. Work, November 15, 1977, Max Fink's personal archive.

60. Matthew Rudorfer, interview by Max Fink, Boca Raton, Fla., February 9, 2004.

61. Max Fink, interview by Edward Shorter and David Healy, Nissequogue, N.Y. October 25, 2002.

62. Jack D. Blaine and Susan M. Clark, "Report of the NIMH-NIH Consensus Development Conference on Electroconvulsive Therapy," *Psychopharmacology Bulletin* 22 (1986): 445–502, quote on 452.

63. [Glen N. Peterson], "Consensus Statement," *International Psychiatric Association for the Advancement of Electrotherapy, Summer Newsletter*, 1985, 6.

64. Richard Weiner, interview by Heather Dichter, Durham, N.C., January 6, 2005.

65. Richard Weiner to Harold Pincus, December 4, 1986, Weiner's personal archive.

66. See APA Joint Reference Committee, "Specification of Charge to Task Force on Development of Safety and Performance Standards for ECT Devices," c. September 1987, app. 10, Richard Weiner's personal archive.

67. Richard Weiner, interview by Heather Dichter, Durham, N.C., January 6, 2005.

68. See APA "News Release," December 21, 1989, quote on 4, Richard Weiner's personal archive,

69. The task force's report was published as *The Practice of Electroconvulsive Therapy: Recommendations for Treatment, Training, and Privileging: A Task Force Report of the American Psychiatric Association* (Washington, D.C.: APA, 1990). On its being sold out, see "Task Force Minutes," May 17, 1990, Richard Weiner's personal archive. A second edition appeared in 2001.

70. Richard Weiner, interview by Heather Dichter, Durham, N.C., January 6, 2005.

71. "ECT Effective Says AMA House," *Psychiatric News,* April 21, 1989, 45.

72. Carl Salzman, editorial, "ECT, Research, and Professional Ambivalence," *AJP* 155 (1998): 1–2.

73. U.S. Department of Health and Human Services, *Mental Health: A Report of the Surgeon General, Rockville, MD* (Washington, D.C.: U.S. Department of Health and Human Services, National Institutes of Health, and National Institute of Mental Health, 1999), quote on 258.

74. Richard M. Glass, "Electroconvulsive Therapy: Time to Bring It out of the Shadows," *JAMA* 285 (March 14, 2001): 1346–1348.

75. World Psychiatric Association, "Position Statement on the Use and Safety of Electroconvulsive Therapy," *Science & Care: Bulletin of the WPA Scientific Sections,* no. 1 (January–March, 2004): 7–11, quote on 10. See also John Geddes, U.K. ECT Review Group, "Efficacy and Safety of Electroconvulsive Therapy in Depressive Disorders: A Systematic Review and Meta-analysis," *Lancet* 361 (March 8, 2003): 799–808.

76. Arthur Zitrin, interview by Edward Shorter, New York, July 11, 2004.

77. Milton Greenblatt et al., "Choice of Somatic Therapies in Depression," *Current Psychiatric Therapies* 25 (1964): 134–142, see table 2, 140.

78. Harold Sackeim, "Memory and ECT: From Polarization to Reconciliation," *JECT* 16 (2000): 87–96, quote on 88.

79. Harold Sackeim, interview by David Healy, Chappaqua, N.Y., July 10, 2004.

80. Joseph Zubin and S. Eugene Barrera, "Effect of Electric Convulsive Therapy on Memory," *Proceedings of the Society for Experimental Biology* 48 (1941): 596–597.

81. Joseph Zubin, "Loss of Familiarity as an Explanation of Autobiographical Memory Loss," *Behavioral and Brain Sciences* 7 (1984): 41–42, quote on 42.

82. Russell D. Lutchman et al., "Mental Health Professionals' Attitudes towards and Knowledge of Electroconvulsive Therapy," *Journal of Mental Health* 10 (2001): 141–150.

83. Donald I. Templer, "ECT and Brain Damage: How Much Risk Is Acceptable?" *Behavioral and Brain Sciences* 7 (1984): 39.

84. John P. J. Pinel, "After Forty-five Years ECT Is Still Controversial," *Behavioral and Brain Sciences* 7 (1984): 30–31, quote on 31.

85. *Doris Hogue v. State Personnel Board of Review,* opinion no. 33373 (Ohio App. 1974), LexisNexis Academic, LEXIS 3141.

86. Ricks Warren, "Electroconvulsive Therapy: Ethical Considerations for Psychologists," *Corrective and Social Psychiatry* 25 (1979): 100–103, quote on 102.

87. Bruce J. Winick, *The Right to Refuse Mental Health Treatment* (Washington, D.C.: American Psychological Association, 1997), 91.

88. It is especially striking that psychologists' hostility to ECT should be maintained during their systematic campaign today to gain prescribing privileges for psychotropic medication (a goal that has been achieved in several U.S. states). Psychologists might argue that medication is a preferred approach, but for them to hold out medication as the holy grail of psychological practice, and at the same time condemn an obviously effective treatment such as ECT, is inconsistent.

89. Richard Weiner, interview by Heather Dichter, Durham, N.C., January 6, 2005.

90. Harold A. Sackeim et al., "Postictal Excitement Following Bilateral and Right-Unilateral ECT," *AJP* 140 (1983): 1367–1368.

91. Harold Sackeim, interview by David Healy, Chappaqua, N.Y., July 10, 2004.

92. See Harold A. Sackeim et al., "Effects of Stimulus Intensity and Electrode Placement on the Efficacy and Cognitive Effects of Electroconvulsive Therapy," *New England Journal of Medicine* 328 (March 25, 1993): 839–846; Sackeim et al., "A Prospective, Randomized, Double-Blind Comparison of Bilateral and Right Unilateral Electroconvulsive Therapy at Different Stimulus Intensities," *Archives of General Psychiatry* 57 (2000): 434.

93. Max Fink is convinced that it is resolved and that it is time for the field to move on. Fink, "Stimulus Titration and ECT Dosing: Move On!" *JECT* 18 (2002): 11–13.

94. Lothar B. Kalinowsky, " 'The New Yorker' on ECT: A Response," (APA) New York State District Branches, *Bulletin* (April–May 1975): 4–5. "What she describes is something that neither I nor several colleagues who unsuccessfully wrote to *The New Yorker* have ever seen" (4).

95. Richard Weiner, interview by Heather Dichter, Durham, N.C., January 6, 2005.

96. Leonard Cammer, "Presentation to the APA Task Force on ECT," May 11, 1976, Max Fink's personal archive.

97. Richard Weiner, interview by Heather Dichter, Durham, N.C., January 6, 2005.

98. Börje Cronholm and Jan-Otto Ottosson, "The Experience of Memory Function after Electroconvulsive Therapy," *British Journal of Psychiatry* 109 (1963): 251–258, quote on 258.

99. Larry R. Squire, "Opinion and Facts about ECT: Can Science Help?" *Behavioral and Brain Sciences* 7 (1984): 34–37, quote on 36.

100. Gina Kolata, "Experts Say Treatments Affect Recall," *New York Times*, October 19, 1988, B3.

101. Lelon A. Weaver Jr., "ECT Damage: Are There More Pressing Problems?" *Behavioral and Brain Sciences* 7 (1984): 39–41, quote on 40.

102. Harold Sackeim, interview by David Healy, Chappaqua, N.Y., July 10, 2004.

103. James L. Levenson and Allan Brock Willett, "Milieu Reactions to ECT," *Psychiatry* 45 (1982): 298–306, quote on 300.

104. Zigmond Lebensohn, "Rough Notes at ECT Hearings, American Psychiatric Association, May 11, 1976," Max Fink's personal archive.

105. Benedict Carey, "Shock Therapy and the Brain," *Los Angeles Times,* November 17, 2003, F1.

106. J. H. Mazkalnins to Glen N. Peterson, January 7, 1986, Max Fink's personal archive. For the story, see Bob Becker, "Experts Are of 2 Minds on Shock," *Cleveland Plain Dealer,* January 5, 1986:1.

107. This potentially mammoth task was facilitated by the ProQuest service that permitted searching all of the newspapers scanned into a large database. We included several articles in Canadian newspapers as well. At the time that we did the search, September 2004, ProQuest incorporated only a few newspapers for the pre-1994 period.

108. Polly Morrice, review of Barbara Esstman's *Night Ride Home, New York Times,* December 21, 1997, BR 17.

109. Bess Liebenson, "Help for Depression Put in the Foreground," *New York Times,* October 6, 1996, CN6.

110. John Horgan, "Science Triumphant? Not So Fast," *New York Times,* January 19, 1998, A17.

111. Vanderbilt University Television News Archive, *ABC Evening News,* February 16, 1987. We are grateful to Andrea Tone for these references.

112. Ibid., *CBS Evening News,* February 3, 1993.

113. Ibid., *ABC Evening News,* July 30, 1996.

114. Stacey Pamela Patton, "Electrogirl: Stacey Patton's Computer Screen Name Is More Than a Joke. It's a Courageous Expression of Hope That Fearsome Electric Shock Treatments May Save Her Life," *Washington Post,* September 19, 1999, F1. Subsequent quotations are all from this source.

115. S. V. Eranti and D. M. McLoughlin, "Authors' Reply" (to criticisms of an article they had written earlier in 2003 in the *British Journal of Psychiatry* 182:8–9), *British Journal of Psychiatry* 183 (2003): 172–173.

116. Anthony Browne, "Shock Therapy Patients to Sue," *Observer,* January 23, 2000.

117. Jacqui Wise, "Shock, Horror or Help? ECT Is a Barbarous Ordeal for Some Patients," *Guardian,* January 21, 1997, T014.

118. National Institute for Clinical Excellence, *Guidance on the Use of Electroconvulsive Therapy,* Technology Appraisal Guidance, no. 59 (London: NICE, 2003), 19–20. The report said ECT should be "used only to achieve rapid and short-term improvement of severe symptoms after an adequate trial of other treatment options has proven ineffective" (5). The report prompted a group of researchers to study specifically quality of life, and found that it "improved as early as 2 weeks after the completion of ECT." See W. Vaughn McCall et al., "Quality of Life and Function after Electroconvulsive Therapy," *British Journal of Psychiatry* 185 (2004): 405–409.

119. Mind, press release, March 26, 2003.

120. "Interpellanza di Tolotti," *Salute,* May 6, 2002, 1. See also Richard Abrams, letter, "Use of ECT in Italy," *AJP* 157 (2000): 840; Bruno Simini, "Electroconvulsive Therapy Is Restricted in Italy," *Lancet* 353 (March 20, 1999): 993; Athanasios Koukopoulos, "ECT: Why So Little in Italy?" *International Journal of Practical Psychiatry and Behavioural Health* 3 (1993): 79–81.

121. Harold Bourne, "Electroconvulsive Therapy Ending Where It Began," *Psychiatric Bulletin* 23 (1999): 505.

122. "ECT Restricted in Italy," *Psychiatric Bulletin* 23 (1999): 505.

123. Christoph Lauber et al., "Can a Seizure Help? The Public's Attitude toward Electroconvulsive Therapy," *Psychiatric Research* 134 (2005): 205–209.

124. Chris Hendry, "ECT Forbidden in Slovenia," *Journal of Addiction and Mental Health* 5 (January/February 2002) p. 2.

125. Tom Bolwig, telephone interview by David Healy, July 17, 2004.

126. G. Gazdag et al., "Rates of Electroconvulsive Therapy Use in Hungary in 2002," *JECT* 20 (2004): 42–44.

127. Kurt Blumenthal, "Insulin, Cardiazol, and Electroshock Treatment in Palestine during the Last Five Years," *AJP* 101 (1945): 332–346. The paper was first given at the Congress of Neurologists and Psychiatrists, April 17, 1942, at Tel Aviv. It is unknown where Blumenthal trained.

128. Alexander I. Nelson, *Electroconvulsive Therapy in Psychiatry, Addictive Medicine, and Neurology* (in Russian) (Moscow: BINOM, Laboratoria Znanij, 2005).

129. Athanasios Koukopoulos, personal communication to Edward Shorter, April 2, 2006.

130. Max Fink, personal communication to Edward Shorter, September 12, 2004.

131. "Critical History—Future Trends," abstract book, First European Symposium on ECT, March 26–29, 1992, Graz, Austria.

132. P. Hofmann et al., "Austrian Psychiatrists' and Neurologists' View and Current Practice on ECT," see abstract book, ibid., 113.

133. T. C. Baghai et al., *Elektrokonvulsionstherapie: Klinische und wissenschaftliche Aspekte* (Vienna: Springer, 2004).

134. A. Conca et al., "Die Elektrokrampftherapie: Theorie und Praxis," *Neuropsychiatrie* 18 (2004): 1–17.

135. Gerhard W. Eschweiler, "Elektrokrampftherapie," *Neuro-Psychiatrische Nachrichten,* November 12, 2003 (online newsletter, downloaded January 10, 2005). The official body was the Wissenschaftlicher Beirat of the Bundesärztekammer.

136. Tom Bolwig, personal communication to "Dear Friends," February 23, 2006.

137. Lerer quoted in Avihai Becker, "The Shocking Truth," http://www.haaretz .com/hasen/pages/ShArt.jhtml?itemNo=324457. Bernard Lerer kindly shared this article with us in an e-mail message of August 3, 2003.

CHAPTER ELEVEN. Magnets and Implants:
New Therapies for a New Century?

1. Sarah H[olly] Lisanby and Thomas E. Schlaepfer, "Magnetic Seizure Therapy of Major Depression," *Archives of General Psychiatry* 58 (2001): 303–305; Sarah H. Lisanby, "Magnetic Seizure Therapy: Development of a Novel Convulsive Technique," in Sarah Lisanby, ed., *Brain Stimulation in Psychiatric Treatment (Review of Psychiatry* 23 [Washington D.C.: American Psychiatric Publishing, 2004]): 67–91; and Thomas Schlaepfer, telephone interview by David Healy, July 17, 2004.

2. Thomas Schlaepfer, telephone interview by David Healy, July 17, 2004.

3. Sarah H. Lisanby et al., "Safety and Feasibility of Magnetic Seizure Therapy (MST) in Major Depression: Randomized Within-Subject Comparison with Electroconvulsive Therapy," *Neuropsychopharmacology* 28 (2003): 1852–1865.

4. Jan-Otto Ottosson, "Experimental Studies of the Motor Action of Electroconvulsive Therapy," *Acta Psychiatrica Scandinavica* 35 (1960): 1–141; J.-O. Ottosson, "Seizure Characteristics and Therapeutic Efficiency in Electro Convulsive Therapy: An Analysis of the Antidepressant Efficiency of Grand Mal and Lidocaine Modified Seizures," *Journal of Nervous and Mental Disease* 135 (1962): 239–251.

5. Anthony T. Barker, "Determination of the Distribution of Conduction Velocities in Human Nerve Trunks" (Ph.D. diss., University of Sheffield, 1976); Anthony T. Barker et al., "Non-invasive Stimulation of Motor Pathways within the Brain Using Time-Varying Magnetic Fields," *Electroencephalography and Clinical Neurophysiology* 61 (1985): S245; Anthony T. Barker, Reza Jalinous, and Ian L. Freeston, "Non-invasive Magnetic Stimulation of the Human Motor Cortex," *Lancet* 1 (1985): 1106–1107; Anthony T. Barker et al., "Clinical Evaluation of Conduction Time Measurements in Central Motor Pathways Using Magnetic Stimulation of the Human Brain," *Lancet* 1 (1986): 1325–1326.

6. Mike J. R. Polson, Anthony T. Barker, and Ian L. Freeston, "Stimulation of Nerve Trunks with Time Varying Magnetic Fields," *Medical and Biological Engineering and Computing* 20 (1982): 243–244.

7. Arsène D'Arsonval, "Dispositifs pour la mesure des courants alternatifs de toutes fréquences," *Counsel of Royal Society for Biology* (Paris) 3 (1896): 450–457; Sylvanus P. Thompson, "Physiological Effect of an Alternating Magnetic Field," *Proceedings of the Royal Society, London (Biology)* 82 (1910): 396–398.

8. Patrick A. Merton and Herbert P. Morton, "Stimulation of the Cerebral Cortex in the Intact Human Subject," *Nature* 285 (1980): 227.

9. Reza Jalinous, "The Use of Time-Varying Magnetic Fields to Stimulate the Human Nervous System: Theory and Practice" (Ph.D. diss., University of Sheffield, 1988).

10. Anthony T. Barker, "History and Basic Principles of Magnetic Nerve Stimulation," in Alvaro Pascual-Leone et al., eds., *Handbook of Transcranial Magnetic Stimulation* (London: Arnold, 2002), 3–70.

11. G. Hoflich et al., "Application of Transcranial Magnetic Stimulation in Treatment of Drug Resistant Major Depression: A Report of Two Cases," *Human Psychopharmacology* 8 (1993): 361–365.

12. T. Zyss, "Deep Magnetic Brain Stimulation—The End of Psychiatric Electroshock Therapy?" *Medical Hypotheses* 43 (1994): 69–74.

13. Amos Fleischmann et al., "The Effect of Transcranial Magnetic Stimulation of Rat Brain on Behavioral Models of Depression," *Brain Research* 699 (1995): 130–132.

14. N. Grisaru et al., "Transcranial Magnetic Stimulation in Depression and Schizophrenia," *European Neuropsychopharmacology* 4 (1994): 287–288; Robert H. Belmaker and Amos Fleischmann, "Transcranial Magnetic Stimulation: A Potential New Frontier in Psychiatry," *Biological Psychiatry* 38 (1995): 419–421.

15. James C. Ballenger and Robert M. Post, "Carbamazepine (Tegretol) in Manic-Depressive Illness: A New Treatment," *AJP* 137 (1980): 782–790; Margaret Harris et al., "Mood Stabilizers: The Archaeology of the Concept," *Bipolar Disorders* 5 (2003): 446–452, with commentary by Paul Grof.

16. David Healy, *Mania* (Baltimore: Johns Hopkins University Press, forthcoming).

17. Harold A. Sackeim et al., "Seizure Threshold in ECT: Effects of Sex, Age, Electrode Placement, and Number of Treatments," *Archives of General Psychiatry* 44 (1987): 355–360.

18. Susan R. Weiss, et al., "Quenching: Inhibition of Development and Expression of Amygdala Kindled Seizures with Low Frequency Stimulation," *NeuroReport* 6 (1995): 2171–2176.

19. Mark S. George, "Why Would You Ever Want To? Toward Understanding the Antidepressant Effect of Prefrontal rTMS," *Human Psychopharmacology* 13 (1998): 307–313; Mark S. George et al., "Changes in Mood and Hormone Levels after Rapid Rate Transcranial Magnetic Stimulation of the Prefrontal Cortex," *Journal of Neuro Psychiatry and Clinical Neurosciences* 8 (1996): 172–180; Mark S. George et al., "Mood Improvement Following Daily Left Prefrontal Repetitive Transcranial Magnetic Stimulation in Patients with Depression: A Placebo Controlled Crossover Trial," *AJP* 154 (1997): 1752–1756.

20. Harold A. Sackeim et al., "Regional Cerebral Blood Flow in Mood Disorders: I. Comparison of Major Depressives and Normal Controls at Rest," *Archives of General Psychiatry* 47 (1990): 60–72; M. S. Nobler et al., "Regional Cerebral Blood Flow in Mood Disorders: III. Effects of Treatment and Clinical Response in Depression and Mania," *Archives of General Psychiatry* 51 (1994): 884–897.

21. Eric M. Wassermann et al., "Seizures in Healthy People with Repeated 'Safe' Trains and Transcranial Magnetic Stimuli," *Lancet* 347 (1996): 825–826; Mark S. George and Eric M. Wassermann, "Rapid Rate Transcranial Magnetic Stimulation (rTMS) and ECT," *Convulsive Therapy* 10 (1994): 251–253.

22. J. D. Martin et al., "Mood Effects of Prefrontal Repetitive High Frequency TMS in Healthy Volunteers," *CNS Spectrums* 2 (1997): 53–68.

23. Mark S. George et al., "Changes in Mood and Hormone Levels after Rapid-Rate Transcranial Magnetic Stimulation (rTMS) of the Prefrontal Cortex," *Journal of Neuropsychiatry and Clinical Neuroscience* 8 (1992): 172–180.

24. Mark S. George, telephone interview by David Healy, September 24, 2004.

25. Ibid.

26. Mark S. George et al., "Daily Repetitive Transcranial Magnetic Stimulation (rTMS) Improves Mood in Depression," *Neuro Report* 6 (1995): 1853–1856.

27. Alvaro Pascual-Leone et al., "Beneficial Effects of Rapid Rate Transcranial Magnetic Stimulation of the Left Dorsolateral Prefrontal Cortex in Drug Resistant Depression," *Lancet* 348 (1996): 233–237.

28. Harold Sackeim, interview by David Healy, Chappaqua, N.Y., July 10, 2004.

29. M. S. Nobler et al., "Regional Cerebral Blood Flow in Mood Disorders: III."

30. Harold A. Sackeim, "Magnetic Stimulation Therapy and ECT," *Convulsive Therapy* 10 (1994): 255–258.

31. Mark S. George and Eric M. Wassermann, "Rapid-Rate Transcranial Magnetic Stimulation (rTMS) and ECT," *Convulsive Therapy* 10 (1994): 251–253.

32. This dynamic has been very visible in organizations such as the American College of Neuropsychopharmacology or the British Association for Psychopharmacology; see David Healy, *The Creation of Psychopharmacology* (Cambridge, Mass.: Harvard University Press, 2002).

33. Harold A. Sackeim, "The Left and Right Wings of ECT," editorial submitted to *JECT* (2004), and later rejected. Sackeim refers to it in his interview.

34. M. S. George et al., "Prefrontal Cortex Dysfunction in Clinical Depression," *Depression* 2 (1994): 59–72.

35. Jose H. Martin et al., "Repetitive Transcranial Magnetic Stimulation for the Treatment of Depression: Systematic Review and Meta-analysis," *British Journal of Psychiatry* 182 (2003): 480–491; Thomas E. Schlaepfer and M. Kosel, "Transcranial Magnetic Stimulation in Depression," in Lisanby, *Brain Stimulation in Psychiatric Treatment,* 1–16.

36. R. H. Belmaker, e-mail interview by David Healy, September 22, 2004.

37. Timothy W. Kneeland and Carol A. Warren, *Pushbutton Psychiatry: A History of Electroshock in America* (Westport, Conn.: Praeger, 2002).

38. American College of Neuropsychopharmacology Workshop on Repetitive Transcranial Magnetic Stimulation (rTMS): A Novel Probe of Mood, Annual General Meeting, Caribe Hilton, San Juan, Puerto Rico, December 9–13, 1996.

39. Marco Bresadola, "Early Galvanism as Technique and Medical Practice," in P. Bertucci and G. Pancaldi, eds., *Electric Bodies: Episodes in the History of Medical Electricity* (Bologna: University of Bologna Press, 2001), 157–180.

40. Edwin Clarke and L. S. Jacyna, *Nineteenth-Century Origins of Neuroscientific Concepts* (Berkeley: University of California Press, 1987).

41. Margaret Rowbottom and Charles Susskind, *Electricity and Medicine: History of Their Interaction* (San Francisco: San Francisco Press, 1984), 19–20 and passim.

42. Richard Hunter and Ida Macalpine, "John Birch" section, in *Three Hundred Years of Psychiatry, 1535–1860* (New York: Carlisle Publishing, 1963), 535.

43. Raffaella Seligardi, "What Is Electricity? Some Chemical Answers, 1770–1815," in Bertucci and Pancaldi, *Electric Bodies,* 181–208.

44. Iwan R. Morus, "Batteries, Bodies and Belts: Making Careers in Victorian Medical Electricity," in Bertucci and Pancaldi, *Electric Bodies,* 209–238; J. Althaus, "On the Therapeutic Use of Electricity by Induction," *Lancet* 2 (1857): 162–164, 187–190.

45. Thomas K. Derry and Trevor I. Williams, *A Short History of Technology* (Oxford: Oxford University Press, 1970), 608–636.

46. Guillaume Duchenne, *De l'electrisation localisée et de son application à la physiologie et à la thérapeutique* (Paris: Baillière, 1855).

47. Emil Du Bois-Reymond, *Untersuchungen über thierische Elektrizität* (Berlin: G. Reimer, 1848).

48. Anonymous, "An Exposure of Electrical Quackery," *Lancet* 1 (1889): 949–950; H. Lewis Jones, "The Application of Electricity in Medical and Surgical Practice," *Lancet* 1 (1900): 695–699.

49. Allan Beveridge and Edward Renvoize, "Electricity and British Psychiatry in the 19th Century," *Journal of Psychopharmacology* 4 (1900): 145–151.

50. Edward Stainbrook, "The Use of Electricity in Psychiatric Treatment during the 19th Century," *Bulletin of the History of Medicine* 22 (1948): 156–177.

51. A. Robertson, "Case of Insanity of Seven Years' Duration: Treatment by Electricity," *Journal of Mental Science* 30 (1884): 54–57; Joseph Wiglesworth, "The Uses of Galvanism in the Treatment of Certain Forms of Insanity," *British Medical Journal* 2 (1887): 506–507; A. H. Newth, "The Value of Electricity in the Treatment of Insanity," *Journal of Mental Science* 24 (1884): 76–82.

52. J. Althaus, *A Treatise on Medical Electricity* (London: Longmans, Green, 1873); Wiglesworth, "The Uses of Galvanism."

53. George M. Beard, "Neurasthenia, or Nervous Exhaustion," *Boston Medical and Surgical Journal* 80 (1869): 217–221.

54. George M. Beard and A. D. Rockwell, *A Practical Treatise on the Medical and Surgical Uses of Electricity, Including Localised and Generalised Electrification* (New York: William Wood, 1871).

55. De Watteville, "Practical Remarks on the Use of Electricity in Mental Illness," *Journal of Mental Science* 30 (1885): 483–488.

56. Beard and Rockwell, *Practical Treatise.*

57. George M. Beard, "The Treatment of Insanity by Electricity," *Journal of Mental Science* 19 (1873): 355–360.

58. H. Lewis Jones, "The Use of General Electrification as a Means of Treatment in Certain Forms of Mental Disease," *Journal of Mental Science* 47 (1901): 245–250.

59. Hector A. Colwell, *An Essay on the History of Electrotherapy and Diagnosis* (London: Heinemann, 1922).

60. Stéphane Leduc, "Production de sommeil et de l'anesthésie générale et locale par les courants intermittents de basse tension," *Archives d'Électricité Médicale* 10 (1902): 617–621; see also James P. Morgan, "The First Reported Case of Electrical Stimulation of the Human Brain," *Journal of the History of Medicine* 37 (1982): 51–64; and Rowbottom and Susskind, *Electricity and Medicine,* 192.

61. Felipe Fregni et al., "Treatment of Depression with Transcranial Direct Current Stimulation," *British Journal of Psychiatry* 186 (2005): 446–447.

62. Ronald Melzack and Patrick D. Wall, "Pain Mechanisms: A New Theory," *Science* 150 (1965): 971–979; R. Melzack and P. D. Wall, *The Challenge of Pain* (Harmondsworth: Penguin, 1982).

63. Such as Alpha Stim 100, a microcurrent stimulator, which aims to normalize the electrical activity of the nervous system and brain. See http://www.alpha stim.com.

64. Melody Petersen, "Madison Avenue Plays Growing Role in Drug Research," *New York Times,* November 22, 2002.

65. A. C. Pandey et al., "Gabapentin in Bipolar Disorder: A Placebo-Controlled Trial of Adjunctive Therapy," *Bipolar Disorder* 2 (2000): 249–255.

66. P. Bailey and F. Bremer, "A Sensory Cortical Representation of the Vagus Nerve," *Journal of Neurophysiology* 1 (1938): 405–412; Harold A. Sackeim, "Vagus Nerve Stimulation," in Lisanby, *Brain Stimulation in Psychiatric Treatment,* 99–136.

67. Jake Zabara, "Inhibition of Experimental Seizures in Canines by Repetitive Vagal Stimulation," *Epilepsia* 33 (1992): 1005–1012.

68. J. Kiffin Penry and J. Christine Dean, "Prevention of Intractable Partial Seizures by Intermittent Vagal Stimulation in Humans: Preliminary Results," *Epilepsy* 31, suppl. (1990): S40–S43.

69. Cyberonics, *Physicians Manual for the NCP Pulse Generator* (Houston, Tex.: Cyberonics, 1998), http://www.vnstherapy.com/depression/hcp/Manuals/default .aspx.

70. Elinor Ben-Menachem et al., "Vagus Nerve Stimulation for Treatment of Partial Seizures: A Controlled Study of Effect on Seizures," *Epilepsia* 35 (1994): 616–626; Adrian Handforth et al., "Vagus Nerve Stimulation Therapy for Partial Onset Seizures: Randomised Active Control Trial," *Neurology* 51 (1998): 48–55.

71. George L. Morris and Wade M. Mueller, "Vagus Nerve Stimulation Study Group (E01–E05): Long-Term Treatment with Vagus Nerve Stimulation in Patients with Refractory Epilepsy," *Neurology* 53 (1999): 1731–1735; Christopher M. De Giorgio et al., "Prospective Long-Term Study of Vagus Nerve Stimulation for the Treatment of Refractory Seizures," *Epilepsia* 41 (2000): 1195–1200; Martin C. Salinsky et al., "Vagus Nerve Stimulation for the Treatment of Medically Intractable Seizures: Results of a One-Year Open Extension Trial," *Archives of Neurology* 53 (1996): 1176–1180.

72. Gerda Elger et al., "Vagus Nerve Stimulation Is Associated with Mood Improvements in Epilepsy Patients," *Epilepsy Research* 42 (2000): 203–210.

73. Mark S. George et al., "Vagus Nerve Stimulation: A New Tool for Brain Research and Therapy," *Biological Psychiatry* 47 (2000): 287–295.

74. A. John Rush et al., "Vagus Nerve Stimulation (VNS) for Treatment-Resistant Depression: A Multi-center Study," *Biological Psychiatry* 47 (2000): 276–286.

75. Jerrold F. Rosenbaum and George R. Heninger, "Vagus Nerve Stimulation for Treatment Resistant Depression," *Biological Psychiatry* 47 (2000): 273–275.

76. Harold S. Sackeim et al., "Vagus Nerve Stimulation (VNS) for Treatment Resistant Depression: Efficacy, Side Effects, and Predictors of Outcome," *Neuropsychopharmacology* 25 (2001): 713–728.

77. Lauren B. Marangell et al., "Vagus Nerve Stimulation (VNS) for Major Depressive Episodes: One-Year Outcomes," *Biological Psychiatry* 51 (2002): 280–287.

78. Harold A. Sackeim, "Vagus Nerve Stimulation," in Lisanby, *Brain Stimulation*, 99–153.

79. Thomas Schlaepfer, telephone interview by David Healy, July 17, 2004.

80. Cyberonics press releases of June 15 and August 12, 2004, as posted on http://www.cyberonics.com, accessed December 2, 2004.

81. *New York Times*, February 4, 2005.

82. Cyberonics, "FDA Advisory Panel Recommends Approval of Cyberonics' Depression Device," press release, June 15, 2004.

83. Anthony Marson et al., "Immediate versus Deferred Antiepileptic Drug Treatment for Early Epilepsy and Single Seizures: A Randomised Controlled Trial," *Lancet* 365 (2005): 2007–2013.

84. R. Meyers, "Surgical Interruption of the Pallidofugal Fibers: Its Effect on Syndrome of Paralysis Agitans and Technical Considerations in Its Applications," *New York State Journal of Medicine* 42 (1942): 317–325.

85. Krishna Kumar, Cory Toth, and Rahul K. Nath, "Deep Brain Stimulation for Intractable Pain: A 15-Year Experience," *Neurosurgery* 40 (1997): 736–746.

86. R. G. Heath and W. A. Mickle, "Evaluation of Seven Years' Experience with Depth Electrode Studies in Human Patients," in E. R. Rameyand and D. S. O'Doherty, eds., *Electrical Studies in the Unanesthetized Brain* (New York: Hoeber, 1960), 214–247.

87. P. Damier, "The Stimulation of Deep Cerebral Structures in the Treatment of Parkinson's Disease," *European Neuropsychopharmacology* 8 (1998): S84; Patricia Limousin, et al., "Electrical Stimulation of the Sub-thalamic Nucleus in Advanced Parkinson's Disease," *New England Journal of Medicine* 339 (1998): 1105–1111.

88. B. P. Beijani et al., "Transient Acute Depression Induced by High Frequency Deep Brain Stimulation," *New England Journal of Medicine* 341 (1999): 1004.

89. Bart Nuttin et al., "Electrical Stimulation in the Anterior Limbs of Internal Capsules in Patients with Obsessive Compulsive Disorder," *Lancet* 354 (1999): 1526.

90. Bart Nuttin, "Brain Implants Show Promise against Obsessive Disorder," *Nature* 419 (2002): 685; Bart Nuttin, "France Wires Up to Treat Obsessive Disorder," *Nature* 417 (2002): 677; Jan Gybels, Paul Cosyns, and Bart Nuttin, "La psychochirurgie en Belgique," *Cahiers du Comité Consultatif National d'Ethique pour les Sciences de la Vie et de la Santé* 32 (2002): 18–21.

91. George Curtis, telephone interview by David Healy, October 23, 2004.

92. Bart Nuttin et al., "Electrical Stimulation of the Brain for Psychiatric Disorders," *CNS Spectrums* 5 (2000): 35–39; Bart Nuttin et al., "Long-Term Electrical Capsular Stimulation in Patients with Obsessive-Compulsive Disorder," *Neurosurgery* 52 (2003): 1263–1274.

93. Luc Mallet et al., "Compulsions, Parkinson's Disease, and Stimulation," *Lancet* 360 (2002): 1302–1304.

94. Ben D. Greenberg, D. L. Murphy, and Steve A. Rasmussen, "Neuroanatomically Based Approaches to Obsessive Compulsive Disorders: Neurosurgery and Transcranial Magnetic Stimulation," *Psychiatric Clinics of North America* 23 (2000): 671–686.

95. Bart Nuttin et al., "Deep Brain Stimulation for Psychiatric Disorders," *Neurosurgery* 51 (2002): 51; Ben D. Greenberg, "Deep Brain Stimulation in Psychiatry," in Lisanby, *Brain Stimulation,* 53–63.

96. J. L. Abelson et al., "Deep Brain Stimulation for the Treatment of Refractory Obsessive Compulsive Disorder (OCD)," presentation at President's Symposium on Anxiety Disorders, New Directions, Novel Approaches, Psychiatric Research Society, Park City, Utah, February 12, 2004; S. F. Taylor et al., "Effects of Sustained Deep Brain Stimulation on Regional Glucose Uptake in Obsessive Compulsive Disorder," *Biological Psychiatry* 55 (2004): 238S.

97. Carolyn Abraham, "Electrical Brain Implants Target Deep Depression," http://www.theglobeandmail.com/servlet/story/RTGAM.20050301.wxhdepresion01/, accessed March 1, 2005.

98. Helen S. Mayberg et al., "Deep Brain Stimulation for Treatment-Resistant Depression," *Neuron* 45 (2005): 651–660.

99. Helen Mayberg, telephone interview by Edward Shorter, August 12, 2005.

100. Alan Baumeister, "The Tulane Electrical Brain Stimulation Program: A Historical Case Study in Medical Ethics," *Journal of the History of the Neurosciences* 9 (2000): 262–278; Robert Heath, *Exploring the Mind-Brain Relationship* (Baton Rouge, La.: Moran Printing, 1996).

101. Xingbao Li et al., "Acute Left Pre-frontal Transcranial Magnetic Stimulation in Depressed Patients Is Associated with Immediately Increased Activity in Pre-frontal Cortical as Well as Sub-cortical Regions," *Biological Psychiatry* 55 (2004): 882–890.

102. Mark S. George et al., "Vagus Nerve Stimulation: A New Tool for Brain Research and Therapy," *Biological Psychiatry* 47 (2000): 287–295.

103. Torsten M. Madsen et al., "Increased Neurogenesis in a Model of Electroconvulsive Therapy," *Biological Psychiatry* 47 (2000): 1043–1049.

104. Joseph K. Belanoff et al., "An Open Label Trial of C-1073 (Mifepristone) for Psychotic Major Depression," *Biological Psychiatry* 52 (2002): 386–392; Philip W. Gold, Wayne C. Drevets, and Dennis S. Charney, "New Insights into the Role of Cortisol and the Glucocorticoid Receptor in Severe Depression," *Biological Psychiatry* 52 (2002): 381–385.

105. David Healy, *Let Them Eat Prozac* (New York: New York University Press, 2004).

106. Ames Delbourgo, "Electrical Humanitarianism in North America: Dr. T. Gale's Electricity or Etherial Fire Considered (1802) in Historical Context," in Bertucci and Pancaldi, *Electric Bodies,* 117–156.

107. Laurence Hirshberg, Sufen Chiu, and Jean Frazier, "Emerging Brain-Based Interventions for Children and Adolescents: Overview and Clinical Perspective," *Child and Adolescent Psychiatry Clinics of North America* 14 (2005): 1–19.

CHAPTER TWELVE. Epilogue: Irrational Science

1. John C. Whitehorn, *One Hundred Years of American Psychiatry, 1844–1944* (New York: Columbia University Press, 1944), 188.

2. J. S. Neki, "Psychiatry in South East Asia," *British Journal of Psychiatry* 123 (1973): 257–261; N. S. Vahia, D. R. Doongaji, and Dilip V. Jeste, "Twenty-five Years of Psychiatry in a Teaching General Hospital in India," *Indian Journal of Psychiatry* 16 (1974): 221–228; G. D. Shukla, "Electroconvulsive Therapy in a Rural Teaching General Hospital in India," *British Journal of Psychiatry* 139 (1981): 569–571.

3. Madhukar H. Trivedi et al., "Clinical Results for Patients with Major Depressive Disorder in the Texas Medication Algorithm Project," *Archives of General Psychiatry* 61 (2004): 669–680.

4. George Bush et al., "Catatonia: Rating Scale and Standardised Examination," *Acta Psychiatrica Scandinavica* 93 (1996): 129–136.

5. Sergio Starkstein et al., "Catatonia in Depression: Prevalence, Clinical Correlates and Validation of a Scale," *Journal of Neurology, Neurosurgery and Psychiatry* 60 (1996): 326–332; Patricia Rosebush et al., "Catatonic Syndrome in a General Psychiatric Inpatient Population: Frequency, Clinical Presentation, and Response to Lorazepam," *Journal of Clinical Psychiatry* 51 (1990): 357–362.

6. B. Mahendra, "Where Have All the Catatonics Gone?" *Psychological Medicine* 11 (1981): 669–671.

7. Max Fink and Michael Taylor, *Catatonia* (Cambridge: Cambridge University Press, 2003); David Healy, *The Creation of Psychopharmacology* (Cambridge, Mass.: Harvard University Press, 2002).

8. David Healy et al., "Service Utilisation in 1896 and 1996: Morbidity and Mortality," *History of Psychiatry* 16 (2005): 27–41; Padmaja Chalassani, David Healy, and Richard Morris, "Incidence and Presentation of Catatonia and Related Motor Syndromes in Two Acute Psychiatric Admission Units in India and the United Kingdom," *Psychological Medicine* 35 (2005): 1667–1675.

9. William J. Bleckwenn, "Production of Sleep and Rest in Psychotic Cases," *Archives of Neurology and Psychiatry* 24 (1930): 365–375.

10. Henri Baruk, J. Launay, and J. Berges, "Experimental Catatonia and Psychopathology of Neuroleptics," *Journal of Clinical & Experimental Psychopathology* 19 (1958): 277–291.

11. Jean Delay, Pierre Pichot, and Thérèse Lemperière, "Un neuroleptique majeur non-phenothiazine et non reserpinique: L'haloperidol dans le traitement des psychoses," *Annales Médico-Psychologiques* 118 (1960): 145–152.

12. Stanley N. Caroff, "Neuroleptic Malignant Syndrome," *Journal of Clinical Psychiatry* 41 (1980): 79–83.

13. Sheldon Gelman, *Medicating Schizophrenia: A History* (New Brunswick N.J.: Rutgers University Press, 1999).

14. Gregory L. Fricchione et al., "Intravenous Lorazepam in Neuroleptic Induced Catatonia," *Journal of Clinical Psychopharmacology* 3 (1985): 338–342.

15. Fink and Taylor, *Catatonia*, 46; Gregory Fricchione, "Neuroleptic Catatonia and Its Relationship to Psychogenic Catatonia," *Biological Psychiatry* 20 (1985): 304–313.

16. John Davis, Stanley Caroff, and Stephen Mann, "Treatment of Neuroleptic Malignant Syndrome," *Psychiatric Annals* 30 (2000): 325–332.

17. The rediscovery of catatonia as a clinical entity had begun in the 1970s. In 1991, Fink and Michael Alan Taylor urged that it be included in *DSM-IV*. See their "Catatonia: A Separate Category for DSM-IV?" *Integrative Psychiatry* 7 (1991): 2–10.

18. U. Osby et al., "Mortality and Causes of Death in Schizophrenia in Stockholm County, Sweden," *Schizophrenia Research* 45 (2000): 21–28; Matti Joukamaa et al., "Schizophrenia, Neuroleptic Medication and Mortality," *British Journal of Psychiatry* 188 (2006): 122–127.

19. The term *cerebroversion* may first have been proposed by Conrad Swartz. Its first use in print was as a synonym for ECT by Jeffrey H. Morse and colleagues in Salem, Virginia. See their letter, *AJP* 148 (1991): 1764. But this word and variants on it, such as *neuroversion* have probably occurred to many. In this case, the use of the word is to describe a process rather than ECT as such, and the first person that I (Healy) heard use it was P. Chalassani in north Wales in 1998.

Index

References to illustrations are in *italics*.

About the Authors

Edward Shorter is the Jason A. Hannah Professor of the History of Medicine in the Faculty of Medicine of the University of Toronto. A well-known author, among his previous books are *The Making of the Modern Family* (1975), *From Paralysis to Fatigue* (1991), and *A History of Psychiatry* (1997).

David Healy studied medicine at the University of Dublin and Cambridge University. He is a professor of psychiatry at Cardiff University; a former secretary of the British Association for Psychopharmacology; and author of more than 140 peer-reviewed articles, 200 other pieces, and 15 books, including *The Psychopharmacologists* (three volumes, 1996–2000), *The Antidepressant Era* (1997), *The Creation of Psychopharmacology* (2002), and *Let Them Eat Prozac* (2004).